VASCULAR ACCESS
IN
CLINICAL PRACTICE

VASCULAR ACCESS
IN
CLINICAL PRACTICE

EDITED BY

SCOTT S. BERMAN

University of Arizona,
Carondelet St. Mary's Hospital, and
the Southern Arizona Vascular Institute
Tucson, Arizona

ILLUSTRATIONS BY FRED ANDERSON

MARCEL DEKKER, INC.　　　　　　　　NEW YORK • BASEL

NKF-DOQI™ Disclaimer

These guidelines are based upon the best information available at the time of publication. They are designed to provide information and assist decision making. They are not intended to define a standard of care, and should not be construed as one. Neither should they be interpreted as prescribing an exclusive course of management. Variations in practice will inevitably and appropriately occur when clinicians take into account the needs of individual patients, available resources, and limitations unique to an institution or type of practice. Every health-care professional making use of these guidelines is responsible for evaluating the appropriateness of applying them in the setting of any particular clinical situation.

NFK-DOQI is a trademark of the National Kidney Foundation, Inc.

ISBN: 0-8247-0768-0

This book is printed on acid-free paper.

Headquarters
Marcel Dekker, Inc.
270 Madison Avenue, New York, NY 10016
tel: 212-696-9000; fax: 212-685-4540

Eastern Hemisphere Distribution
Marcel Dekker AG
Hutgasse 4, Postfach 812, CH-4001 Basel, Switzerland
tel: 41-61-261-8482; fax: 41-61-261-8896

World Wide Web
http://www.dekker.com

The publisher offers discounts on this book when ordered in bulk quantities. For more information, write to Special Sales/Professional Marketing at the headquarters address above.

Current printing (last digit):
10 9 8 7 6 5 4 3 2 1

PRINTED IN THE UNITED STATES OF AMERICA

Foreword

Those who work with their hands are laborers;
Those who work with their heads are craftsmen;
Those who work with their hands, their heads and their hearts are artists.
—Sebastiani Winery

The field of dialysis access and its complications has become huge over the past decade. According to the last count in 1998, it is estimated that over 300,000 patients in the United States are on some form of dialysis—hemodialysis in 60% of these patients, renal transplants in approximately 25%, and peritoneal dialysis in 9%. The cost of revising failed or failing dialysis access graft exceeds $500 million per year. Strategic planning with subsequent publication by the National Kidney Foundation Dialysis Outcomes Quality Initiatives (NKF-DOQI)–Clinical Practice Guidelines for Vascular Access has made the art of doing procedures on these patients into a science with expected plans of attack and outcomes. Overall, I think this is a good thing.

Many vascular surgeons are true experts in this field of dialysis access, and this book is one of the best I have read that unleashes all the knowledge from those who actually do the work. The chapters are written with the true philosophy of those who live and breathe dialysis access surgery and the descriptions of "how I do it" are nicely written and easily followed. At the end of each chapter is a modified outline of the NFK-DOQI–Clinical Practice Guidelines for Vascular Access on the chapter topic with down-to-earth recommendations and approaches to the problems in dialysis access. The depth and breadth of this book are also reflected in the inclusion of excellent chapters on the historical perspective of dialysis, preoperative evaluation of the renal failure patient, anesthesia considerations, and information on new horizons for biomaterials that will be important to even further improve patency of dialysis grafts and therefore also renal failure patient quality of life.

I am delighted to have been chosen to write this foreword for a most important book that will teach us the labor and craft of dialysis work and give us the philosophy of how to be artists as well.

Julie Ann Freischlag, M.D.
Professor and Chief, UCLA Division of Vascular Surgery
Director, UCLA Gonda (Goldschmied) Vascular Center
Los Angeles, California

Preface

Vascular Access in Clinical Practice was conceived during my training in both general surgery and vascular surgery. As a senior resident and fellow, I was often charged with the establishment of vascular access for hemodialysis and long-term venous access. Although there were a plethora of reference texts on surgical techniques, vascular access often received little if any attention in the broad scope of general or vascular surgery. I was disappointed at the lack of practical information available about access techniques.

The concept of a "how to" text evolved simultaneously with the development of my large practice of hemodialysis patients in the Southwest. Establishing, and—often more vexing—maintaining, vascular access became a daily challenge. It became apparent to me that many techniques applied in this patient group were passed along by word of mouth through training programs, and more recently through a biennial conference devoted to hemodialysis access organized by Ohio State University under the guidance of Mitchell Henry, M.D. As a regular attendee at that symposium, I witnessed firsthand the thirst for tips and knowledge regarding vascular access that existed in the community of healthcare providers who care for the end-stage renal disease patient.

What started as a simple "how to" reference has evolved into a comprehensive manual. The contributors all have experience caring for large numbers of hemodialysis patients on a regular basis, and the chapters include not only published tehcniques but also some well-known yet not well-publicized tricks of the trade such as use of the pneumatic tourniquet for access construction and revascularizatrion for access-related steal.

The text begins with an overview of hemodialysis. The next chapters in Part I are devoted to preoperative assessment and anesthetic techniques for access surgery. These are followed by chapters that are devoted to hemodialysis access fistulae and grafts and describe surveillance techniques and salvage techniques, both surgical and nonsurgical. The section on hemodialysis concludes with a discussion of the pathophysiology of access failure at cellular and biochemical levels.

Part II, which covers dialysis access complications, begins with a chapter devoted to central venous access catheters specifically used for hemodialysis. The subsequent chapter discusses accessing fistulae, grafts, and catheters and provides information regarding the care of these sites. A chapter follows on the complications of dialysis access fistulae and grafts. The section's final chapter examines biomaterials used for access devices. Part III is devoted entirely to central venous access catheters used for nondialysis indications. This section outlines catheter selection, placement techniques, and complications. In Part IV the text concludes with three chapters devoted to peritoneal dialysis and includes catheter placement techniques and complications.

I have attempted to minimize redundancy throughout the text by careful use of cross-referencing of other chapters rather than repetition of previously covered material.

As this text evolved, so too has the treatment of access surgery by the medical profession. The National Kidney Foundation's publication of the Dialysis Outcome Quality Initiative (NKF-DOQI) provided insight into the state of the art of dialysis access and, moreover, established goals for all access surgeons in managing this difficult clinical problem. I have incorporated and referenced the DOQI guidelines throughout the text where appropriate to provide the reader with a practical method of correlating the text information within the context of national guidelines. Thanks to these national standards, vascular access surgery has been elevated in stature in the scope of practice of general and vascular surgery. The attention that access surgery now receives at U.S. and international surgery meetings is evidence of this change.

My commitment to this field is the product of my experience as as surgical resident and vascular fellow. Two surgeons, Roger T. Gregory and Marc H. Glickman, instilled in me the challenge of excellence in the care of dialysis patients and the concept of applying vascular surgery principles to the clinical problems presented by the hemodialysis patient, at a time when that approach was not embraced readily by the surgical community.

This work could not have been accomplished without the efforts of the contributors. A special thanks to Beth Campbell, formerly of Quality Medical Publishing, for her confidence in this project, and Brian Black at Marcel Dekker, Inc., for his persistence and drive to complete this project. It is my hope that this work will serve to motivate others to view vascular access not as ''a work order'' but as a clinical challenge equal in magnitude and intellectual enthusiasm to other problems addressed by the healthcare community.

Scott S. Berman

Contents

Contributors

Scott S. Berman, M.D.   Professor of Biomedical Engineering and Assistant Professor of Clinical Surgery, The University of Arizona; Chief, Section of Vascular Surgery, Carondelet St. Mary's Hospital; and Director of Vascular and Endovascular Surgery, The Southern Arizona Vascular Institute, Tucson, Arizona

W. Bradford Carter, M.D.   Associate Professor, Division of Surgical Oncology, Department of Surgery, The University of Maryland, Baltimore, Maryland

John Daller, M.D.   Assistant Professor, Department of Surgery, University of Texas Medical Branch, Galveston, Texas

Luke S. Erdoes, M.D.   Vascular Associates, Chattanooga, Tennessee

Kenneth Fox, M.D.   Pediatric Cardiovascular Surgeon, Children's Hospital of Austin/Cardiothoracic and Vascular Surgeons, Austin, Texas

Andrew T. Gentile   Clinical Assistant Professor of Surgery, Department of Vascular Surgery, Southern Arizona Vascular Institute, The University of Arizona Health Sciences Center, Tucson, Arizona

Dan Ihnat, M.D.   Fellow, Section of Vascular Surgery, University of Arizona, Tucson, Arizona

Sam H. James, M.D.   Associate Professor of Clinical Medicine, Section of Nephrology, Department of Medicine, The University of Arizona Health Sciences Center, Tucson, Arizona

Bruce E. Jarrell, M.D.   Chairman, Department of Surgery, The University of Maryland, Baltimore, Maryland

John M. Marek, M.D.   Assistant Professor, Department of Surgery, University of New Mexico School of Medicine, Albuquerque, New Mexico

Joseph L. Mills, M.D.   Associate Professor and Chief, Section of Vascular Surgery, Department of Surgery, The University of Arizona Health Sciences Center, Tucson, Arizona

Rudy Mounia, R.N.   Product Manager, IMPRA Inc., Tempe, Arizona

Mark P. Ramirez, M.D.   Santa Rita Anesthesiology, Tucson, Arizona

Donald J. Roach, M.D.   Interventional Radiologist, Radiology Limited, Tucson, Arizona

Stephen J. Ruffenach, D.O.   Clinical Assistant Professor, Section of Nephrology, Department of Medicine, The University of Arizona Health Sciences Center, Tucson, Arizona

Mark Sarfati, M.D.   Assistant Professor, Division of Vascular Surgery, The University of Utah, Salt Lake City, Utah

Thomas Stejskal, M.D.   Chief, Section of Radiology, Carondelet St. Mary's Hospital, and Director of Vascular and Interventional Radiology, The Southern Arizona Vascular Institute, Tucson, Arizona

Alex Westerband, M.D., FACS   Chief of Vascular Surgery, Southern Arizona Veterans Affairs Heath Care Systems, and Assistant Professor of Clinical Surgery, The University of Arizona Health Sciences Center, Tucson, Arizona

Stuart K. Williams, Ph.D.   Professor and Chair, Department of Biomedical Engineering, The University of Arizona, Tucson, Arizona

To Christi and Alex for untiring love and patience,
to Morris and Naomi for unconditional confidence,
and to the patients with end-stage renal disease who inspire us to persist.

I

Vascular Access for Hemodialysis

1

An Overview of Hemodialysis

Sam H. James and Stephen J. Ruffenach
The University of Arizona Health Sciences Center,
Tucson, Arizona

A HISTORICAL PERSPECTIVE OF HEMODIALYSIS

The foundation of the science of dialysis—the knowledge on which it is based—was laid by the Scottish scientist Thomas Graham, who coined the term *dialysis* (1). Graham used this word to describe a phenomenon he observed—that of the separation of crystalloids from colloids by passage through a semipermeable membrane composed of albumin-covered parchment. In 1854 he predicted that his findings relating to osmosis and semipermeable membranes could be applied to medicine. Such applications were indeed attempted by many clinicians in the decades that followed. Although hemodialysis did not become a viable clinical tool for the treatment of renal failure until the 1960s, the first clinical dialysis was performed on animals by the German physician George Haas in 1914. His research in dialysis continued and, in October 1924, he was credited with the first dialysis on a clinically uremic human (2). With the help of an understanding of the basic physical principles of dialysis, the early pioneers were able to meet the challenges of producing semipermeable membranes across which blood could be purified and of developing an extracorporeal system through which the blood could circulate without clotting. Thereafter, the research revolved around elaborating the physics of dialysis as well as improving the dialysis membrane. Dialysis machines were constantly being improved, with particular attention to safety of the dialysis procedure.

Today, with the widespread use of microprocessors, dialysis machines have become technically advanced. Membrane technology has resulted in the discovery of new semipermeable membranes that are more biocompatible and have improved permeability properties. The advent of new dialyzers and improved machinery has shortened the length of dialysis from 12 h down to $2^{1}/_{2}$ to 4 h per session. As a result of these refinements, it is now possible to extend the dialysis procedure to a broader spectrum of patients with renal failure. Integrated physiological monitoring combined with refined vascular access techniques have led to improved clinical experiences and outcomes for the stable end-stage renal disease (ESRD) patient and made it possible to dialyze the critically ill renal failure patient who was undialysable in the past.

BASIC PHYSICS OF HEMODIALYSIS

Hemodialysis employs the basic principles of diffusion and ultrafiltration to achieve the goal of replacing renal function. Diffusion is a consequence of random thermal motion of molecules, leading to the passive transfer of solute across semipermeable membranes without net solvent transfer. The net direction of movement of solute molecules across semipermeable membranes relies on the existence of a *concentration* gradient and is in the direction of higher concentration to lower concentration of the same solute. Ultrafiltration, on the other hand, is the movement of solvent with some of its contained solutes across the semipermeable membrane in response to a *pressure* gradient applied across the membrane. Solvent, otherwise known as ultrafiltrate, will move out of the blood compartment, where the pressure is higher, into the dialysate compartment, where the pressure is lower. Thus, hemodialysis waste products are removed by diffusion, whereas fluid is removed by ultrafiltration. In addition, solute drag is a process whereby a small but significant portion of solute moves passively with the solvent out of the blood compartment, contributing to the dialysis process.

THE HEMODIALYSIS PROCESS

The dialysis machine controls the flow of blood in one chamber and the flow of dialysate in the other. The currently available dialyzers (artificial kidneys) are composed of two compartments, one for blood and the other for dialysate, separated by a semipermeable membrane. The rate of flow in both compartments is set at optimal rates to process a specific volume of blood and maximize the use of the dialysate solution. By measuring pre- and postdialyzer solute concentrations, the amount of solute removed can be assessed and the adequacy of dialysis calculated. Each patient requires different amounts of dialysis, depending on factors such as body size, muscle mass, metabolic rate (urea generation), and the amount of food eaten. The dialysis prescription, which identifies a desired degree of solute removal, is tailored to each patient's needs. The volume of blood processed, the speed of processing, and the time on dialysis differ from patient to patient and are based on the patient's needs, vascular access performance, desires, and tolerances.

The transmembrane pressure across the semipermeable membrane from the blood compartment to the dialysate compartment can be manipulated by the hemodialysis process. By so doing, one can calculate with accuracy the amount of fluid that will be removed before dialysis is commenced. Removal of solute from the blood compartment employs the principle of diffusion—whereby the solute moves down its concentration gradient out of the blood compartment into the dialysate compartment across the semipermeable membrane. In order to maximize solute removal, several factors must be controlled (3). First, blood and dialysate should flow in countercurrent directions in order to improve the efficiency of solute removal by maintaining an optimal concentration gradient throughout the dialyzer (Figure 1.1). Membranes of different permeabilities exist. High-flux dialyzers have the highest permeability thus allowing the most efficient removal of solute. Membrane selection will affect the clearance of different-size molecules, which will also have a bearing on the clearance of medications and exogenous toxins. Other factors of importance include blood dialysate flow rates, the concentration gradient of the solute between the blood and the dialysate compartments, the surface area of the membrane, the distance solute travels from the blood to the dialysate compartment, and, last, the temperature of the two fluids. A high dialysate temperature may create a thermal barrier to solute clearance. All of the above factors relate to the diffusibility of solute molecules from the blood compartment into the dialysate compartment.

It is clear from the above discussion that the performance of vascular access is crucial if dialysis is to be effective. With the advent of high-flux bicarbonate dialysis, it is possible to process more blood in a shorter time while maintaining adequacy of dialysis. Furthermore, better pumps, tubing, and needles have made it possible to increase blood flow rates from 250 mL/min to approximately 500 mL/min, so that similar volumes of blood can be processed in a shorter period of time. This allows patients to spend less time on dialysis and yet still achieve treatment of equal adequacy. The demand for higher blood flow rates has also called for improved vascular access and the rejection of what was previously considered adequate. Despite the advances in the hemodialysis process, vascular access has lagged behind and continues to be a major limiting factor in the treatment of chronic dialysis patients.

Blood flow rates seen with radiocephalic fistulas range from 150 to 600 mL/min, whereas prosthetic bridge grafts achieve blood flows on the order of

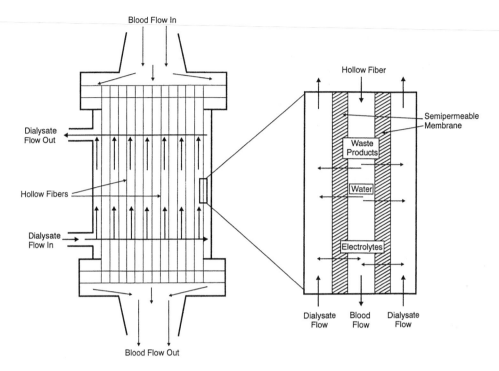

FIGURE 1.1   Hollow-fiber dialyzer (inset: single fiber with direction of movement of water and solute).

800 to 1600 mL/min (4). One can easily see how this wide variation in access flow rates can affect the efficiency of dialysis. No matter how rapid and efficient the dialysis process becomes, access flow rates must be maximal to support proficient treatments. Access grafts, which are on the low end of flow rates to maintain patency (<300 mL/min), provide inadequate dialysis and are often more detrimental to maintaining effective renal replacement therapy than an occluded access site.

MANAGEMENT OF ACUTE RENAL FAILURE

In managing a patient who has acute renal failure, one must determine the cause of the renal failure. Specifically, one must attempt to reverse the pathological process that led to the renal failure. Typically, the cause involves a combination of factors such as hypovolemia, hypotension, infection, and or exposure to a nephrotoxin. Provided that the patient is not at any immediate risk, conservative medical management to correct the underlying pathology should be initiated. At the same time, attention should be directed to other complications of renal failure, such as electrolyte, acid-base, and volume disturbances. Failure to respond to conservative measures should result in the patient being placed on dialysis. Indications for dialytic intervention can be absolute or relative (5,6) (Table 1.1). An absolute indication, if present, is a basis for initiating dialysis. ''Relative indications'' may justify the initiation of dialysis if several exist simultaneously or if, individually, they are severe and unresponsive to medical management.

The presence of uremia, particularly when manifest by neurological signs, is an indication to initiate immediate dialysis. Features include altered mental status, asterixis, hypersomnolence, seizure, and coma. These neurological manifestations are the effects of toxin accumulation on neuronal and neuromuscular activity. Uremia can cause platelet dysfunction, resulting in a hypocoagulable state (7). Patients who have pericarditis are at risk of intrapericardial hemorrhage. The inflammatory process may cause blood vessel disruption. The hypocoagulable state of uremia may result in extensive intrapericardial bleeding. Pericardial tamponade should always be considered in uremic patients who develop unexplained hypotension.

Disorders of fluids and electrolytes often provide indications for immediate dialysis. Fluid retention refractory to diuretic therapy, particularly when manifest by pulmonary edema, requires immediate dialytic intervention. If unresponsive

TABLE 1.1   Indications for Initiating Dialysis

Absolute indications
  Central nervous system
    Altered mental status
    Asterixis
    Neuromuscular irritability
    Somnolence
    Coma
    Seizures
  Pericarditis
  Hemorrhage
  Symptomatic fluid overload (pulmonary edema),
      unresponsive to diuretic therapy
  Toxin and drug overdose
Relative indications
  Hyperkalemia
  Acidosis
  Hyponatremia
  Nausea and vomiting

to routine medical management, potassium levels above 7 mmol/L, severe acid-base disturbances, hyponatremia, hyperuricemia, and protracted nausea and vomiting are all relative indications for dialysis (see Table 1-1). Serum potassium levels frequently rise in acute renal failure. Potassium will be released from damaged cells and will shift out of cells when acidosis is present. Failure of the kidneys to excrete potassium adds to the rise in serum levels.

The cause of acute renal failure frequently contributes to metabolic acidosis. When severe, acidosis interferes with normal metabolic processes. Dialysis is not indicated if the acidosis can be corrected with treatment of the underlying condition and the serum bicarbonate level remains above 10 mmol/L.

The use of markedly elevated blood urea nitrogen (BUN) as an indication for the initiation of dialysis remains controversial. Creatinine and BUN are sentinel molecules; when elevated, they indicate the presence of high concentration of other more diverse and difficult-to-measure molecules that induce uremia. Although most clinicians are reluctant to let a BUN rise to a level greater than 100 mg/dL, there are clinical settings where marked azotemia (elevated BUN and creatinine) can be found without uremia or other indications for dialysis. In considering dialysis, the patient's catabolic rate should be noted, as well as the ability of the dialysis process to remove nitrogenous waste products. The frequency of dialysis will depend on the above as well as on the need to remove fluid and electrolytes and to correct acid-base disturbances.

Continuous renal replacement therapy has evolved in the treatment of intensive care unit patients who develop acute renal failure. With the advent of improved dialyze membrane technology as well as the need to dialyze hemodynamically unstable patients, continuous arteriovenous hemofiltration was introduced in the late seventies. This allows for clearance by convection with large volume exchange on an ongoing basis. Solute and water removal take place at a slow rate, thus preventing the hemodynamic instability usually associated with hemodialysis. The process relies on natural blood flow between an artery and a vein to circulate the blood through the dialyzer. Subsequently dialysate has been added to the system—as with conventional dialysis—flowing countercurrent to the blood, also at a markedly reduced rate. As a result, the clearance obtained with the addition of diffusion to the existing convection of the hemofiltration process has markedly enhanced clearance. The process is known as *continuous arteriovenous hemodialysis*. Most recently, simple machines have been developed that allow the process to be performed on venous blood alone—i.e., *continuous venovenous hemodialysis*.

The advantage of the continuous renal replacement therapies is that we are now able to dialyze hemodynamically unstable patients and to remove fluid as needed. The process is ongoing and changes can be made according to the patient's changing condition and the therapy required. Electrolyte and acid-base disturbances can be corrected immediately. Large-volume therapies can be administered without overloading the patient. Despite major advances in the management of seriously ill patients with multiorgan failure, the mortality from acute renal failure has not diminished. This is mainly because renal failure occurs in the setting of serious illnesses to which the patients ultimately succumb.

THE ROLE OF HEMODIALYSIS IN OVERDOSES

Overdose of certain medications and ingestion of various toxins are known to be treatable with acute dialysis (8). The use of dialysis should depend on the severity of intoxication. The decision to initiate dialysis should be based on the following criteria (9):

1. Progressive patient deterioration despite intensive care
2. Development of coma with severe intoxication and midbrain dysfunction
3. Impairment of normal drug excretory function
4. Intoxication with agents producing metabolic and/or delayed effects
5. Intoxication with an intractable drug that can be removed at a greater rate than by nitrogenous elimination

Substances that are highly protein-bound, or lipid-soluble, have a high volume of distribution, or are of large molecular size are not easily amenable to removal by dialysis. In the mid-1960s, it was noted that the use of hemoperfusion with a charcoal column was effective in absorbing intoxicants from the blood, often doing so more efficiently than standard dialysis.

MANAGEMENT OF CHRONIC RENAL FAILURE

In chronic renal failure, dialysis should be commenced when the patient begins to develop uremic symptoms that are not readily reversible by conservative medical management. Symptoms that begin to interfere with the patient's quality of life and the ability to function productively are indications that dialysis is imminent. In general, patients should be started on the chronic dialysis program before the ravages of advanced renal failure take their toll. The benefits of early dialysis are to prevent uremic complications such as malnutrition, peripheral neuropathy, and renal osteodystrophy.

The body is able to adapt to chronic renal insufficiency at the expense of losing muscle mass, which is the source of creatinine. Decreasing protein intake will limit the buildup of other nitrogenous metabolites. By so doing, the serum creatinine and BUN are held at relatively lower levels. In the long term, this adaptive process is extremely detrimental, as poor nutritional status during dialysis is a major predictor of a poor outcome (10,11). Dialysis is frequently a stepping-stone to renal transplantation. Malnourished patients are at greater risk of an adverse outcome following renal transplantation than well-nourished patients, who have better-preserved tissues and immune systems.

In chronic renal failure, metabolic complications will be detected when the glomerular filtration rate drops below 30 mL/min. Problems with fluid, electrolytes, and acid-base disturbances need to be addressed on an ongoing basis. Should anemia develop before ESRD sets in, iron deficiency should be corrected and the patient started on erythropoietin. Once the glomerular filtration rate drops below 20 mL/min, dialysis is impending. This is the ideal moment to establish vascular access. Once the patient becomes symptomatic for uremia, dialysis can be started through the newly established vascular access. Patients with diabetes, who constitute a large proportion of those on any dialysis program, develop symptoms at a lower level of serum creatinine and need to be dialyzed earlier than nondiabetics. As a general rule, dialysis should be started when the serum creatinine reaches 10 mg/dL. However, the acceptable range for the commencement of dialysis is wide, as it depends on many variables besides uremia.

Once begun on dialysis, several aspects of the ESRD patient require simultaneous management. The new fistula must be assessed for adequacy of blood flow. This is a simple process where both arterial and venous pressures are continually measured by the dialysis machine. The pressures may vary depending on the blood flow rate. If blood is pumped out of the fistula faster than the natural blood flow can enter the fistula, measured machine arterial pressure will drop and/or the fistula will collapse, further impeding blood flow out of the fistula. The dialysis machine may alarm before the fistula collapses once the arterial pressure monitor senses a drop in pressure beyond the set pressure safety limits. Poor arterial flow can be overcome by either repositioning badly placed fistula needles or by lowering the blood flow rate. Native fistulae that are small and have inadequate blood flows may mature with repeated use. The fistula should be used cautiously at first, with smaller needles and slower pump speeds. Over the ensuing weeks to months, the fistula enlarges and blood flow increases secondary to hypertrophy of the inflow artery. Needle size and pump flow rates can be progressively increased until the desired pump flow rates are achieved. These manipulations are less common when prosthetic bridge grafts serve as the access, since graft collapse is unlikely. Over time, however, hypertrophy of the inflow artery of a prosthetic graft may indeed result in improved fistula flow rates as the access matures.

Elevated venous pressures imply fistula outflow obstruction and may occur at any time. However, unexplained elevation of venous pressure may occur as a result of small-diameter or poorly placed venous needles. Clotting in the extracorporeal circulation or kinking of the lines may also result in high venous pressures. Once these causes of high venous pressure in the mechanical circuit have been excluded, the vascular access should be evaluated for patency of the venous outflow tract. Evaluation and management of this problem are addressed elsewhere in the text.

By means of urea kinetics, it is possible to estimate the adequacy of dialysis (3,12). The dialysis prescription is monitored using urea kinetics on at least a quarterly basis. Changes are made to provide the patient with sufficient dialysis to maintain a positive nitrogen balance. Underdialyzed patients are uremic and have insufficient nutritional intake. As a result, they develop a negative nitrogen balance, which is associated with a poor outcome. Careful attention must be paid to the patient's nutritional needs.

Several other aspects of the ESRD patient's care need to be addressed over the long term. Hypertension, fluid overload, and anemia are three parameters where good control ensures cardiac protection. This becomes of paramount importance, as cardiac complications are the greatest cause of morbidity and mortality in dialysis patients (13). Renal osteodystrophy and lipid abnormalities are ongoing problems and require evaluation and treatment throughout the duration of dialysis (14–16).

It is common for ESRD patients managed on hemodialysis to be on a wide variety of chronic and acute medications. Adjusting the prescription of drugs having a renal route of elimination or active metabolites excreted via the renal route is an important responsibility in managing dialysis patients. While serum levels for some drugs, such as aminoglycosides and cardiac glycosides, are readily available, most medication must be managed by consulting standard references (17).

While the patient's impaired renal status can lead to drug accumulation or affect typical clinical responses, dialysis can lead to rapid drug elimination. In hemodialysis, there are a wide variety of dialyzers that have different clearance rates for different phamacological agents. Drug clearance is dependent on blood and dialysate flow rates, dialyzer surface area, pore size of the dialyzer, and the time spent on dialysis. Recently, high-efficiency or high-flux dialyzers have come into more common use. These dialyzers offer greater rates of drug elimination due to convection, given their larger pore size. While higher drug clearance rates can be expected, patients tend to be on dialysis for shorter periods of time with high-flux dialyzers; therefore clearance rates tend to be similar to those found on non–high-flux dialyzers.

Fundamentally, a knowledge of the impact of declining renal function on prescribed drugs as well as the ability of dialysis to reduce serum drug levels is of crucial importance. Standard reference texts are a required part of the dialysis unit (18).

CONCLUSION

Dialysis is not a complete substitute for native renal function. However, dialysis has evolved over the last 30 years into a safe and sophisticated procedure that is acceptable to both patient and doctor. The intention is to provide adequate renal replacement therapy that will significantly enhance patient survival without overwhelmingly compromising the patient's lifestyle. Undoubtedly the current success of dialysis is one reason why the kidney has become such a successfully transplanted organ. Dialysis, which provides the bridge between ESRD and transplantation, maintains and improves the patient's physical condition, thus ensuring the best possible outcome.

With the improved ability to provide dialysis, the number of patients receiving renal replacement therapy, in both the acute and chronic situations, has increased. Moreover, patients who were previously considered undialyzable are being included in many dialysis programs. The elderly, who were excluded from dialysis in the early days, presently constitute a major proportion of the dialysis population. By the end of 1992, the U.S. Renal Data System had documented 255,000 patients on dialysis in the United States. The incidence of ESRD was 214 cases per million population, with 899 and 914 per million in the 70-to-74 and 75-to-79 age groups, respectively (19). These numbers are a testimony to the impact of dialysis on health care in this country.

REFERENCES

1. Graham T. Osmotic force. Phil Trans R Soc Lond 144:177–228, 1854.
2. Benedum J. Pioneer of dialysis, George Haas (1886–1971). Med Hist J 14:196–217, 1979.
3. Sargent JA, Gotch FA. Principles and biophysics of dialysis. In Maher JF, ed. Replacement of Renal Function by Dialysis, 3rd ed. Norwell, MA: Kluwer Academic Publishers; 1989:87–143.
4. Oates CP, William ED, McHugh MI. The use of Diasonics DRF400 duplex ultrasound scanner to measure volume flow in arteriovenous fistulae in patients undergoing hemodialysis: an analysis of the measurement uncertainties. Ultrasound Med Biol 16:571, 1990.
5. Rose BD, Black RM. Manual of Clinical Problems in Nephrology. Boston: Little, Brown, 1988:371–379.
6. Cronin RE. The patient with acute azotemia. In Schrier RW, ed. Manual of Nephrology Diagnosis and Therapy. Boston: Little, Brown; 1981:137–150.
7. Eberst ME, Berkowitz LR. Hemostasis in renal disease: pathology and management. Am J Med 96:168–179, 1994.
8. Henry JA. Specific problems of drug intoxication. Br J Anaesth 58:223–233, 1986.
9. Winchester JF. Poisoning: Is the role of the nephrologist diminishing? Am J Kidney Dis 13:171–183, 1989.
10. Lowrie EG, Lew NL. Death risk in hemodialysis patients: the predictive value of commonly measured variables and an evaluation of death rate differences between facilities. Am J Kidney Dis 15:458–482, 1990.
11. Avram MM, Mittman N, Bonomini L, et al. Markers for survival in dialysis: a seven-year prospective study. Am J Kidney Dis 26:209–219, 1995.
12. Hakim RM, Depner TA, Parker TF. Adequacy of hemodialysis. Am J Kidney Dis 20:107–123, 1992.

13. Rostand SG, Rutsky EA. Cardiac disease in dialysis patients. In Nissenson AR, Fine RN, Gentile DE, eds. Clinical Dialysis, 3rd ed. Norwalk, CT: Appleton & Lange; 1995:652–698.

14. Malluche H, Faugere M-C. Renal bone disease 1990: an unmet challenge for the nephrologist. Kidney Int 38:193–211, 1990.

15. Llach F. Secondary hyperparathyroidism in renal failure: the trade-off hypothesis revisited. Am J Kidney Dis 25:663–679, 1995.

16. Chan MK. Lipoprotein metabolism in dialysis patients. In Nissenson AR, Fine RN, Gentile DE, eds. Clinical Dialysis, 3rd ed. Norwalk, CT: Appleton & Lange, 1995: 699–713.

17. Piafsky DM. Disease induced changes in the serum binding of basic drugs. Clin Pharmacokinet 5:245–262, 1980.

18. Bennet WM, Golper TA. Drug usage in dialysis patients. In Nissenson AR, Fine RN, Gentile DE, eds. Clinical Dialysis, 3rd ed. Norwalk, CT: Appleton & Lange; 1995:806–826.

19. US Renal Data System (USRDS). USRDS 1995 Annual report, Bethesda, Md: In Incidence and causes of treated ESRD. Am J Kidney Dis 26(4,S2):S39–S50, 1995.

2

Anesthetic Considerations

Mark P. Ramirez
Santa Rita Anesthesiology, Tucson, Arizona

Scott S. Berman
The University of Arizona, Carondelet St. Mary's Hospital, and The
  Southern Arizona Vascular Institute, Tucson, Arizona

Patients with end-stage renal disease (ESRD) who need to undergo anesthesia for dialysis access placement are therapeutic challenges by virtue of their numerous pathophysiological abnormalities (1). With the continuing growth of the ESRD population, more and more patients are requiring surgical procedures to establish or maintain dialysis access. The American Society of Anesthesiologists (ASA) Physical Status Classification of these patients is usually 3 (severe systemic disease, not incapacitating) and often 4 (severe systemic disease that is a constant threat to life), which indicates that extra care and vigilance are needed in providing anesthetic care to these patients. The anesthetic technique will vary between patients and no single approach (general vs. regional) has yet proven consistently superior over the other (2,3). Newer, shorter-acting hypnotics, muscle relaxants, and inhaled volatile agents as well as improvements in intraoperative monitoring allow for an individualized approach. Some surgeons are comfortable injecting local anesthetic into the operative site, thereby producing a field blockade, whereas others prefer a motionless field and an amnestic patient, which often requires a regional technique or a general anesthetic. Moreover, some anesthesiologists are adept at placing supraclavicular blocks for the upper extremity,

15

while others find that the small but significant risk of pneumothorax is prohibitive. Patients with chronic illness are sometimes quite anxious and demand to "be put to sleep," subsequently refusing regional techniques. The "best" approach is what works safely for the patient, surgeon, and anesthesiologist.

ANESTHETIC CONCERNS

Renal Impairment

In anuric patients, with the exception of insensible losses, the elimination of fluid is entirely dependent upon dialysis. Hypertension, hypervolemia, and edema will result from excess sodium intake. Hyponatremia will follow excessive water intake. A patient who is overdialyzed may be relatively hypovolemic when anesthesia commences but may quickly develop pulmonary edema with minimal amounts of intravenous fluids (e.g. 500 mL). Patients with ESRD have limited physiological reserves. Chronic congestive heart failure is relatively common, but perioperative manifestations are minimized if hemodialysis has occurred 12 to 24 h prior to surgery.

Serum potassium levels are highly variable, though hypokalemia is uncommon in ESRD patients. Large potassium losses can occur from vomiting, diarrhea, or nasogastric suctioning. The usual acceptable lower limits of serum potassium for elective surgery (3.0 meq/L) are arbitrary generalizations (4). The previously conjectured concerns of intraoperative ventricular arrhythmias associated with hypokalemia have been called into question by prospective studies (5,6). Other factors that impact the significance of hyokalemia include concomitant medications (e.g., digitalis), acid-base balance, and electrocardiogram abnormalities. Recall that potassium administration is not always a benign exercise and that 0.5% of patients receiving this therapy may suffer significant morbidity and mortality from iatrogenic hyperkalemia (7). There are no absolute rules dictating the management of these ESRD patients. Individual judgment must be exercised in each situation.

More often, hyperkalemia exists in ESRD patients and is exacerbated by chronic metabolic acidosis. Many of these individuals generally tolerate serum potassium levels in excess of 6 meq/L without sequelae. However, the general recommendation suggests that elective surgery be postponed if the serum potassium exceeds 5.5 meq/L (8). Up to one-third of patients with chronic renal failure may require treatment for significant hyperkalemia within 24 h of a major surgical procedures (9). Electrocardiographic abnormalities, which are often seen first, include the appearance of tall, thin T waves. Later changes include PR interval prolongation, ST segment depression, QRS interval lengthening, disappearance of the P wave, and finally ventricular fibrillation (10). Elective surgical cases can

TABLE 2.1 Emergent Treatment of Hyperkalemia

Indication Onset	Treatment	Mechanism	
Severe progressive hyperkalemia	Calcium chloride 1–2 g IV over several minutes	Antagonizes K ion effect upon neuromuscular membranes	Immediate, but lasts only 5–10 min
Severe to moderate hyperkalemia	Glucose (1 amp D50) with 10–15 U of regular insulin IV	Shifts K ion into cells	5 min, effect lasts several hours
	Sodium bicarbonate 50–100 meq IV	Shifts K ion into cells	Within minutes

allow for treatment via dialysis, but emergent surgery in a hyperkalemic patient requires emergency treatment (Table 2.1).

Treatment of hyperkalemia with calcium salts should be cautiously undertaken and only during monitoring of the patient's heart rhythm, particularly if digitalis has been administered, since toxic dysrhythmias may develop. If necessary, the injection may be repeated in 5 to 10 min. It is important to remember that calcium infusions provide only temporary benefit and that other forms of therapy for hyperkalemia are essential. Calcium infusion will help protect against the conduction abnormalities and arrhythmias of potassium excess but will not affect the serum levels of the ion. Treatment with sodium bicarbonate is effective by forcing potassium intracellularly through its buffering capacity; however, the consequent fluid overload in patients prone to congestive heart failure and pulmonary edema, due to the attendant sodium load with bicarbonate infusions, limits their use in treating hyperkalemia. Glucose and insulin therapy may reduce serum potassium by 1 to 2 mmol/L within 30 min, and bicarbonate may be added to enhance this effect. The cation exchange resin kayexalate is mentioned for only completeness, since this mode of therapy works far too slowly for an emergent situation.

Disorders of phosphate elimination and calcium balance affect the skeletal and muscular systems of ESRD patients. Since the kidney is no longer able to synthesize vitamin D, absorption of calcium from the gastrointestinal tract is poor. Phosphate elimination is reduced because of renal dysfunction. Together these stimuli cause parathyroid gland hyperplasia and calcium resorption from the bones, leading to renal osteodystrophy. The syndrome of renal osteodystrophy includes osteoporosis, osteomalacia, and joint deformities. These maladies place

ESRD patients at risk for fractures secondary to poor positioning on the operative table. Hyperphosphatemia can result in metastatic calcification in muscle tissue, and cutaneous deposition may result in significant pruritus. The treatment for chronic hypocalcemia and hyperphosphatemia consists respectively of oral calcium supplements and oral phosphate binders such as aluminum hydroxide. Aggressive treatment can occasionally produce phosphate depletion syndrome, causing muscular weakness, rhabdomyolysis, paresthesias, hemolysis, platelet abnormalities, and ventilatory insufficiency.

Hypermagnesemia may be seen in uremia and is more common in patients taking magnesium-based antacids and purgatives. High levels can interact with anesthetic agents and muscle relaxants to produce prolonged neuromuscular blockade and subsequent difficulty with neuromuscular reversal. This, in turn, can result in respiratory compromise, apnea, and aspiration after extubation in the immediate postoperative period.

Cardiovascular Abnormalities

Accelerated atherosclerosis is not uncommon in ESRD patients who are maintained on chronic dialysis (11). This leads to manifestations of coronary, cerebrovascular, and peripheral vascular disease. Associated risk factors often seen in ESRD patients include hypertension, diabetes mellitus, and altered lipid metabolism. Myocardial ischemia is common and may be silent. A high index of suspicion should be reserved for these patients and appropriate preoperative evaluation and intraoperative management should be directed toward reducing complications related to coronary artery disease. Hypertension is almost universally present in this population. It can result from fluid overload or increased renin levels; patients can also develop sudden hypertension during intubation or significant hypotension after the induction of general anesthesia with resultant myocardial ischemia (12).

Hematological Abnormalities

Normochromic normocytic anemia is very commonly seen in ESRD patients, though the incidence of this problem has been reduced with the widespread use of recombinant erythropoietin. There is an associated increased incidence of hypertension and arteriovenous fistula thrombosis related to erythropoietin usage (13). Since the anemia of renal failure is of gradual onset, compensatory mechanisms such as increased cardiac output and rightward shift of the oxyhemoglobin dissociation curve facilitate oxygen delivery to tissues. Cardiac output increases because of an increase in stroke volume without tachycardia (14). Anemia decreases blood viscosity, thereby decreasing systemic vascular resistance. Tissue oxygenation is maintained even with hematocrits in the 20 to 25% range. Coagulopathies may be present in these patients. Large heparin doses administered prior to hemodialysis may continue to circulate at the time of surgery. Defects in platelet function manifest as poor aggregation and can be partially corrected by dialysis.

Neurological Abnormalities

Central nervous system (CNS) dysfunction can range from subtle personality changes to myoclonus and seizures. Dialysis itself is associated with a disequilibrium syndrome, dementia, and progressive intellectual impairment (15). Some patients develop a behavior pattern that is passive-aggressive and manipulative. Peripheral neuropathy is common and has been used as a firm indication to begin dialysis. It can progress to flaccid quadriplegia if treatment is delayed.

Gastrointestinal Complications

Peptic ulcer disease is seen in up to 25% of patients with renal failure and is not eliminated by renal replacement therapy. Patients with ESRD frequently have increased gastric juice volumes and delayed gastric emptying times that make them prone to aspiration if there is a loss of protective airway reflexes (16). Chronic viral hepatitis is very common and universal precautions should be strictly enforced to prevent disease transmission.

Pharmacological Considerations

Numerous drugs used in the practice of anesthesia are eliminated by the kidneys. Their dosing, therefore, must be reduced to avoid prolonged or adverse effects. Moreover, the response of ESRD patients to these agents is extremely variable due to the complex interplay between changes in excretion, low pH, serum protein binding, and volume of distribution. As anemia results in an increased cardiac output, many drugs exert their effects much more quickly, since flow to the brain is increased. Some drugs have metabolites that can result in significant toxicity. Examples include meperidine, which is transformed into normeperidine; high levels of this can cause CNS irritability and seizures. Morphine metabolites (glucuronides) are active directly on the CNS and can accumulate after repeated dosing. This may result in a prolonged effect and may contribute to respiratory depression (17). The half-life of pancuronium, a neuromuscular blocker, is prolonged as much as fourfold; its increased duration of action can lead to respiratory compromise if not fully reversed (18). Careful titration of induction agents such as thiopental and propofol is needed, since they can cause significant vasodilatation and myocardial depression in selected patients. Severe hypotension and cardiac arrest can result, especially in patients with volume depletion or left ventricular dysfunction. Significant decreases in dosage are still effective with drugs that are protein-bound (e.g., thiopental), since many uremic patients suffer from hypoalbuminemia. Less drug is bound to protein and thus available to reach receptor sites. Cardiovascular and CNS toxicity of local anesthetics such as lido-caine and bupivicaine are increased by acidosis, hypercarbia, or prior administra-tion of a drug such as cimetidine—conditions that are commonly encountered in ESRD patients and which will slow elimination. Symptoms can range from light-headedness and tinnitus to seizures and cardiac arrest.

PREOPERATIVE EVALUATION

Whether regional or general anesthesia is planned, a thorough review of the pa-tient's past anesthetic experience should always be obtained. A bedside evalua-tion should concentrate on pulmonary, cardiac, neurologic, renal, and pharmaco-logical history. Dialysis records are useful for documentation of "dry weight." Ideally, dialysis should be conducted 12 to 24 h prior to surgery. Previous anes-thesia records are often available and are essential in order to avoid unpleasant surprises at the time of surgery. A directed physical examination of the patient's airway, heart, lungs, and neurological function can be performed in a few min-utes. Attention is paid to the presence of hypertension, orthostasis, and mental status changes as well as neuropathies, pulmonary compromise such as rales or effusions, and cardiac function to detect overt heart failure. Evidence of bruising or petechiae is also sought. Chest radiograph reports and electrocardiograms add to the physical exam. Particular attention is paid to hemoglobin, platelet count, coagulation studies, glucose, potassium, creatinine, BUN, sodium, and total CO_2. It is helpful to review ionized calcium, phosphate, and magnesium levels if avail-able. Patients should be NPO for 6 to 8 h, but should be provided with their regular cardiac and antihypertensive medications on schedule with small sips of water. Since gastric volumes can be increased, consideration of adding H_2 antagonists (or omeprazole) and intestinal motility agents (metoclopramide or cisapride) to the preanesthetic drug regimen is helpful in reducing the risk of pulmonary aspiration. If pulmonary edema, pneumonia, severe uncontrolled hy-pertension, congestive heart failure, severe hyperglycemia, hyperkalemia, coagu-lopathy, or severe anemia are detected, it is usually better to delay the surgical procedure and optimize the patient's condition if at all possible, particularly for an elective procedure.

ANESTHETIC PROCEDURES

General Anesthesia

General anesthesia may be used for vascular access of the upper and lower ex-tremity or for patients who require peritoneal dialysis access procedures. A reli-able intravenous line is established in the extremity opposite the operative site for patients undergoing upper extremity surgery. A crystalloid solution free of potassium is usually a good choice. Some practitioners prefer 5% dextrose with water, but this is not useful if lost blood is to be replaced with crystalloid or for the replacement of preoperative volume deficits. Moreover, administration of dextrose may contribute to perioperative hyperglycemia in ESRD patients with brittle diabetes. The anesthesia machine, monitors, and the availability of suction are checked, and appropriate medications are drawn up in advance. It is useful to have drugs available to treat hypertension, hypotension, bradycardia, and arrythmias. An antianxiety premedication such as midazolam can be given. The standard ASA monitors are applied [e.g., electrocardiogram (ECG), pulse oximeter, automated blood pressure cuff, end-tidal carbon dioxide, temperature probe]. The use of a five-lead ECG system with a lead at the V_5 location should be considered to monitor the left ventricle for ischemia. The simultaneous display of leads II and V_5 allows for the detection of up to 90% of ischemic episodes (19). The patient is given 100% oxygen for several minutes via the anesthesia machine circuit with a tight mask fit to eliminate the inspiration of room air. One should consider the use of cricoid pressure at this point to reduce the risk of aspiration. An induction (sleep) dose of thiopental, propofol, or etomidate is given. Muscle paralysis for intubation can be accomplished with shorter-acting drugs such as succinylcholine, mivacurium, or the intermediate-duration agents atracurium, rocuronium, and vecuronium. Atracurium has the advantage of not accumulating after repeat dosing. In contrast, the tendency of vecuronium to accumulate if used for maintenance suggests that caution should be exercised with the use of this drug (20). Succinylcholine will result in a 0.5- to 1-meq increase in serum potassium when administered, but it can be used safely if the patient's potassium is within normal limits; moreover, it is not associated with the dangerous elevations in potassium levels that are seen in patients with burns, neuromuscular disorders, closed head injuries, and denervation injuries (21). Maintenance of anesthesia is achieved with nitrous oxide, oxygen, and a volatile agent such as isoflurane. A narcotic such as fentanyl can be added to augment the maintenance regimen and provide some postoperative pain relief; fentanyl appears to be a good choice because of its elimination by the liver and its rapid tissue redistribution. Neuromuscular blockade should be followed with a twitch monitor. At the conclusion of surgery, the blockade can be reversed if needed and the patient extubated when awake enough to protect the airway against aspiration. Postoperative pain can be controlled with small doses of fentanyl (e.g., 25 µg) in the postanesthesia care unit. Hypertension can be a problem in this setting but frequently responds to intravenous labetalol or other short-acting intravenous agents. With strict attention to detail and an understanding of the altered physiology of this patient population, a properly conducted general anesthetic is a reasonable technique that can be applied safely.

Regional Anesthesia

Aside from general anesthesia, several other approaches are available when it is necessary to provide surgical anesthesia for the creation of arteriovenous fistulae. The use of local anesthetics (LA) is appealing in these patients, since access procedures are often performed on an outpatient basis. Postoperative pain relief is excellent with this approach. A regional technique may allow for less hemodynamic variability and reduce the risk of aspiration. However, no technique is perfect. The evaluation and preparation must be as diligent as for general anesthesia. Preexisting neurological deficits should be well documented in the anesthesia record. Regional anesthesia should not be considered if the patient refuses the technique despite educational efforts, local infection at the injection site, or systemic coagulopathy. The increased use of sedatives with a partially effective block may render a patient apneic or may prolong the recovery, which is longer than for a formal general anesthetic. Sedation and analgesia may easily become unconscious sedation with an unprotected airway and increase the risk of aspiration and hypoxia. The anesthesiologist must always be prepared to provide general anesthesia if regional anesthesia proves inadequate. While a regional block is being administered, the patient should be monitored with pulse oximetry, ECG, and noninvasive blood pressure monitoring. Functional intravenous access must be present. Emergency drugs to treat seizures and cardiac arrest as well as to manage the airway must be available. Airway adjuncts such as bag, mask, suctioning apparatus, and a supply of oxygen are essential. Adequate preparation can help prevent an unexpected complication from becoming an anesthetic disaster.

For the less common, unconventional dialysis access procedures such as those in the lower extremity, local/regional anesthetic techniques apply as well. Specific regional methods include spinal and epidural techniques. A detailed discussion of these methods is beyond the scope of this chapter. However, interested readers are referred to the available reports and texts for a comprehensive review (22,23).

Local Anesthetics

Commonly available agents are classified as amino esters or amino amides. All local anesthetics produce blockade of nerve impulses by inhibiting the influx of sodium ions, which precludes depolarization, thereby preventing conduction. Examples of amino ester local anesthetics are cocaine, procaine, tetracaine, and chloroprocaine. They are metabolized by plasma and hepatic cholinesterases and produce metabolites related to paraaminobenzoic acid (PABA). PABA is the usual culprit in allergic reactions when amino esters are employed. Most nerve blockade is carried out using one of the amino amides: lidocaine, bupivacane, mepivacaine, ropivacaine, etidocaine, or prilocaine. The amino amides undergo only hepatic metabolism; therefore allergic reactions to these agents are very rare and are usually due to preservatives (methylparaben) contained in multidose vials (24). Methylparaben-free formulations are readily available for regional anesthesia. Vasoconstrictors (epinephrine or phenylephrine) are added to local anesthetic solutions, which prolongs their duration of action and limits systemic absorption. Some susceptible patients may develop significant tachycardia or hypertension when these additives are absorbed. The use of vasoconstrictors in conjunction with LAs is contraindicated in proximity to end arteries of the distal extremities.

Systemic toxicity of LAs affects the central nervous system (CNS) and the cardiovascular system (Table 2.2). It most often results from an inadvertent intravascular injection or the administration of an excessive dose to tissues at the surgical site. Seizures probably result from a selective depression of inhibitory centers in the CNS, allowing excitatory centers to predominate (25). Very low doses (e.g., 1 to 3 mL) accidentally injected into an artery lead to seizures more readily than venous injections. This is the result of retrograde flow in the arterial system, which allows local anesthetic to enter the cerebral circulation (26). Toxicity is enhanced by acidosis, hypercarbia, or drugs that tend to slow the elimination of local anesthetics. Seizure potential is reduced by the concomitant use of benzodiazepines and barbiturates. Seizures can be rapidly treated with thiopental while supporting the patient's ventilation. Cardiac toxicity is less common than CNS toxicity but more difficult to treat. Local anesthetic agents affect the conduction system of the heart by blocking sodium channels. Bupivicaine toxicity is much more severe than that due to other LAs because its relatively slow dissociation and accumulation at these sites (27). As a result, resuscitation from bupivicaine-mediated cardiac arrest can be extremely difficult. Administration of local anesthetics in divided doses during the performance of nerve blocks will allow for the early recognition and avoidance of serious toxicity.

Specific Regional Techniques

The sensory innervation of the upper extremity is supplied by the nerve roots C5 to T1 and at times by C4 and T2. The five roots combine to form three trunks, which are accessible at the scalene triangle of the neck. The trunks divide into anterior and posterior divisions, which then unite to form three cords, each of which, in turn, has two terminal branches supplying the arm.

Adequate surgical anesthesia may be obtained with the following:

- Infiltration of local anesthetic
- Peripheral nerve blockade
- Brachial plexus blockade
- Axillary block

TABLE 2.2 Toxicity and Management of Local Anesthetic

	Symptoms	Therapy	Cause, Prevention, Peculiarities
CNS stimulation, moderate intoxication	Restlessness, agitation, tremors, tinnitus, metallic taste, muscle twitches	O_2 by mask, sedation with thiopental 25–50 mg or midazolam 2–4 mg	Monitor dose, aspirate before injection, consider using epinephrine LA solutions, repositioning the needle, and divided dosing; maintain verbal contact with patient, ask for warning symptoms
	Nausea, vomiting	Droperidol 0.625 mg or ondansetron 4 mg	
	Seizures	Sedation, ventilation, intubation if prolonged	
CNS and CVS depression, severe intoxication	Speech disturbances, disorientation, unconsciousness, apnea	O_2 by mask, ventilation; consider intubation	Avoid intravenous LA injection
	Bradycardia, hypotension	O_2 by mask, atropine, ephedrine	Have patient monitors in place, emergency drugs ready; airway equipment and suction immediately available
	Asystole	CPR	
Allergic reactions	Erythema, urticaria, bronchospasm, analphalaxis	Epinephrine, antihistamine, H_2 blocker, corticosteroids	Use preservative-free LA solutions (methylparaben-free)

Abbreviations: CNS, central nervous system; CVS, ; LA, .
Source: Modified from Ref. 34.

TABLE 2.3 Agents Used for Local Anesthesia

Agent	Concentration	Duration (hours) Without Epinephrine	Duration (hours) with Epinephrine	Dosage Range[a]
Lidocaine	0.5–1.0%	0.5–2	1–3	Up to 50 mL
Mepivacaine	0.5–1.0%	0.5–2	1–3	Up to 50 mL
Bupivacaine	0.25–0.5%	2–4	4–8	Up to 45 mL

[a] Maximum recommended dosage for 70-kg patient using the higher-concentration solution containing epinephrine.
Source: Adapted from Ref. 35.

Local Anesthesia

Simple infiltration of local anesthetics (Table 2.3) to the operative site is used frequently at some institutions for the placement of arteriovenous (AV) fistulas in the wrist and forearm. It is often supplemented by intravenous narcotics, barbiturates, and benzodiazepines during monitored anesthesia care (MAC). Local anesthesia may produce a moving surgical field due to incomplete relief of intraoperative pain, requiring larger doses of intravenous agents and additional infiltration. This, in turn, can result in "unconscious sedation," with the increased risk of pulmonary aspiration and prolonged recovery in the postanesthesia care unit. Despite these limitations, very effective peripheral access surgery using local anesthesia alone can be accomplished with obvious patient care and cost advantages (28). Local anesthesia combined with MAC is also the method of choice for placing tunneled long-term dialysis catheters.

Peripheral Nerve Blockade

The musculocutaneous and medial antebrachial cutaneous nerves can be blocked by peripheral infiltration. This technique has been described as well received by patients and surgeons for the creation of AV fistulas in the forearm (29). For both peripheral and brachial plexus nerve blocks, narrow-gauge (22 to 25 gauge) short-bevel needles should be used to minimize nerve trauma, which can result in postblock neuropathy (30). About 5 to 7 mL of local anesthetic is placed in the proximal coracobrachialis muscle, lateral and deep to the axillary sheath, which accomplishes adequate blockade of the musculocutaneous nerve (Figure 2.1). The medial antebrachial cutaneous nerve is anesthetized by injecting an additional 10 mL subcutaneously as a half ring on the medial aspect of the forearm, about one-half to two-thirds the distance from the shoulder to the elbow. This procedure is described as relatively simple to perform and avoids the need for high doses of local anesthetics.

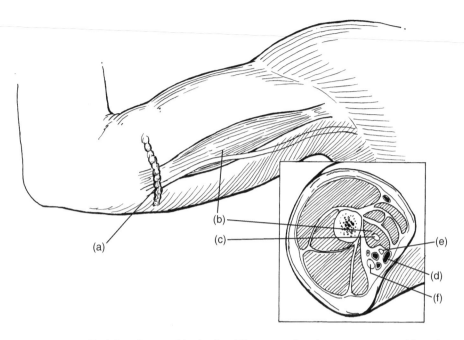

FIGURE 2.1 Peripheral nerve blockade of the musculocutaneous nerve achieved by injecting local anesthetic into the coracobrachialis muscle and of the medial antebrachial cuaneous nerve by injecting a ring subcutaneously along the medial arm. (a) subcutaneous ring, (b) coraco-brachialis muscle, (c) musculocutaneous nerve, (d) basilic vein, (e) median nerve, (f) medial brachial cutaneous nerve.

Brachial Plexus Blockade

The superficial location of the brachial plexus in the scalene triangle provides easy access to surgical anesthesia of the upper arm, elbow, forearm, and radial aspect of the hand. The anesthetic agent can be delivered at a point where the three trunks are close together as they pass over the first rib, resulting in a rapid onset of reliable blockade (Figure 2.2). The pulse of the subclavian artery is palpated and a short-bevel, $1^1/2$-in., 22-gauge needle is advanced caudally and laterally until paresthesias are noted by the patient. After negative aspiration, 30 to 40 ml of a local anesthetic solution such as 1.5% mepivacaine or 0.5% bupivacaine is injected in 5-mL increments while carefully observing for signs of toxicity. The risk of pneumothorax (0.6 to 6.0%) limits its use in outpatients and in patients with preexisting pulmonary compromise (31). This usually develops over 24 h and a chest radiograph taken earlier may not show any evidence of a prob-

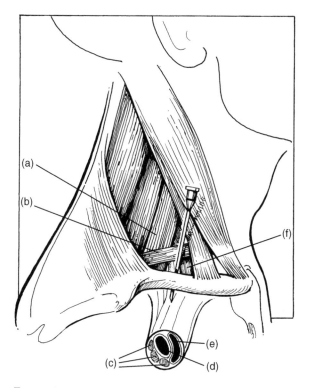

FIGURE 2.2 Technique for supraclavicular brachial plexus blockade. (a) Middle scalene muscle, (b) omohyoid muscle, (c) brachial plexus, (d) subclavian artery, (e) subclavian vein, (f) anterior scalene muscle.

lem. The main advantage of the supraclavicular approach is that it allows for surgical procedures on the upper arm, forearm, and hand.

Axillary Block

Blockade of branches of the brachial plexus as they pass through the axilla provides anesthesia of the forearm and hand. This technique is limited to patients who can abduct their arm to 90 degrees or more. The axilla and inner aspect of the upper arm is cleansed with antiseptic solution. The pulsation of the axillary artery is located at the anterior axillary wall (Figure 2.3). A 22-gauge, short-bevel, $1^1/2$-in. needle is introduced slightly above the pulsation; when the needle penetrates the axillary sheath, a click or pop is often felt by the anesthesiologist. At times, paresthesias are noted, which are used by some to signal an adequate

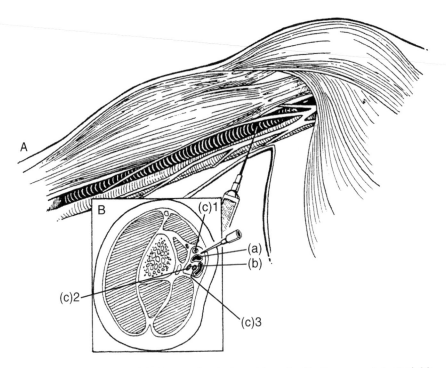

FIGURE 2.3   A. Axillary block anesthesia is achieved with the arm abducted 90 degrees while maintaining pressure on the axillary artery. B. Perivascular infiltration of the local anesthetic achieves nerve block through the proximity of the median, radial, and ulnar nerves to the vascular structures. (a) Axillary artery, (b) axillary vein, (c) brachial plexus cords: 1. lateral; 2. posterior; 3. medial.

endpoint. If the axillary artery is penetrated, the needle is advanced slightly through its posterior wall, which is still contained within the axillary sheath. After negative aspiration, 30 to 40 mL of local anesthetic is incrementally injected. Anesthesia is often incomplete at the mid- to upper arm. In addition, a separate peripheral block of the musculocutaneous nerve (which supplies the lateral arm region) may be needed since this nerve is spared as often as 25% of the time with the axillary approach (32). To reduce the discomfort of pneumatic tourniquets (if chosen for use during the access procedure), the intercostobrachial nerve should be blocked by a subcutaneous infiltration of local anesthetic in a half-ring fashion high up on the arm's axillary side. Depending upon which local anesthetic is used, loss of sensation will be noted within 10 to 15 min, though complete surgical anesthesia may take twice as long. Axillary blocks avoid the risk of pneumothorax and are relatively easy to perform with a high rate of success. The previously reported decreased duration of brachial plexus blocks in renal failure patients has not been a consistent finding in other studies (33). Complications associated with axillary blocks include hematoma, nerve injury, intravascular injection, and arterial/venous insufficiency.

CONCLUSION

Just as surgical access procedures must be tailored to the individual patient's needs, so too must the anesthetic technique chosen match the requirements of the individual patient. ESRD patients represent unique challenges to anesthesia personnel because of their altered physiology and comorbid conditions. Careful attention to detail preoperatively should allow for provision of an anesthetic that maximizes patient comfort without compromising patient safety.

REFERENCES

1. Brenner B, Lazarus M. Chronic renal failure. In Isselbacher K, Braunwald E, Wilson J, et al, eds. Harrison's Principles of Internal Medicine, 13th ed. New York: McGraw-Hill; 1994:1274–1281.
2. Seltzer J. Is regional anesthesia preferable to general anesthesia for outpatient surgical procedures on an upper extremity? (editorial.) Mayo Clin Proc 66:544–547, 1991.
3. Bode RH Jr, Lewis KP, Zarich SW, et al. Cardiac outcome after peripheral vascular surgery. Anesthesiology 84:3–13, 1996.
4. Wong, KC. Cations and the Mechanisms of drug actions. In Annual Refresher Course Lectures. Park Ridge, IL: American Society of Anesthesiologists, 1991.
5. Vitez TS, Soper LE, Wong KC, Soper P. Chronic hypokalemia and intraoperative dysrhythmias. Anesthesiology 63:130–133, 1985.
6. Hirsch IA, Tomlinson DL, Slogoff S, Keats AS. The overstated risk of preoperative hypokalemia. Anesth Ann 67:131–136, 1988.
7. Burke GR, Gulyassay PF. Surgery in the patient with renal disease and related electrolyte disorders. Med Clin North Am 63:1191–1203, 1979.
8. Weir PHC, Chung FF. Anesthesia for patients with chronic renal disease. Can Anaesth Soc J 31:468, 1984.
9. Brenowitz JB, Williams CD, Edwards WS. Major surgery in patients with chronic renal failure. Am J Surg 134:765, 1977.
10. Marriott HJL. Practical Electrocardiography, 7th ed. Baltimore: Williams & Wilkins; 1977:308–309.
11. Lindner A, Charra B, Sherrard DJ, Scribner BH. Accelerated atherosclerosis in prolonged maintenance hemodialysis. N Engl J Med 290:697, 1974.
12. Goldman L, Caldera DL. Risk of general anesthesia and elective operation in the hypertensive patient. Anesthesiology 50:285, 1979.

13. Casati S, Passerini P, Campise MR, et al. Benefits and risks of protracted treatment with human recombinant erythropoietin in patients having haemodialysis. Br Med J 295:1017, 1987.

14. Varat M, Adolph R, Fowler N. Cardiovascular effects of anemia. Am Heart J 83: 415–426, 1976.

15. Fraser CL, Arieff AI. Nervous system complications in uremia. Ann Intern Med 109:143–153, 1988.

16. McConnell JB, Stewart WK, Thjodleifsson B, Wormsley KG. Gastric function in chronic renal failure: Effects of maintenance hemodialysis. Lancet 1:1121, 1975.

17. Chauvin M, Sandouk P, Scherrmann JM, et al. Morphine pharmacokinetics in renal failure. Anesthesiology 66:327–331, 1987.

18. McLeod K, Watson M, Rawlins M. Pharmacokinetics of pancuronium in patients with normal and impaired renal function. Br J Anaesth 48:341, 1976.

19. London MJ, Hollenberg M, Wong MG, et al. Intraoperative myocardial ischemia: Localization by continuous 12 lead electrocardiography. Anesthesiology 69:232–241, 1988.

20. Pollard B, Doran B. Should vecuronium be used in renal failure? (letter.) Can J Anaesth 36:602, 1989.

21. Miller RD, Way WL, Hamilton WK, Layzer RB. Succinylcholine induced hyperkalemia in patients with renal failure? Anesthesiology 36:138, 1972.

22. Cavino BG, Scott DB, Lambert DH. Handbook of Spinal Anesthesia and Analgesia. Philadelphia: Saunders; 1994.

23. Brown DL. Regional Anesthesia and Analgesia. Philadelphia: Saunders; 1996.

24. Nagel J, Fuscaldo J, Fireman P. Paraben allergy. JAMA 237:1594, 1977.

25. de Jong RH, Robles R, Corbin R. Central actions of lidocaine synaptic transmission. Anesthesiology 30:19, 1969.

26. Aldrete JA, Romo-Salas F, Arora S, et al. Reverse arterial blood flow as a pathway for central nervous system toxic responses following injection of local anesthetics. Anesth Analg 57:428, 1978.

27. Clarkson CW, Hondeghem LM. Mechanism for bupivicaine depression of cardiac conduction: Fast block of sodium channels during the action potential with slow recovery from block during diastole. Anesthesiology 62:396, 1985.

28. Didlake R, Curry E, Rigdon EE, et al. Outpatient vascular access surgery: Impact of a dialysis-unit based surgical facility. Am J Kidney Dis 19:39–44, 1992.

29. Eldredge SJ, Sperry RJ, Johnson JO. Regional anesthesia for arteriovenous fistula creation in the forearm: A new approach. Anesthesiology 77:1230–1231, 1992.

30. Selander D, Dhuner KG, Lundberg G. Peripheral nerve injury due to injection needles used for regional anesthesia. Acta Anaesth Scand 21:182–188, 1977.

31. Abram SE, Hogan QH. Complications of nerve blocks. In Benumof JL, Saidman LJ, eds. Anesthesia and Perioperative Complications. St. Louis: Mosby–Year Book; 1992:52–76.

32. Vester-Andersen T, Christians C, Sorensen M, et al. Moller K. Perivascular axillary block II: Influence of injected volume of local anesthetic on neural blockade. Acta Anaesthesiol Scand 27:95, 1983.

33. Beauregard L, Martin R, Tetrault J. Brachial plexus block and chronic renal failure. Can J Anaesth 56:941, 1987.
34. Hoerster W, Kreuscher H, Hiesel HChr: Regional Anesthesia. St Louis: Mosby Year-Book; 1990:49–50.
35. Firestone L, Lebowitz P, Cook C. Clinical Anestheisa Procedures of the Massachusetts General Hospital. Boston: Little, Brown; 1988:189.

3

Preoperative Evaluation

John M. Marek
University of New Mexico School of Medicine, Albuquerque,
New Mexico

Scott S. Berman
The University of Arizona, Carondelet St. Mary's Hospital, and
The Southern Arizona Vascular Institute,
Tucson, Arizona

The 1998 report of the U.S. Renal Data System indicates that nearly 300,000 Americans are currently being treated for end-stage renal disease (ESRD) (1). New cases of ESRD have increased dramatically over the past decade to over 41,000 per year of late (1). The annual mortality rate among dialysis patients remains high due to the advanced age and frequent comorbid conditions present; however, improvements in technology and patient care have extended the number of years patients receive dialysis. This patient population clearly represents a challenge to the physician who has the task of placing a well-functioning dialysis access route. Thoughtful patient evaluation and planning prior to an access procedure may lessen patient morbidity and discomfort and offer the maximal opportunity for a successful outcome and prolonged, uninterrupted access.

Currently 60% of ESRD patients are being treated with hemodialysis, 25% have a functioning renal transplant, and 9% perform peritoneal dialysis. Important decisions regarding hemodialysis versus peritoneal dialysis are discussed in subsequent chapters. While renal transplantation remains the optimal treatment for most patients, the limited availability of donor organs leaves the majority of

ESRD patients in need of temporary or permanent hemodialysis. Regardless of the eventual primary renal replacement therapy chosen, the majority of patients will require a period of hemodialysis. This chapter focuses on the preoperative evaluation of patients requiring hemodialysis. Sections are devoted to the evaluation of patients undergoing placement of dialysis catheters and/or arteriovenous (AV) fistulae as well as to considerations in the pediatric population.

EVALUATION OF THE PATIENT FOR DIALYSIS CATHETER PLACEMENT

A detailed discussion of issues revolving around temporary and long-term hemodialysis catheters appears in Chapter 7. A brief overview is presented in the ensuing section. Catheter placement is indicated in patients with acute renal failure requiring temporary dialysis and for ESRD patients while permanent fistulas mature or during complications of their primary renal replacement therapy. A subset of patients—including adults who have exhausted permanent fistula options and young children—may be entirely dependent on these catheters for hemodialysis access. Indeed, due to the many inherent problems with prosthetic arteriovenous fistulae, some authors have advocated the use of tunneled Permcath-type catheters when an autologous fistula is not feasible (2,3).

In planning any dialysis access procedure, consideration must be given to the type of permanent renal replacement therapy planned for the patient and when that therapy will be ready for use. There are many approaches to this clinical problem. Our own approach is summarized in the algorithm appearing in Figure 3.1. If an ESRD patient requires immediate dialysis access, a percutaneous temporary catheter is usually placed at the bedside, preferably via an internal jugular vein. If prolonged access will be needed in this patient, a decision is made regarding the suitability of constructing an autogenous AV fistula. Patients with favorable anatomy for a native fistula have a tunneled catheter placed at the time of fistula construction to provide a bridge for dialysis until the fistula has matured. Similarly, if an ESRD patient requires dialysis within a few weeks and an autologous fistula or peritoneal catheter is planned, a tunneled dialysis catheter should be placed at the same time as the fistula. However, if a prosthetic bridge graft, which can be accessed in 10 to 14 days, is planned, a temporary percutanous catheter will suffice if needed. Overall, thoughtful planning of the temporary and permanent replacement therapy will decrease unnecessary procedures as well as patient discomfort.

Preoperative evaluation of patients who require the insertion of hemodialysis access catheters may reduce the incidence of procedural complications and improve catheter function, as detailed in Chapter 16. Patients often require placement of a temporary percutaneous catheter on an urgent basis, and this may limit the extent of preoperative testing. However, a brief history and physical may

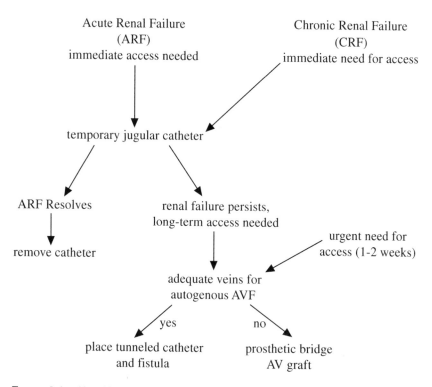

FIGURE 3.1 Algorithm for decisions regarding temporary and long-term hemodialysis access.

prove extremely helpful. Many dialysis patients have complicated medical histories with multiple prior access attempts and failures. The history and physical examination should focus on the items listed in Table 3.1. Mansfield et al. (4) conducted a prospective randomized study of subclavian vein catheterization and noted that prior major surgery in the region, body habitus, and prior catheterizations were associated with failed attempts and increased complications. Patients with prior catheter insertions should be questioned carefully regarding their clinical course with the device. If there is clinical evidence of venous thrombosis (catheter malfunction, arm edema), insertion at that site should be avoided in the absence of preoperative venography or a venous duplex exam (5,6) (Figure 3.2). Patients who have had catheters removed for infection are at a higher risk for ipsilateral venous thrombosis. Patients with arm edema related to prior axillary node dissection should not have placement in the ipsilateral subclavian vein, as thrombosis will further exacerbate arm swelling. Placement in the area of a prior

TABLE 3.1   Preoperative Evaluation for Placement of Hemodialysis Access
Catheters

Vascular access history
  Prior sites used
  Prior central venous thrombosis
  Prior catheter infections
  Other catheter complications (pneumo- or hemothorax)
Avoidance of potential anatomic pitfalls
  Body habitus
  Cervical or mediastinal adenopathy
  Chest wall tumors
  Prior chest or breast surgery
  Known venous anomalies
  Rotation flaps as part of head and neck or breast reconstructive surgery
Complete blood count and electrolytes
Coagulation studies if clinically indicated

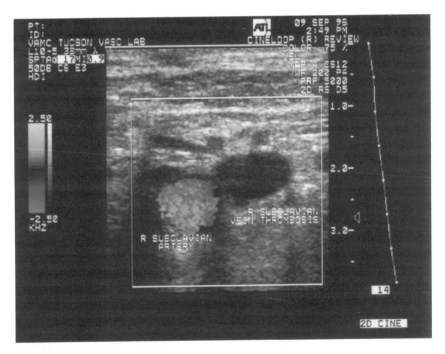

FIGURE 3.2   Venous duplex scan demonstrating subclavian vein thrombosis in
patient with prior subclavian dialysis line.

breast reconstruction (autologous or prosthetic) or an area that has received radiation therapy should be avoided.

The traditional subclavian approach has been reported to cause subclavian vein stenosis or occlusion in up to 50% of dialysis patients (7–10). This may result in venous obstruction and arm edema as well as the loss of the arm for a future permanent access fistula. Placement of the catheter in the jugular system via the right internal or external jugular has a lower incidence of stenosis and has become the preferred method in renal failure patients. We feel, as do other authors, that the subclavian vein approach for the insertion of a dialysis catheter should be abandoned in all but a select group of patients (7). Specifically, patients in whom upper extremity access has been abandoned because of inadequate arterial inflow to maintain a patent fistula or in whom peripheral venous sites have been exhausted yet have a preserved central venous system are suitable for subclavian vein catheter placement. Another group of patients to consider for subclavian vein insertion are those with poor cardiac function (ejection fraction <20%) in whom dialysis is provided on a compassionate basis and survival beyond 2 years is limited.

The only preoperative laboratory studies necessary prior to catheter insertion are a complete blood count, including the platelet count and electrolytes, to evaluate metabolic abnormalities. Coagulation studies should be performed if the patient is receiving anticoagulation (warfarin or intravenous heparin), has a history of bleeding disorders, or has completed a dialysis treatment just prior to the procedure. A chest x-ray should be obtained preoperatively to identify mass lesions, assess the patient for pulmonary edema, and serve as a baseline for postoperative comparison. Ideally, patients are dialyzed the day prior to any operative procedures.

Relative contraindications to catheter placement are few and generally include sepsis or new, unexplained fevers. Fevers of unknown origin or known sepsis should delay placement, if possible, to prevent contamination and subsequent infection of the catheter. If necessary a temporary percutaneous catheter may be placed at the bedside; once the sepsis resolves, a tunneled catheter can be placed. If a previous catheter is the suspected source of sepsis, the line should be removed and the patient treated with several days of antibiotics prior to placement of a new catheter. Neutropenia (<1000 absolute neutrophil count) in oncology patients should lead to consideration of postponing catheter placement due to the increased risk of infection in this circumstance. Thrombocytopenia is not an absolute contraindication, as patients can undergo transfusion during or immediately prior to catheter placement. We recommend platelet transfusion for patients with platelet counts less than 50,000/mL (1 U of single-donor or 10 U of random-donor platelets) within 2 h of catheter insertion. Repeat platelet counts are usually unnecessary after catheter placement unless otherwise indicated.

TABLE 3.2   Preservation of Veins for AV Access

1. Arm veins suitable for placement of vascular access should be preserved regardless of arm dominance. Arm veins, particularly the cephalic veins of the nondominant arm, should not be used for venipuncture or intravenous catheters. The dorsum of the hand should be used for intravenous lines in patients with chronic renal failure. When venipuncture of the arm veins is necessary, sites should be rotated.
2. Instruct hospital staff, patients with developing ESRD (creatinine >3 mg/ dL), and all patients with conditions likely to lead to ESRD to protect the arms from venipuncture and intravenous catheters. A Medic Alert bracelet should be worn to inform hospital staff to avoid IV cannulation of essential veins.
3. Subclavian vein catherization should be avoided for temporary access in all patients with chronic renal failure due to the risk of central venous stenosis.

Source: Modified from Ref. 11, p. 30.

EVALUATION OF THE PATIENT FOR HEMODIALYSIS FISTULA PLACEMENT

Preoperative assessment of the patient referred for permanent dialysis access may be the most important factor in providing a properly functioning arteriovenous fistula. The rate of loss of renal function in patients with chronic renal failure is usually predictable. Patients with creatinine clearance values of 10 mL/min or less are almost certain to need dialysis within 3 months. This interim period should be used for assessment of the patient's general condition and to determine which mode of dialysis to use. Permanent vascular access should be established early in patients selected for hemodialysis, since maturation time is needed before the system is usable, particularly if an autologous fistula is constructed (Tables 3.2 to 3.4).

The decision as to whether a particular ESRD patient is a candidate for long-term dialysis usually rests with the patient, the family, and the nephrologist or internist. Some authors believe that long-term dialysis should not be offered to patients with incurable malignancies, those with severe multisystem problems, or elderly, debilitated patients. Clearly this may be a difficult decision and is patient-specific. Once a decision is made to proceed with long-term dialysis, a thorough history and physical should be performed. In addition to evaluating a patient's general condition, specific attention is directed to those items appearing in Table 3.2 as recently reported by the National Kidney Foundation in their Dialysis Quality Outcome Initiative (11). The preoperative evaluation for placement of AV fistula focuses upon a determination of the optimal type of fistula, the site for placement, and avoidance of complications of fistula placement (Table 3.5).

TABLE 3.3 Timing of Access Placement

1. Patients should be referred for surgery to attempt construction of a primary AV fistula when their creatinine clearance is <25 mL/min, their serum creatinine level is >4 mg/dL, or within 1 year of an anticipated need for dialysis. The patient should be referred to a nephrologist prior to the need for access to facilitate chronic renal failure treatment and for counseling about modes of ESRD care, including hemodialysis, peritoneal dialysis, and renal transplantation.
2. A new primary fistula should be allowed to mature for at least 1 month, and ideally for 3 to 4 months, prior to cannulation.
3. Dialysis AV grafts should be placed at least 3 to 6 weeks prior to an anticipated need for hemodialysis in patients who are not candidates for primary AV fistulae.
4. Hemodialysis catheters should not be inserted until hemodialysis is needed.

Source: Modified from Ref. 11, p. 31.

TABLE 3.4 Access Maturation

1. A primary AV fistula is mature and suitable for use when the vein's diameter is sufficient to allow successful cannulation but not sooner than 1 month, and preferably 3 to 4 months, after construction.
2. The following procedures may enhance maturation of AV fistulae: (a) Fistula hand-arm exercise (e.g., squeezing a rubber ball with or without a lightly applied tourniquet) will increase blood flow and speed maturation of a new native AV fistula. (b) Selective obliteration of major venous side branches will speed maturation of a slowly maturing AV fistula. (c) When a new native AV fistula is infiltrated (i.e., presence of hematoma with associated induration and edema), it should be rested until swelling is resolved.
3. Polytetrafluoroethylene (PTFE) dialysis AV grafts should not routinely be used until 14 days after placement. Cannulation of a new PTFE dialysis AV graft should not routinely be attempted, even 14 days or longer after placement, until swelling has gone down enough to allow palpation of the course of the graft. Ideally, 3 to 6 weeks should be allowed prior to cannulation of a new graft.
4. Patients with swelling that does not respond to arm elevation or that persists beyond 2 weeks after dialysis AV access placement should receive a venogram or other noncontrast study to evaluate central veins.
5. Cuffed and noncuffed hemodialysis catheters are suitable for immediate use and do not require maturation.

Source: Modified from Ref. 11, p. 32.

TABLE 3.5 Preoperative Evaluation for Placement of
Arteriovenous Fistulae or Grafts

Vascular access history
  Prior fistula placements and etiology of failure
  Prior subclavian vein cannulation
  Symptoms of potential central venous stenoses (arm edema)
Avoidance of potential complications
  Arterial system
    Pulse physical examination
    Allen test
    Blood pressure and Doppler studies
    Arteriography if clinically indicated
  Venous system
    Venous physical examination
    Venography or venous Duplex if clinically indicated
Complete blood count and electrolytes
Coagulation or hypercoaguability studies if clinically indicated

---

The patient's history should be evaluated for prior central venous catheter placements or arm edema, which may suggest central venous stenosis or occlusions. Many of these stenoses or occlusions remain asymptomatic until a fistula is placed in the ipsilateral arm, and subsequent arm edema, high venous pressures, and fistula failure result (Figure 3.3). Any prior fistula procedures as well as the reasons for failure should be noted. Patients with multiple prior fistula failures without obvious etiology may be hypercoagulable and warrant long-term anticoagulation following fistula placement. Additional considerations in planning an autologous or prosthetic fistula as well as access in the pediatric population are discussed separately (Table 3.6).

EVALUATION OF VENOUS ANATOMY

Adequate venous outflow is critical in obtaining a properly functioning AV fistula. Stenosis at the venous anastomosis or in the venous outflow of an extremity AV fistula accounts for over 80% of access failures. Percutaneous catheters in the subclavian vein have been used for temporary hemodialysis for the past 20 years. Surratt et al. (5) performed upper extremity venography in 43 patients (62 extremities) prior to placement of a permanent vascular access graft. A 40% incidence of significant subclavian vein stenosis or occlusion was found in patients with prior or existing temporary dialysis catheters in the subclavian vein. No stenoses were found in patients without a history of dialysis catheters in the subclavian vein. The authors concluded that the subclavian vein should be evalu-

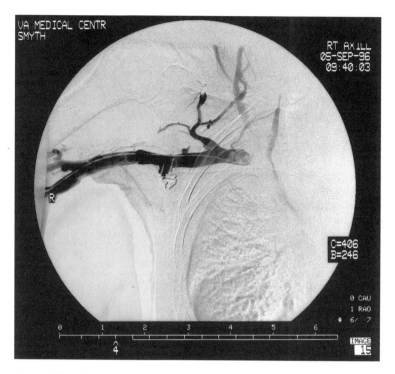

Figure 3.3 Venography demonstrating subclavian vein occlusion in a patient who developed arm edema and arteriovenous graft failure.

Table 3.6 Patient History and Physical Examination Prior to Permanent Access Selection

---

1. To determine the type of access most suitable for an ESRD patient, a history must be taken and physical examination of the patient's venous, arterial, and cardiopulmonary systems must be performed.
2. Diagnostic evaluation should be performed when indicated based on patient history or physical examination.

Source: Modified from Ref. 11. p. 18.

TABLE 3.7 Diagnostic Evaluation Prior to Permanent Access Selection

1. Venography prior to placement of access is indicated in patients with the following: (a) edema in the extremity in which an access site is planned; (b) collateral vein development in any planned access site; (c) differential extremity size if that extremity is contemplated as an access site; (d) current or previous subclavian catheter placement of any type in venous drainage of planned access; (e) current or previous transvenous pacemaker in venous drainage of planned access; (f) previous arm, neck, or chest trauma or surgery in venous drainage of planned access; (g) multiple previous accesses in an extremity planned as an access site.
2. Additional or alternate imaging techniques are indicated in selected cases where multiple previous vascular accesses have been placed or when residual renal function makes contrast studies undesirable. Appropriate techniques include (a) Doppler ultrasound (evidence) and (b) magnetic resonance imaging.
3. Arteriography or Doppler examination is indicated when arterial pulses in the desired access location are markedly diminished.

Source: Modified from Ref. 11, p. 20.

ated preoperatively in any patient with a history of subclavian vein catheterization. Furthermore, they encouraged the use of sites other than the subclavian vein for temporary hemodialysis access (Table 3.7).

The "gold standard" for evaluation of central venous stenoses remains contrast venography. Duplex screening has been performed, but may miss lesions particularly in the portion of the vein behind the clavicle. Knudson et al. (12) evaluated 91 patients with suspected upper extremity venous thrombosis and found the sensitivity of venous duplex was 78% with a specificity of 92%. They noted four cases of isolated superior vena cava or proximal innominate vein obstruction that were missed by color Doppler imaging. Duplex scanning can also be effectively applied to assess the peripheral venous circulation prior to access placement (13). This is particularly important in patients with a prior history of intravenous drug abuse, poorly visualized venous structures despite tourniquet application, or those who have sustained recent and multiple venipunctures. Duplex mapping can document the size and patency of the cephalic and basilic veins, the principal outflow sites for forearm bridge and autogenous AV fistulae. Stenoses or occlusions in these structures, which may not be readily apparent without ultrasound imaging, will lead to failure of any access that relies on their outflow. Moreover, the availability of this information can guide access placement, so that the best chance at access patency is achieved at the initial procedure. Stenosis or occlusion in the cephalic and basilic vein virtually eliminates the

TABLE 3.8 Selection of Permanent Vascular Access and Order of Preference for Placement of AV Fistulae

---

1. The order of preference for placement of AV fistulae in patients requiring chronic hemodialysis is (a) a wrist (radial-cephalic) primary AV fistula (evidence) and (b) an elbow (brachial-cephalic) primary AV fistula.
2. If it is not possible to establish either of these types of fistula, access may be established using (a) an arteriovenous graft of synthetic material (e.g., PTFE) (evidence) or (b) a transposed brachial-basilic vein fistula.
3. Cuffed tunneled central venous catheters should be discouraged as permanent vascular access.

Source: Modified from Ref. 11, p. 22.

option of a wrist or forearm AV access and should guide the surgeon to either an upper arm access configuration or use of the contralateral extremity (Table 3.8).

Autogenous AV Fistulas

The Brescia-Cimino radial artery–cephalic vein fistula remains the first choice for long-term hemodialysis because of superior long-term patency rates and decreased fistula complications. However, a large number of dialysis patients have inadequate vessels or flow to maintain a Cimino fistula (14,15). Findings on physical examination that favor the use of a Cimino include a strong radial pulse as well as a cephalic vein that is continuous from the wrist to the elbow. The cephalic vein may be well developed at the wrist but may drain into a number of smaller forearm veins or be sclerotic from prior venipunctures, resulting in inadequate length of vein for dialysis or failure to mature. The continuity of the cephalic vein may be tested by percussion of the vein at the wrist and gentle palpation at the elbow for a transmitted fluid wave (16). This may be performed with a tourniquet placed in the upper arm. If continuity is in question, a venous duplex study may be performed. Distal arterial ischemia is rare with a Cimino fistula; however, the potential for this complication exists. Symptomatic ischemia distal to an autogenous or prosthetic fistula has been reported to occur in 3 to 7% of patients (17,18). Patients with diabetes appear to be at an increased risk for ischemia distal to a fistula (19). Blood pressure should be measured in each arm and compared to detect any proximal arterial stenoses, indicated by a gradient of 20 mmHg or more between extremities. Occult subclavian artery stenoses or occlusions are more commonly seen on the left. We perform Doppler evaluation of digital artery flow with and without radial artery compression. Disappearance of digital flow with radial artery compression signifies an incomplete palmar arch and excludes the use of a Cimino fistula. The Allen test may also be used to evaluate ulnar and radial artery patency as well as the continuity of the palmar arch. Preference is given to the patient's nondominant hand, but an autogenous fistula in either arm is superior to a prosthetic fistula. Proper selection is important, so that multiple procedures may be avoided in the patient who is unlikely to develop a useful Cimino fistula after careful preoperative evaluation.

We have had good success with the upper arm cephalic vein–brachial artery autogenous fistula. The upper arm cephalic vein is frequently not subjected to multiple intravenous lines and blood draw attempts as are the forearm veins and offers an excellent autogenous conduit for access (20). It may similarly be evaluated by venous duplex scanning or percussion along its course with a tourniquet in place near the axilla. In many patients, this has become our primary fistula of choice. For reasons that are not clear, there is a higher incidence of clinically significant steal with antecubital autogenous fistulae. This complication is addressed in detail in Chapter 12.

Recently there has been renewed interest in the use of the brachial artery–basilic vein fistulae (21). This type of fistula comprises the transposition of the basilic vein from the medial upper arm to the subcutaneous tissue overlying the biceps muscle with an end-to-side anastomosis between the basilic vein and the brachial artery at the elbow (see Chapter 4). Two-year patency rates of 70 to 80%, with relatively few complications, are now being reported. Coburn and Carney (22) recently compared patency and complication rates between the brachial arteriovenous fistula and polytetrafluorethylene (PTFE). In a retrospective review of 59 basilic vein AV fistulae and 47 PTFE AV bridge grafts, they noted significantly superior primary patency rates for the basilic vein transposition fistulae (90% at 1 year and 86% at 2 year vs. 70% at 1 year and 49% at 2 years). Similar results have recently been reported by Matsuura et al. (23).

Prosthetic AV Grafts

The expanded polytetrafluoroethylene (ePTFE) graft was first used as a bridge conduit in 1976 and is currently the most popular method of establishing long-term dialysis access (24). Criteria for placement of ePTFE grafts are failure of autogenous fistula, lack of adequate superficial veins for an autogenous fistula, or deeply embedded veins, as are usually found in obese patients. The most common reason for lack of superficial veins is multiple prior intravenous cannulations.

The majority of the preoperative assessment for placement of a prosthetic AV graft is similiar to that for an autogenous fistula; however, the options for graft placement are generally larger. Multiple variations of prosthetic fistula configurations have been described from the simple forearm straight or loop fistula, upper arm and neck fistulae, as well as fistulae constructed in the thigh. The specific details of bridge graft construction are reviewed in Chapter 5. In patients with recently thrombosed prosthetic grafts, thrombectomy, and revision should be considered before moving to a new access site.

If upper extremity access sites have been exhausted, the thigh may be used. Preoperative evaluation should include measurement of an ankle-brachial pressure index (ABI). If the ABI is less than 0.75 or the patient has symptoms of claudication or leg ischemia, further evaluation including arteriography should precede graft placement.

CONSIDERATIONS IN THE PEDIATRIC PATIENT

Each year, three to five children per million develop chronic renal failure. The ultimate goal for renal replacement therapy is transplantation, which is less expensive and offers a superior quality of life compared with maintenance dialysis.

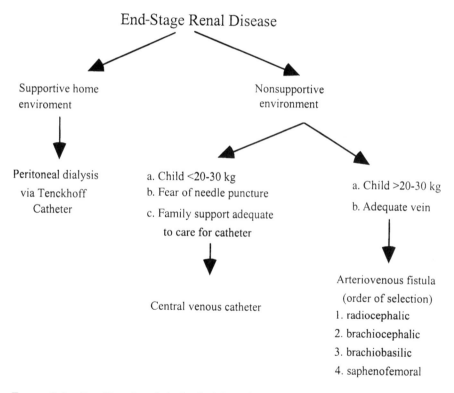

FIGURE 3.4 Algorithm for dialysis decisions in the pediatric population. (From Ref. 25.)

Unfortunately, 70% of children with renal failure will require dialysis for short periods while awaiting transplantation, and 23%, who are ineligible for transplantation or following failed transplantation will require long-term dialysis (25). This small group of children represents a difficult dialysis access problem.

Success of a dialysis access procedure in children is determined by the size of the child, length of time on dialysis, and prior use of access sites. Peritoneal dialysis via a Tenckhoff catheter is the preferred dialysis modality; however, this is dependent upon a supportive home environment. In patients who fail peritoneal dialysis or in whom it is inappropriate, hemodialysis becomes necessary. Tunneled catheters have gained increased popularity in children, especially those in whom transplantation is likely or until a functioning fistula can be constructed. In older children who will likely require long-term dialysis, an autogenous fistula may be constructed beginning at the most distal site possible in the upper arm. Prosthetic ePTFE grafts have been shown to function poorly in children, especially those less than 30 kg in weight, and should be reserved for use following the failure of other modalities. Lumsden et al. (25) present a useful algorithm to this difficult clinical problem (Figure 3.4).

REFERENCES

1. United States Renal Data System. 1998 Annual data report. Am J Kidney Dis 32(Suppl 1), 1998.
2. McDowell DE, Moss AH, Vasilakis C, et al. Percutaneously placed dual-lumen silicone catheters for long-term hemodialysis. Am Surg 59:569–572, 1993.
3. Moss AH, Vasilakis BS, Holley JL, et al. Use of a silicone dual-lumen catheter with a dacron cuff as a long-term vascular access for hemodialysis patients. Am J Kindey Dis 16:211–215, 1990.
4. Mansfield PF, Hohn DC, Fornage BD, et al. Complications and failures of subclavian-vein catheterization. N Engl J Med 331:1735–1738, 1994.
5. Surratt RS, Picus D, Hicks ME, et al. The importance of preoperative evaluation of the subclavian vein in dialysis access planning. Am J Roentgenol 156:623–625, 1991.
6. Haire WD, Lynch TG, Lieberman RP, Edney JA. Duplex scans before subclavian vein catheterization predict unsuccessful catheter placement. Arch Surg 127:229–230, 1992.
7. Cimochowski GE, Worley E, Rutherford RE, et al. Superiority of the internal jugular over the subclavian access for temporary dialysis. Nephron 54:154–161, 1990.
8. Shillinger F, Schillinger D, Montagnac R, et al. Post catheterization vein stenosis in haemodialysis: Comparative angiographic study of 50 subclavian and 50 internal jugular accesses. Nephrol Dial Transplant 6:722–724, 1991.
9. Clark DD, Albina JE, Chazan JA. Subclavian vein stenosis and thrombosis: A potential serious complication in chronic hemodialysis patients. Am J Kidney Dis 15:265–268, 1990.
10. McNally PG, Brown CB, Moorhead PF, Raferty AT. Unmasking subclavian vein

obstruction following creation of arteriovenous fistulae for haemodialysis: A problem following subclavian line dialysis? Nephrol Dial Transplant 1:258–260, 1987.

11. NKF-DOQI Clinical Practice Guidelines for Vascular Access. New York: National Kidney Foundation; 1997:18–33.

12. Knudson GJ, Wiedmeyer DA, Erickson SJ, et al. Color doppler sonographic imaging in the assessment of upper extremity deep venous thrombosis. Am J Roentgenol 154:399–403, 1990.

13. Silva MB Jr, Hobson RW II, Pappas PJ, et al. A strategy for increasing use of autogenous hemodialysis access procedures: Impact of preoperative noninvasive evaluation. J Vasc Surg 27:302–307, 1998.

14. Kherlakian GM, Roedersheimer LR, Arbaugh JJ, et al. Comparison of autogenous fistula versus expanded polytetrafluoroethylene graft fistula for angioaccess in hemodialysis. Am J Surg 152:238–243, 1986.

15. Ogden DA. Comparing vascular access methods. Trans ASAIO 29:782–794, 1983.

16. Hamiov M. The peripheral subcutaneous arteriovenous fistula. In Hamiov M, ed. Vascular Access: A Practical Guide. New York: Futura, 1987:41–57.

17. Mattson WJ. Recognition and treatment of vascular steal secondary to hemodialysis prostheses. Am J Surg 154:198, 1987.

18. Zibari GB, Rohr MS, Landreneau MD, et al. Complications from permanent hemodialysis vascular access. Surgery 104:681, 1988.

19. Connolly JE, Brownell DA, Levine EF, McCart PM. Complications of renal dialysis access procedures. Arch Surg 119:1325–1328, 1984.

20. Bender MH, Bruyninckx CM, Gerlag PG. The brachiocephalic elbow fistula: A useful alternative angioaccess for permanent hemodialysis. J Vasc Surg 20:808–813, 1994.

21. Dagher FJ, Gelber R, Ramos E, et al. The use of basilic vein and brachial artery as an A-V fistula for long term hemodialysis. J Surg Res 20:373–376, 1976.

22. Coburn MC, Carney WI. Comparison of basilic vein and polytetrafluorethylene for brachial arteriovenous fistula. J Vasc Surg 20:736–743, 1994.

23. Matsuura JH, Rosenthal D, Clark M, et al. Transposed basilic vein versus polytetrafluoroethylene for brachial-axillary arteriovenous fistulas. Am J Surg 176:219–21, 1998.

24. Baker LD, Johnson JM, Goldfarb D. Expanded polytetraflouroethylene (ePTFE) subcutaneous arteriovenous conduit: An improved vascular access for chronic hemodialysis. Trans ASAIO 22:272–277, 1976.

25. Lumsden AB, MacDonald MJ, Allen RC, Dodson TF. Hemodialysis access in the pediatric patient population. Am J Surg 168:197–201, 1994.

4

Autogenous Hemodialysis Access Techniques

Luke S. Erdoes

Vascular Associates, Chattanooga, Tennessee

Scott S. Berman

The University of Arizona, Carondelet St. Mary's Hospital, and
  The Southern Arizona Vascular Institute,
  Tucson, Arizona

Fifty years since the development of hemodialysis (1), a dependable method of chronic access to the circulation remains elusive. An optimal angioaccess should allow high flow, be easy to cannulate, not create distal hypoperfusion, and last indefinitely. Few would argue that autogenous arteriovenous (AV) fistulae come closest to this standard. This is also the view of the National Kidney Foundation Kidney Disease Outcomes Quality Initiative, as cited throughout this text. The following is both a technical and philosophical look at autogenous access for hemodialysis.

Basic principles of angioaccess apply to both autogenous AV fistulae and nonautogenous bridge grafts. The nondominant upper extremity should be used first, and each access should be constructed as distally as possible. The upper extremity is preferable to the lower, since upper extremity fistulae are easier to cannulate and more convenient for the patient; in addition, arterial inflow is more often preserved. The upper extremity is also less prone to infection than the lower extremity, particularly if a groin incision is used (2). Autogenous fistulae are preferred as initial conduits over any prosthetic bridge graft. Despite this dictum, an "all autogenous" policy, similar to lower extremity infrainguinal arterial bypass, is foolhardy. The nature of any angioaccess dictates eventual failure, and many patients will require hemodialysis for 15 or more years, necessitating multiple access procedures.

ANATOMY

The superficial venous anatomy of the upper arm is depicted in Figure 4.1, though many variations exist. The cephalic vein originates in the hand, courses through the anatomic snuffbox, and passes on the radial side of the wrist up the forearm. The basilic vein is quite medial and posterior in the forearm. Veins in the antecubital fossa are by definition quite variable in their distribution. There is usually a median cubital vein connecting both the cephalic and basilic systems. The cephalic vein continues in the upper arm, courses between the brachioradialis and biceps muscles into the deltopectoral groove, and eventually drains into the axillary vein. The basilic vein passes just superior to the medial epicondyle and continues up the arm either as the true basilic vein, overlying the brachial artery, or as the brachial vein when it courses with the brachial artery. The basilic and/ or brachial veins become the axillary vein at or near the level of the pectoralis minor muscle. Several perforating veins connect the superficial to the deep brachial system. A relatively constant perforator is present at or just below the antecubital crease connecting the median cubital vein to the deep brachial system.

It is imperative to assess hand perfusion prior to constructing any forearm access. This is easily done at the bedside with the Allen test. Normally the ulnar artery is the dominant supply to the hand and is continuous with the superficial palmar arch. The radial artery continues into the deep palmar arch, and there are connections via collaterals between the superficial and deep arches. If a patient either has a dominant radial artery or has had prior injury to the ulnar artery, extreme care is necessary in constructing an AV access fistula, particularly if distal radial artery ligation is contemplated. Severe hand ischemia may ensue and be very difficult to treat.

VARIATIONS OF AUTOGENOUS ARTERIOVENOUS FISTULAE

Brescia-Cimino Fistula

The fistula from the radial artery to cephalic vein at the wrist, first described by Brescia and Cimino (3), revolutionized hemodialysis by providing a durable, long-lasting conduit for angioaccess. It is the optimal first access in patients with

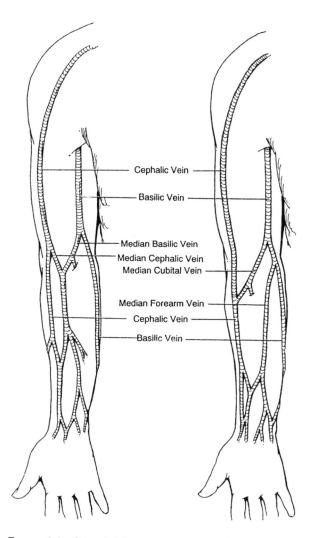

FIGURE 4.1 Superficial venous anatomy of the arm.

suitable venous anatomy and is the "workhorse" of autogenous AV fistulae at the wrist (3,4). Prior to creating this fistula, the cephalic vein and medial forearm veins must be carefully assessed. These veins are commonly used for phlebotomy or intravenous lines. It is common to locate a patent cephalic vein at the wrist, only to find it occluded or discontinuous in the forearm. But it is always preferable to utilize the best cephalic vein to construct this fistula, regardless of extremity dominance, especially if an autogenous fistula is possible in the dominant arm and only a nonautogenous bridge graft in the nondominant arm.

The Brescia-Cimino fistula is best constructed by using a longitudinal incision placed between the cephalic vein and the radial artery at the wrist (Figure 4.2). A transverse incision on the radial side of the wrist is also possible. Local anesthesia and local heparinization are usually all that is necessary. It is also reasonable to use regional nerve block anesthesia and do the anastomosis with proximal tourniquet control, thereby avoiding excessive dissection, mobilization, and clamping of the delicate vessels. The cephalic vein is mobilized first and its

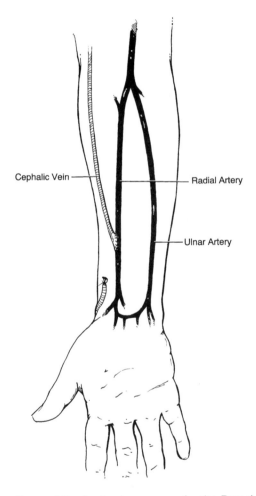

Figure 4.2 Anatomic exposure for the Brescia-Cimino fistula.

patency and quality assessed. If the vein is continuous and at least 3 mm in diameter, it is well founded to perform the procedure. Enough cephalic vein is mobilized to assure a gentle curve and course in the forearm and a tension-free anastomosis. Delicate technique, usually with the aid of loupe magnification and 6-0 or 7-0 monofilament suture, is mandatory, and only gentle distention of the vein using papavarine solution is performed. Upon completion of the anastomosis, the suture should be tied under arterial pressure and there should be an easily palpable thrill in the outflow vein. A pulse in the outflow vein is suggestive of outflow obstruction or fistula thrombosis.

Many variations in anastomotic technique have been reported, including end vein to side artery, side vein to side artery (with or without distal arterial ligation), end artery to end vein, or even end artery to side vein (4) (Figure 4.3a to d). The side-to-side anastomosis is easy to construct, yet it may result in venous hypertension of the hand (5). An anastomosis from the end radial artery to end cephalic vein minimizes the chance of arterial steal and venous hypertension, yet it results in lower fistula flows (6). The technique of end artery to side vein is the most difficult and results in relatively low flows. Most surgeons prefer the anastomosis from the end cephalic vein to the side radial artery, since it minimizes venous hypertension in the hand and produces reliably higher flow rates (7). As an alternative technique, the anastomosis is constructed in a side-to-side fashion, making it technically the easiest to construct. After flow is established and a thrill is palpated in the proximal vein, the distal vein is ligated to eliminate the pathway for venous hypertension. This modified technique preserves the continuity between the distal vein, artery, and proximal vein, permitting access to immediately

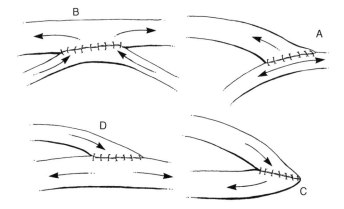

FIGURE 4.3 Options for the anastomoisis of a Brescia-Cimino fistula. A. End vein to side artery. B. Side vein to side artery. C. End artery to end vein D. End artery to side vein.

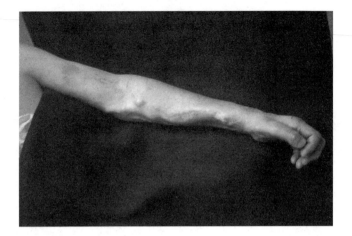

FIGURE 4.4 Patient with a patent Brescia-Cimino fistula, which has provided uninterrupted access for 22 years.

explore a poorly functioning fistula for possible etiologies without having to open the artery, vein, or anastomotic suture line.

The fistula is allowed to mature for 6 to 8 weeks prior to puncture. Occasionally longer periods for maturation are required to allow sufficient "arterialization" of the vein, but if little venous distention is present at 6 weeks, either revision or an alternate access site is usually required. Having the patient perform repetitive hand exercises such as squeezing a ball or a similar-sized compressible object may facilitate development of the outflow vein (8).

Patency rates of 80% at 1 year and 40 to 70% at 3 years have been reported (9–12), and some Brescia-Cimino fistulae have functioned well for a decade or more (Figure 4.4). Arterial steal is unusual, but enlargement or aneurysm formation of the outflow veins can occur, resulting in significant pain, cosmetic deformity, central embolism, and even loss of the access.

Snuffbox Fistulae

There are possible advantages to an even more distal radial cephalic arteriovenous fistula created in the anatomic snuffbox (Figure 4.5). The cephalic vein and radial artery are in very close proximity, and the vein is usually of excellent quality at this level. A side-to-side or end-to-side anastomosis is easily performed with minimal mobilization of the artery and vein. If necessary to improve flow or control vascular steal, the distal radial artery can be ligated (assuming a patent ulnar system). Utilization of the cephalic vein in the snuffbox may facilitate sec-

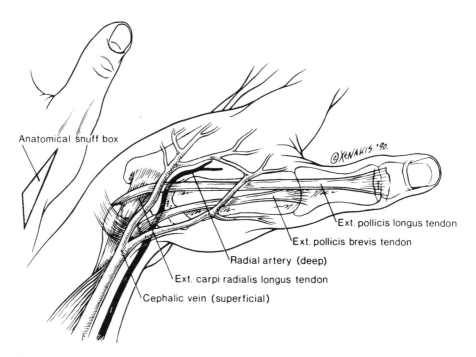

Anatomical snuff box

©XENAKIS '90.

Ext. pollicis longus tendon

Ext. pollicis brevis tendon

Radial artery (deep)

Ext. carpi radialis longus tendon

Cephalic vein (superficial)

FIGURE 4.5 Arterial and venous anatomy of the anatomic snuffbox. (From Ref. 15.)

ondary procedures either at the wrist or in the forearm. Patency rates for snuffbox fistulae approach 80% at 1 year (13–15). There is a significant immediate failure rate, however, usually due to technical failures or an inadequate outflow vein. Despite the early failures, construction of this most distal fistula, through its effect on the subcutaneous cephalic vein in the forearm and upper arm, may facilitate later creation of a traditional Brescia-Cimino fistula at the wrist or of a brachio-cephalic antecubital fistula.

Ulnar Artery or Basilic Vein Forearm Fistulae

There is no inherent reason why the ulnar artery cannot be used to create a fistula at the wrist, but anastomosis from the ulnar artery to the basilic vein in the forearm produces a fistula that is very difficult to cannulate because of the medial and posterior course of the basilic vein. One can mobilize the forearm basilic vein and transpose it to the ulnar or radial artery via a subcutaneous tunnel. This should not be a primary option because extensive dissection is needed to transpose the vein and only a short segment of the vein is then available for cannulation.

Upper Extremity Saphenous Vein Fistulae

Several investigators have utilized the greater saphenous vein transposed to the arm to function as an arteriovenous conduit (16). This method has appeal, since the greater saphenous vein is durable when used for arterial bypass, so it would seem reasonable that it would function well for dialysis access. However, the long-term results have been disappointing. Patency in the range of 40% is reported at 3 years, and a separate leg incision is required (16). For this reason most surgeons reserve the saphenous vein for lower extremity autogenous arteriovenous fistulae (described later).

Reverse Arteriovenous Fistulae

A reverse arteriovenous fistula has been described which allows for the use of veins around the antecubital fossa (17). In this fistula the basilic vein in the upper arm is sewn side to side to the brachial artery. Valves in the antecubital veins are mechanically rendered incompetent and the more cephalad basilic vein is plicated (Figure 4.6). This fistula requires at least 4 to 5 cm of good-quality antecubital vein for cannulation. The venous outflow for a reversed fistula is mainly via perforating veins draining into the deep brachial veins. It is important to preserve as many perforating branches as possible for this fistula. This procedure is rarely if ever indicated, since it is inferior to transposed basilic vein fistulae (as described below) and requires instrumentation to lyse valves. Adequate plication of the basilic vein is difficult and may result in thrombosis or inadequate fistula flow.

Antecubital Arteriovenous Fistulae

Once the options for an autogenous AV fistula in the forearm have been exhausted, arterial-to-venous connections in and around the antecubital fossa are necessary. The AV fistula from the brachial artery to the cephalic vein has been described by several authors (18–25). A side-to-side fistula was initially described by Cascardo et al. (21) in 1970 (Figure 4.7a). This resulted in a high incidence of steal. Gracz et al. (22) described the more popular technique of end vein to side artery (Figure 4.7b) in 1977. The median cubital vein at or just below the antecubital fossa is utilized and an attempt is made to isolate the perforating branch of this vein to use for an end-to-side anastomosis to the brachial artery. A deeper anastomosis was felt to be protected from inadvertent puncture, and the relatively small anastomosis might protect against the development of steal or high output congestive heart failure. Recent reports by Bender et al. (19,25) provide their experience with this fistula—a reported a 93% patency at 1 year and 80% at 3 years. This is in contrast to 76% and 65% patency for Brescia-

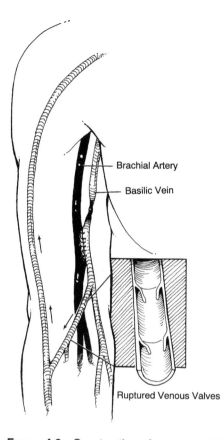

Brachial Artery

Basilic Vein

Ruptured Venous Valves

FIGURE 4.6 Construction of a reverse AV fistula with side-to-side brachiobasilic anastomosis, plication of the proximal basilic vein, and valve lysis of the antecubital veins.

Cimino wrist fistulas and 69% and 62% patency for nonautogenous bridge grafts at 1 and 3 years, respectively.

Many patients have undergone repeated venipuncture in the median cubital vein, and the perforating branch is often obliterated. In these patients the cephalic vein may be used just above the antecubital crease and sewn to the brachial artery. Some mobilization of the vein is required for this technique. Very often a nonautogenous forearm bridge fistula may be placed, which effectively "matures" the upper arm cephalic vein while the bridge is used for dialysis access. When the bridge fistula fails, there should be sufficient cephalic vein to create

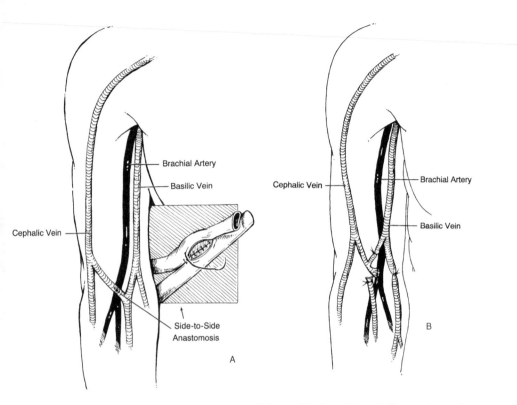

Figure 4.7 Antecubital AV fistula. A. Side-to-side brachiocephalic anastomosis. B. End-to-side anastomosis using the perforating branch of the antecubital vein.

a fistula from the brachial artery to the cephalic vein (Figure 4.8). Because the cephalic vein is already arterialized by functioning as the outflow for the bridge graft, fistula maturation time is decreased and often a secondary upper arm fistula vein can be cannulated after only 1 to 2 weeks.

Transposed Basilic Arteriovenous Fistula

Should the cephalic vein prove to be unusable in the upper arm, the next choice of access is the transposed basilic AV fistula (26–29). Because the basilic vein in the upper arm is deep and usually not visible, it remains relatively protected from harmful venipuncture and is usually a relatively large conduit. The basilic vein is quite thin yet is usable in almost all patients. Preoperative duplex imaging or venography is recommended to assure patency of the basilic vein and to confirm adequate outflow via the axillary/subclavian venous system. Axillary or su-

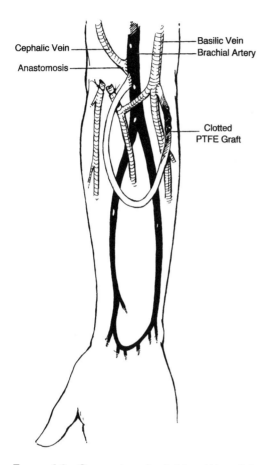

Cephalic Vein

Anastomosis

Basilic Vein

Brachial Artery

Clotted PTFE Graft

FIGURE 4.8 Conversion of a bridge AV graft into an upper arm brachiocephalic fistula.

praclavicular block or even local anesthesia may be utilized; however, due to the extent of dissection and necessary tunneling, most patients require a general anesthetic for this operation.

The basilic vein is mobilized at the level of the medial epicondyle and traced cephalad to its confluence with the axillary vein (Figure 4.9). Care is taken to avoid injury to the overlying cutaneous nerves and the underlying median nerve. Side branches are tied and divided and the vein is gently distended with papaverine solution. The brachial artery is exposed, usually through a separate incision just above the antecubital crease and a very superficial subcutaneous tunnel is created between the brachial artery incision and the most cephalad por-

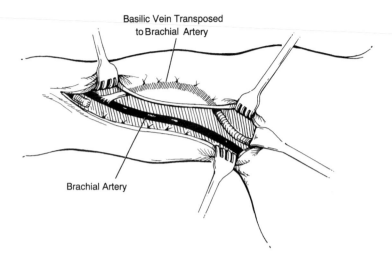

Basilic Vein Transposed
to Brachial Artery

Brachial Artery

FIGURE 4.9   Anatomy and mobilization of the basilic vein for construction of a transposed basilic AV fistula.

tion of the basilic vein. An anastomosis from the end vein to side artery is performed. Postoperative arm swelling is common but usually resolves after several weeks. As with other primary autogenous AV fistulae a maturation time of 6 to 8 weeks is necessary.

Patency rates of 69 to 81% and 49 to 57% at 1 and 3 years, respectively, have been reported (25–29). The most common site of postoperative venous stenosis is in the basilic vein just caudad to the axillary vein, where it goes from a deep plane to the superficial tunnel (27). A transposed basilic fistula does not preclude the future creation of an upper arm bridge graft from the brachial artery to the basilic or axillary vein. The converse is not true; an upper arm bridge graft usually damages the basilic/axillary vein junction and makes tunneling of a transposed basilic vein problematic. Thus, autogenous AV fistulae in the upper arm are usually indicated prior to the placement of upper arm bridge grafts. Furthermore, venous revision of a forearm bridge graft should usually not be performed above the antecubital crease, since such revision damages the upper arm veins and areas for soft tissue tunnels and severely limits future autogenous options. A transposed fistula from the brachial vein to the brachial artery has been reported (18). However, the brachial veins are usually too small or have multiple branch points, precluding the effective construction of this type of fistula.

Lower Extremity Arteriovenous Fistulae

The lower extremity is less desirable than the upper extremity for autogenous AV fistula formation because of more infectious complications, inconvenient po-

sitioning, and a higher incidence of lower extremity vascular occlusive disease
(2). Despite these drawbacks, with the increasing number of dialysis patient-years
and the aging of the dialysis population, the legs must be utilized more frequently
as chronic access sites.

The saphenous vein may be transposed using the saphenofemoral junction
as outflow. The arterial anastomosis may be to the common femoral artery, resulting in a loop, or to the superficial femoral artery, creating a curvilinear fistula
(Figure 4.10 a and b). As the superficial femoral artery is often diseased, the
common femoral artery is more commonly used for fistula inflow. If the saphenous vein is unusable or absent in the thigh, the more distal vein can be utilized.
Patency, however, is probably the same or even worse than a prosthetic bridge

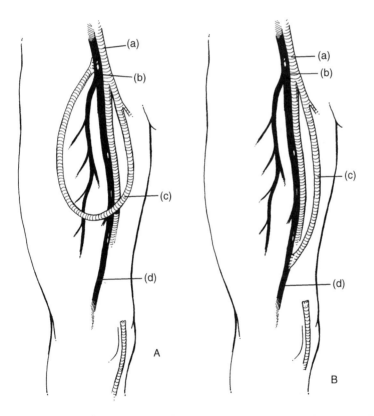

FIGURE 4.10 Options for configuring an autogenous saphenous vein leg fistula.
A. Loop configuration with the arterial inflow from the common femoral artery. B.
Curvilinear configuration with the arterial inflow taken from the distal superficial
femoral artery. (a) Common femoral vein, (b) common femoral artery, (c) greater
saphenous vein, (d) popliteal artery.

graft in the groin, and the distal leg wound used for vein harvest may also become problematic. The contralateral saphenous vein should not be harvested, since it would obviously be better used in a groin fistula in the extremity where it is already present. Due to the relatively infrequent application of leg autogenous AV fistulae for chronic access, series of such patients have not been reported.

CONCLUSION

Available techniques of autogenous AV fistula formation have been discussed, and a rational strategy of successive hemodialysis access placement has been suggested. Whenever feasible, autogenous AV fistulae are preferred over prosthetic bridge grafts. No access procedure should preclude or hinder subsequent procedures. A functional access is a lifeline for the dialysis patient, and it is the responsibility of the surgeon to create the best and most durable access possible.

REFERENCES

1. Kolff WJ, Berk HTJ, terWelle M, et al. The artificial kidney: A dialyzer with a great area. Acta Med Scand 117:121–131, 1944.
2. Bennion RS, Hiatt JR, Williams RA, et al. A randomized, prospective study of pre-operative antimicrobial prophylaxis for vascular access surgery. J Cardiovasc Surg 26:270–275, 1985.
3. Brescia MJ, Cimino JE, Appel K, Hurwich BJ. Chronic hemodialysis using veni-puncture and a surgically created arteriovenous fistula. N Engl J Med 275:1089–1092, 1966.
4. Wilson SE, ed. Vascular Access Surgery, 2nd ed. Chicago, Year Book Medical, 1988:204.
5. Bennion RS, Williams RA. The radiocephalic fistula. Contemp Dial 3:12–16, 1982.
6. Johnson G, Dart CH, Peters RM, Steele F. The importance of venous circulation in arteriovenous fistula. Surg Gynecol Obstet 123:995–1000, 1966.
7. Anderson CB, Etheridge EE, Harter HR, et al. Local blood flow characteristics of arteriovenous fistulas in the forearm for dialysis. Surg Gynecol Obstet 144:531–533, 1977.
8. Moran MR, Enriquez AA, Boyero MR, et al. Hand exercise effect in maturation and blood flow of dialysis arteriovenous fistulas. Angiology 35:641–644, 1984.
9. Palder SB, Kirkman RL, Whittemore AD, et al. Vascular access for hemodialysis. Ann of Surg 302:235–239, 1985.
10. Cantelmo NL, LoGerfo FW, Menzoian JO. Brachiobasilic and brachiocephalic fis-tulas as secondary angioaccess routes. Surg Gynecol Obstet 155:545–548, 1982.
11. Kheriakian GM, Roedersheimer LR, Arbaugh JJ, et al. Comparison of autogenous fistula versus expanded polytetrafluoroethylene graft fistula for angioaccess in hemo-dialysis. Am J Surg 152:238–243, 1986.
12. Riordan S, Frawley J, Gray L, Niesche J. Primary access surgery for long-term haemodialysis. Aust NZ J Surg 64:763–767, 1994.

13. Bonalumi U, Civalleri D, Rovida S, et al. Nine years experience with end-to-end arteriovenous fistula at the "anatomical snuffbox" for maintenance hemodialysis. Br J Surg 69:486–488, 1982.

14. Mehigan JT, McAlexander RA. Snuffbox arteriovenous fistula for hemodialysis. Am J Surg 143:252–253, 1982.

15. Patterson RB. The "snuffbox" radiocephalic fistula: An autogenous alternative. In Sommer BG, Henry ML, eds. Vascular Access for Hemodialysis II. Chicago: WL Gore, 1991:213–217.

16. May J, Harris J, Fletcher J. Long-term results of saphenous vein graft arteriovenous fistulas. Am J Surg 140:387–390, 1980.

17. Giacchino JL, Geis WP, Buckingham JM, et al. Vascular access: Long-term results, new techniques. Arch Surg 114:403–409, 1979.

18. Gessaroli M, Faggioli GL, Freyrie A, Gargiulo M. Regarding The brachiocephalic elbow fistula: A useful alternative angioaccess for permanent hemodialysis. J Vasc Surg 22:195–196, 1995.

19. Bender MHM, Bruyninckx CMA, Gerlag PGG. The brachiocephalic elbow fistula: A useful alternative angioaccess for permanent hemodialysis. J Vasc Surg 20:808–813, 1994.

20. Criado E, Marston WA, Keagy BA. Basilic vein to brachial artery arteriovenous fistula for hemodialysis access. Surgical Rounds:17–25, 1993.

21. Cascardo S, Acchiardo S, Beven EG, et al. Proximal arteriovenous fistulas for haemodialysis when radial arteries are unavailable. Proc Eur Dial Transplant Assoc 7:42–46, 1970.

22. Gracz KC, Ing TX, Soung L, et al. Proximal forearm fistula for maintenance hemodialysis. Kidney Int 11:71–74, 1977.

23. Elcheroth J, DePauw L, Kinnaert P. Elbow arteriovenous fistulas for chronic haemodialysis. Br J Surg 81:982–984, 1994.

24. Dunlop MG, Mackinlay JY, McLJenkins A. Vascular access: Experience with the brachiocephalic fistula. Ann R Coll Surg Engl 68:204–206, 1986.

25. Bender MHM, Bruyninckx CMA, Gerlag PGG. The Gracz arteriovenous fistula evaluated. Results of the brachiocephalic elbow fistula in haemodialysis angioaccess. Eur J Vasc Surg 10:294–297, 1995.

26. Dagher FJ, Gelber RL, Ramos EJ, Salder J. The use of basilic vein and brachial artery as an A-V fistula for long term hemodialysis. J Surg Res 20:373–376, 1976.

27. LoGerfo FW, Menzoian JO, Kumaky DJ, Idelson BA. Transposed basilic vein-brachial arterio-venous fistula. Arch Surg 113:1008–1010, 1978.

28. Rivers SP, Scher LA, Sheehan E, et al. Basilic vein transposition: An underused autologous alternative to prosthetic dialysis angioaccess. J Vasc Surg 18:391–397, 1993.

29. Matsuura JH, Rosenthal D, Clark M, et al. Transposed basilic vein versus polytetrafluoroethylene for brachial-axillary arteriovenous fistulas. Am J Surg 176:219–221, 1998.

5

Construction of Prosthetic Arteriovenous Grafts for Hemodialysis

Scott S. Berman
The University of Arizona, Carondelet St. Mary's Hospital, and
The Southern Arizona Vascular Institute,
Tucson, Arizona

No discussion of establishing chronic vascular access for hemodialysis with prosthetic grafts could commence without emphasizing the one observation that has persisted throughout the medical literature for the last 30 years: Autogenous native arteriovenous (AV) fistulae have performed best in maintaining uninterrupted access for hemodialysis—better than any other configuration—since their first description by Brescia et al. in 1966 (1). All patients who have chronic renal insufficiency and are in need of chronic vascular access for hemodialysis should be considered for construction of a native fistula prior to placement of a prosthetic graft. With the availability and effectiveness of long-term central venous dialysis catheters (see Chapter 7), even patients who present with an acute need for renal replacement therapy can be maintained via this access route, allowing for the creation and maturation of a native arteriovenous fistula. (Table 5.1).

Unfortunately, many patients with renal insufficiency are not candidates for autogenous fistula construction. Oftentimes autogenous venous sites have been exhausted by repeated phlebotomy in the chronically ill patient. With a large percentage of dialysis patients suffering from diabetes mellitus, distal arterial circulation is inadequate to support a native fistula at the wrist. An aging dialysis population contributes to this imbalance in the use of native fistulae due to the

Table 5.1   Goals of Access Placement—Maximizing Primary AV Fistulae

1.   Primary AV fistulae should be constructed in at least 50% of all new pa-
     tients electing to receive hemodialysis as their initial form of renal replace-
     ment therapy. Ultimately, 40% of prevalent patients should have a native
     AV fistula.
2.   Patients should be reevaluated for possible construction of a primary AV
     fistula after failure of every dialysis AV access.
3.   Each center should establish a database to track the types of accesses cre-
     ated and the complications rates.

Source: Modified from Ref. 2.

misconception that autogenous fistulae function poorly in the elderly (3). Furthermore, elderly dialysis patients conceivably do not require long-term access routes
based upon expected short actuarial dialysis survival. Moreover, a nihilistic atti-
tude on the part of access surgeons contributes to the underutilization of autogenous access sites. Along with less common justifications, these arguments result
in autogenous fistula construction for roughly 20% of dialysis patients in the
United States (4,5). By contrast, roughly 80 to 90% of dialysis patients in Europe
receive an autogenous fistula as their first mode of chronic access (6,7).

HISTORICAL PERSPECTIVE

Nonautogenous devices were the earliest types used to obtain access to the circulation for hemodialysis. Nearly two decades passed from the time that Kolff, et
al. (8) described a useful dialyzer until Quinton et al. (9) devised their external
shunt, which provided a consistent way to access the circulation and implement
dialysis therapy. The original Scribner shunt consisted of Teflon tubing inserted
into a peripheral artery and vein. This was soon modified by the use of Silastic
tubing with Teflon ends secured within the selected vessels. A number of similar
externalized shunts were developed, including the Allen-Brown, Thomas, and
Buselmeier shunts (10–12). Each modification attempted to either improve the
efficiency of placement and function of the shunt or to prolong the life of the
shunt in a particular location. These external shunts were the mainstays of dialysis
access through the appearance of the Brescia-Cimino fistula and until the introduction of both the bovine carotid artery graft and the expanded polytetrafluorethylene (ePTFE) graft in the mid 1970s (13,14).

      Bovine xenografts and ePTFE grafts gained rapid acceptance as secondary
routes of vascular access for patients with failed or inadequate sites for Brescia-
Cimino fistulae. Other prosthetic materials introduced for access conduits around

this time included Dacron and human umbilical vein allografts (15,16). Neither of these materials ever realized the success of bovine xenografts and ePTFE for dialysis access. Dacron grafts were associated with high thrombogenecity, which is not tolerated well in the small-diameter conduits used for vascular access. Human umbilical vein grafts are essentially preserved collagen tubes, which are plagued by degeneration and aneurysm formation.

Bovine xenografts have not changed appreciably since their introduction for use as dialysis access conduits. Like the umbilical vein graft, bovine grafts behave as preserved collagen tubes and are susceptible to aneurysmal degeneration. An abundance of literature, including randomized prospective studies, has demonstrated the superiority of ePTFE AV grafts over bovine xenografts in regards to cost, primary patency, secondary patency, and infection rate (17–21). The use of bovine grafts for dialysis access has markedly diminished over the last decade, but they are still favored by some surgeons as the graft of choice.

Recent advancements in the field of vascular access include attempts to develop needle-less implantable ports for the chronic dialysis patient. Two devices had transient periods of popularity in attempting to achieve this goal. Both models, the Hemasite and the DiaTap, consisted of implanted AV grafts connected to external tubes with membranes for needle cannulation, thus sparing the patient the discomfort of repeated needle sticks. As one might intuitively expect, both of these devices suffered from significant infection rates, a high incidence of thrombosis, substantial cost, and technical difficulties that quickly extinguished interest in their use (22,23).

The last 5 years have witnessed the introduction of new prosthetic grafts for dialysis access comprising various configurations and modifications of ePTFE, Silastic, Dacron, and carbon (24–27). Descriptions of these new prosthetics appear later in this chapter, and a detailed discussion of biomaterials used for vascular access is presented in Chapter 9. All share the common goal of achieving a less thrombogenic graft with improved patency rates and better healing characteristics to permit reliable, prolonged, uninterrupted access for chronic dialysis.

GENERAL PRINCIPLES

Preoperative Management

Evaluation

Patients in need of a prosthetic access for hemodialysis have either failed attempts at creating autogenous AV fistulae or are not considered candidates for an autogenous fistula for anatomical or physiological reasons. Urgent need for dialysis should not mandate placement of a prosthetic graft in a patient who would otherwise benefit from construction of an autogenous fistula, since central venous catheters can provide interim access while a native fistula develops (28). A detailed description of the patient's preoperative assessment for dialysis access appears in Chapter 3.

Briefly, the patient's general medical condition should be as optimal as possible, with stable electrolyte concentrations and no overt fluid overload. The nondominant extremity is usually chosen for access placement to avoid depriving the patient of use of the dominant arm during the dialysis sessions. In patients with underlying arterial occlusive disease, such as those with diabetes, ischemic neuropathy following fistula placement can sometimes lead to loss of the hand—a complication that is somewhat better tolerated in the nondominant extremity. Preexisting conditions—such as central venous obstruction, lymphedema, or severe arterial insufficiency due to proximal obstruction—may preclude the use of one extremity versus the other. A careful preoperative physical examination with palpation of all pulses, measurement of blood pressure, Allen's test, Doppler interrogation of the wrist and hand, and a careful neurological examination of both upper extremities is imperative. This provides an opportunity to detect physiological problems that may change the operative strategy and to establish a preoperative baseline should the patient develop circulatory or neurological deficits after access construction.

Examination of the upper extremity veins with a tourniquet in place is helpful in selecting possible sites for venous outflow. If antecubital and upper arm veins are not palpable with a tourniquet in place, venous mapping using duplex Doppler is a simple way to assess the size and patency of basilic and cephalic trunks—a maneuver that may minimize the time usually spent searching for an adequate outflow site (29). This technique is also helpful in the not uncommon circumstance when the patient has had repeated phlebotomy in the chosen extremity prior to its selection as an access site. These patients' arms are often covered with ecchymoses from prior phlebotomies and intravenous lines, making clinical assessment of venous patency difficult. Duplex mapping is also helpful in patients who have had previous access grafts in that extremity or in those with a prior history of intravenous drug abuse.

Anesthesia

Most access procedures can be safely performed by a variety of anesthetic techniques. Local or regional anesthesia is satisfactory for forearm grafts. When dissection in the axilla is required for upper arm grafts, supraclavicular intrascalene blocks can provide effective anesthesia, but general anesthesia is often employed. Moreover, regardless of anesthetic technique, most vascular access operations can be performed on an outpatient basis. Patients are typically observed in a postanesthesia care unit for 1 to 2 h postoperatively prior to discharge (30). It is conceivable that placement of an access graft may be accomplished completely under local anesthesia without the added cost of using an anesthesiologist or nurse anesthetist to monitor the patient. Given the multitude of comorbid medical conditions and advanced age that our dialysis population possesses, we have not adopted this approach. However, this technique may be appropriate in selected young patients with limited medical problems undergoing uncomplicated access surgery. Our preference is to use general anesthesia for graft placement unless contraindicated by comorbid cardiopulmonary conditions. With the advent of the laryngeal mask anesthetic technique and because most graft procedures can be completed in 60 to 90 min, we have not appreciated a significant difference in immediate postoperative anesthetic or cardiopulmonary complications with this approach.

Site Preparation

Preparation of the operative site for graft placement is subject to individual variation. A dictum that we frequently apply is "Never let the operation be limited by the prep and drape." In this regard, for all upper extremity access procedures, the hand, arm, and axilla are included in the sterile prep and drape. With this approach, the surgeon is prepared to deal with any unexpected anatomy or complications that may develop during AV graft placement. The surgical procedure can be altered as necessary without fear of compromising the sterile field. This small detail may have paramount implications when one is dealing with prosthetic grafts and infectious complications. The hand is included in the prep and drape to permit sterile Doppler interrogation after fistula construction, which allows for immediate intervention should vascular compromise be discovered. The axilla is included to allow placement of the sterile tourniquet in the above-elbow position and access to the axillary vein if needed for venous outflow if more proximal veins are found to be inadequate.

Drug Regimen

The use of perioperative antibiotics, though intuitive, has not been clearly shown to reduce risk of infection in prosthetic AV access grafts (31,32). The common practice of administering a single dose of intravenous antibiotics active against gram-positive organisms derives from the well-documented reduction in infection rates when applied to elective vascular reconstructions (33,34). The first-generation cephalosporin antibiotic cefazolin has favorable pharmacokinetics for effective prophylaxis and is usually administered 1 h prior to surgery (35). In patients with a significant allergy to this drug, a single dose of intravenous vancomycin is substituted.

The use of heparin during the placement of dialysis fistulae has not been studied in any significant detail. Since uremic patients are presumed to be in a relatively antithrombogenic state, intravenous heparin is not uniformly employed in access surgery, unlike other vascular reconstruction procedures. However, as a minimum, local infusion of heparin solution into arteries, veins, and graft conduits is typically applied to prevent local formation of thrombus in these structures while flow is interrupted. With respect to dialysis access surgery, systemic heparin is more consistently utilized during thrombectomies and revision procedures because of the presumed thrombogenic nature of the graft surface once thrombectomy is accomplished. Despite the known deficits in platelet aggregation caused by uremia, studies have shown that some patients with chronic renal failure exist in a relatively hypercoagulable state (36). This is not unexpected, given the elevations in thrombogenic factors such as fibrinogen and plasminogen activator inhibitor that have been documented in some patients with diabetes.

General Surgical Techniques

Suturing

The selection of suture material and placement technique are subject to the discretion of the individual surgeon. Like other aspects of access surgery, many decisions find their origin in basic vascular surgery preferences. Significant healing of polymer and biological prostheses at the anastomosis is largely maintained by the suture line; therefore a nonabsorbable material is commonly selected. Polypropylene sutures have been available for a long time and have a track record of effectiveness in cardiovascular surgery. Their established history and availability from a multitude of manufacturers also tend to make them less costly than newer materials. Recent modifications include the swagging on of a smaller-diameter needle than the suture itself in an effort to limit bleeding at the suture line by filling the needle hole with a larger-diameter suture material. The introduction of ePTFE suture by W.L. Gore and Associates (Flagstaff, AZ) provides an alternative to polypropylene for vascular anastomosis. This suture offers ease of handling and strength; with smaller needles, its hemostatic properties are similar to those of its polypropylene counterparts. The major disadvantage of the ePTFE suture is higher cost compared with polypropylene. In the past few years, the availability of a nonpenetrating titanium clip for vascular anastomoses has expanded the options of AV access construction, with a reduction in anastomotic bleeding and better healing compared with surtures, as demonstrated in an animal model of AV grafts (Figure 5.1) (37).

Various techniques for suturing vascular anastomoses have been reported, from the triangulation method originally described by Alexis Carrell to the use of a single suture for the entire anastomosis (Figure 5.2). As with the selection of sutures, specific technique is often directed by surgeon preference. Whereas the triangulation technique is helpful in surgical training programs to nicely demonstrate apposition and avoid technical errors in placement, the single-suture parachute technique is often preferred by accomplished surgeons who switch their focus to expediency. One cautionary note deserves mention. When the single-suture method is chosen, the suture knot should be secured after flow has been

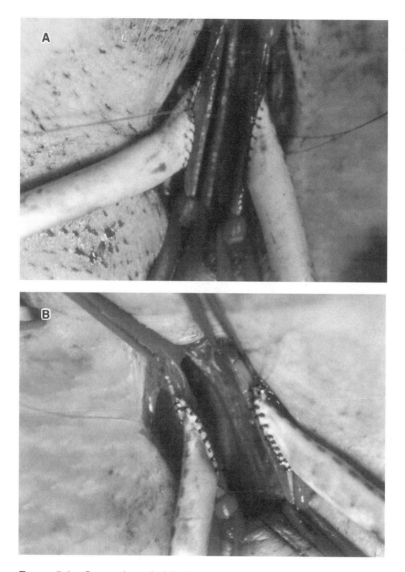

FIGURE 5.1   Gross views (original magnification) of AV fistulas joined to the native vessel with suture (A) or vascular closure system clips (B) shown at implantation (time, T = 0), before release of the vascular loops. The suture holes associated with the conventional anastomoses allowed blood to flow freely for the first several minutes after the release of the loops (C), whereas hemostasis was achieved almost instantaneously on release of vessel loops in the anastomoses constructed with the clips (D). (From Ref. 37.)

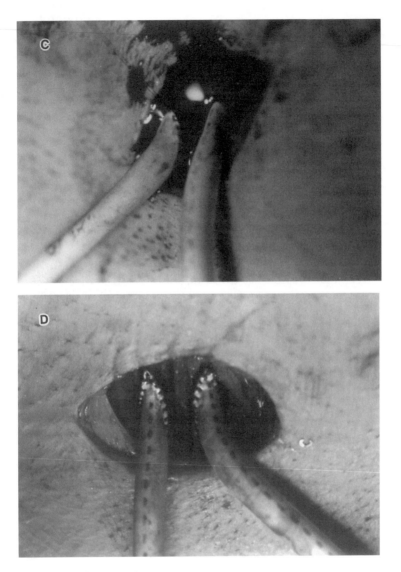

FIGURE 5.1 Continued.

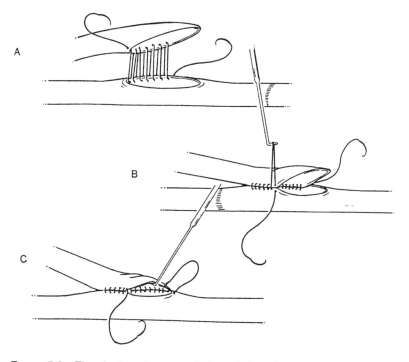

FIGURE 5.2 The single-suture parachute technique for vascular anastomosis. The anastomosis is begun at the side, traversing toward the heel without applying full tension to the suture after each throw (A). Once the heel of the anastomosis is completed, full tension is applied with the aid of a nerve hook (B). The toe end of the anastomosis is completed (C).

established and under full distention of the anastomosis to avoid narrowing due to a purse-string effect of the single stitch. Prior to establishing flow in the AV graft, vigorous backbleeding and flushing of the artery, vein, and graft should be performed to avoid immediate failure caused by thrombus that may have formed in these structures during flow stagnation despite the presence of local or systemic heparinization.

Vascular Control

The technique of vascular control during the placement of an access graft is deserving of some discussion. Traditionally, vascular clamps were used to occlude the native artery and vein while anastomoses were completed. Careful selection of delicate vascular clamps is imperative to avoid trauma to the native arterial and venous structures, which may compromise immediate and long-term fistula function. Local alternatives to clamps include the use of silastic vascular tapes. All these forms of "clamp" control have been shown to cause trauma to the vascular endothelium, which may affect immediate and long-term results (38,39). As an alternative, atraumatic vascular control of the vessels of the upper extremity can be obtained through the use of exsanguination with an Esmarch bandage and a sterile pneumatic tourniquet (40). However, this technique is limited in its application to grafts placed from the antecubital fossa and distally, since tourniquet application is effective only up to the proximal humeral level (Figure 5.3). Use of the pneumatic tourniquet eliminates the need for circumferential dissection of the venous outflow structure, thereby avoiding disruption of the vasa vasorum. This technique permits the use of less than ideal inflow arteries with calcification in their walls, but adequate lumen size and flow, by avoiding the traumatic crushing of these delicate vessels with clamps. In addition, the tourniquet technique provides a bloodless field without the cumbersome presence of vascular clamps, making anastomotic suturing easier.

The specific technique is as follows: Dissection of the arterial inflow proceeds as usual. The venous outflow vein is exposed only on its anterior and minimally on its lateral aspects for an appropriate length. The selected graft is tunneled into place, making sure there are no twists or kinks. Sterile cast padding and a pneumatic tourniquet are snugly applied to above the elbow. The limb is exsan-

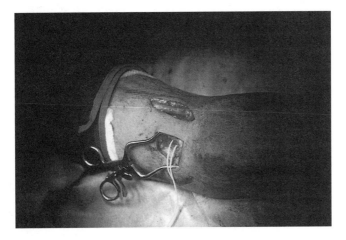

FIGURE 5.3 Use of the sterile pneumatic tourniquet for vascular control. In this picture, the tourniquet technique is used in the construction of an antecubital native AV fistula. The cephalic vein above a failed forearm loop AV graft has matured and is transposed over to the brachial artery. The tourniquet is placed in the proximal upper arm, eliminating the need for clamp application to either the vein or the artery.

guinated with the Esmarch bandage and the tourniquet is inflated up to 250 to 300 mmHg. The arterial and venous anastomoses are performed in the usual manner. The final suture knots on each are not secured, allowing a space for backbleeding and flushing. The tourniquet is released while digital pressure occludes the brachial artery. Flushing and backbleeding maneuvers are completed. Flow is established through the graft as sutures are securely tied. It is important to remove the cast padding and tourniquet completely from the arm before assessing the fistula, as even their uninflated compression can impede venous outflow. The sterile tourniquet technique has become the author's standard method not only for forearm prosthetic grafts but also for radiocephalic and brachiocephalic native fistulae and all revisional surgery distal to the upper humerus. Over a period of 18 months, this technique was used in over 100 access procedures. There have been no major complications related to the use of the tourniquet and early primary patency has been equivalent to that of traditional methods. Whether this technique of vascular control will affect long-term patency remains to be determined. For primary access construction, systemic heparin is not used with this technique; however, patients with thrombosed grafts are routinely heparinized with 3000 U intravenously prior to tourniquet inflation.

Graft Tunneling

Graft tunneling is another critical component of access construction, with technical nuances that deserve mention. The goal of the access surgeon is to provide a useful AV graft so that the nurses or technicians at the dialysis unit will be able to access it reliably and easily three times a week. This requires that the graft be positioned just under the skin and be free of placement complications. Additionally, providing an adequate length of usable graft may enable the dialysis unit staff to avoid having to access the same site repeatedly, thereby limiting aneurysm formation. To meet these goals, graft positioning and tunneling become crucial steps in access surgery. The length of graft chosen is somewhat limited by the anatomical site of insertion. For any chosen location, as long a graft as possible that still avoids kinking should be placed to provide as much usable length as is practical. The subcutaneous tunnel should fit snugly around the abluminal surface of the graft without creating kinks. Since every patient has different skin characteristics, the depth of the tunnel must be determined for each case individually. For patients with very thin skin, the grafts often rest immediately on top of the musculofascial layer. Conversely, in patients with generous subcutaneous fat, the graft is positioned within the subcutaneous layer close to the dermis. A snug fit is facilitated by the use of commercially available tunneling devices specifically designed for graft placement, such as the Kelly-Wick (Impra Inc., Tempe, AZ). These devices ensure a snug apposition of the graft to the surrounding tissue, which will limit the formation of perigraft seromas and permit early usage of the graft, if necessary, with minimal complications (41,42).

The timing of tunneling the graft is left to the surgeon's discretion. Many surgeons perform the arterial anastomosis first, then tunnel the graft under arterial pressure to minimize the chance of kinking. Once tunneled, the graft should be irrigated free of blood with heparin solution prior to performing the venous anastomosis; otherwise thrombosis of the stagnant column of blood will ensue. We prefer to tunnel the graft prior to performing either venous or arterial anastomoses. The available prosthetic grafts are marked with lines to facilitate tunneling without twists or kinks. In the forearm, we use the tourniquet technique exclusively and construct both anastomoses before any flow is established. With this technique, attention to detail in tunneling the graft must be exercised; however, this method spares the graft surface from exposure to stagnant blood. There are many possible variations in these steps, all of which achieve the same end result; the surgeon will usually apply the routine that has become consistent and comfortable for him or her.

Configuration

The configurations of the arterial and venous anastomoses are another poorly studied area of access surgery. Since 80% of access graft failures involve hyperplasia and narrowing at the venous outflow, a long, oblique anastomosis seems desirable to accommodate these changes and prevent thrombosis. An easy way to obtain a gentle obliquity in the graft limb is to use a curved hemostat to mark a bevel 1.5 to 2 cm in length and provide a surface to cut against with a scalpel. The arterial anstomosis, on the other hand, should be as small as possible while still providing adequate flow rates and without causing ischemia from excessive steal from the distal extremity. This goal can usually be met either by using the graft uncut and squared on end at the arterial limb or cutting a short bevel in the graft limb with a small hemostat.

COMMON INSERTION SITES AND TECHNIQUES (TABLE 5.2)

Forearm Bridge AV Grafts

These grafts have become the most common style of prosthetic access and include both a loop and straight configuration (Figure 5.4). There is great debate over the advantages of one pattern versus the other. One argument in favor of utilizing the straight graft as the first choice for prosthetic access contends that by utilizing the most distal artery, the longevity of the forearm access site is prolonged, since a loop graft can be placed at a later time if needed. However, in one of the only comparisons of these two graft configurations using ePTFE, reported by Schmidt and Field (43), only 1 of the 62 patients receiving straight grafts was successfully converted to a loop graft when the straight graft failed. This is not unexpected,

TABLE 5.2 Type and Location of Dialysis AV Graft Placement

1. If a primary AV fistula cannot be established, a synthetic AV graft is the next preferred type of vascular access.
2. Polytetrafluoroethylene (PTFE) tubes are preferred over tubes made of other synthetic materials.
3. There is no convincing evidence to support tapered over uniform tubes, externally supported over unsupported grafts, thick- versus thin-walled configurations, or elastic versus nonelastic material.
4. Grafts may be placed in straight, looped, or curved configurations. Designs that provide the most surface area for cannulation are preferred.
5. Location of graft placement is determined by each patient's unique anatomical restriction, the surgeon's skill, and the anticipated duration of dialysis.

Source: Modified from Ref. 2.

since pathology at the arterial limb of an access graft is not the usual source of failure. No clear advantage has been demonstrated in terms of either primary or secondary patency for loop versus straight forearm grafts. In large series of both bovine and ePTFE forearm bridge fistulae, primary patency on the order of 60% at 12 months has been reported whether a straight or looped configuration was being considered (17–19, 43–46). Similarly, secondary patency rates approaching 80 to 90% are usually achieved with ePTFE grafts in these locations, slightly lower rates being attained with bovine xenografts. The limiting factor in selecting one format over the other is often the availability of suitable inflow arteries and outflow veins. In our practice, the overwhelming majority of patients needing access procedures have diabetes and therefore have poor or overtly diseased distal arteries, thereby precluding the use of a straight forearm fistula.

Many of the basic principles of graft construction have already been discussed above, under "General Principles." More details are provided below, under "Loop Forearm Fistula." These apply to subsequent sections as well, describing other anatomic configurations of prosthetic AV grafts, but are not repeated there. Those discussions are limited to anatomic exposures and special considerations for placement as well as comments regarding functional outcomes.

Loop Forearm Fistula

This access graft is constructed between the brachial artery or one of its major branches and a superficial vein in the antecubital fossa (Figure 5.5). This graft arrangement is the most common form of prosthetic access and is usually constructed using one of the ePTFE graft materials. As with other forearm access procedures, local, regional, and general anesthesia may be employed as deemed appropriate by the operating team. A careful preoperative assessment is con-

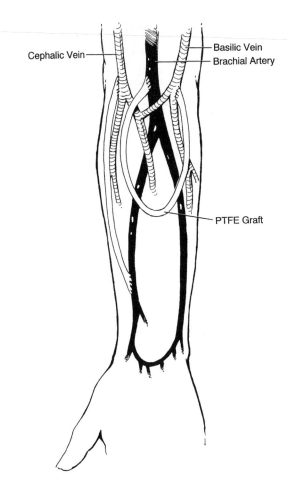

FIGURE 5.4 Forearm bridge AV graft shown in both a loop and straight configuration.

ducted with attention to arm blood pressure, hand perfusion, and venous anatomy with a tourniquet in place. Preoperative duplex mapping is selectively utilized when venous anatomy and patency are not readily apparent by physical examination.

To assist with tunneling, the skin incisions and course of the graft are marked out on the skin after prepping and draping. It is helpful to keep the loop of the graft on the flat volar surface of the forearm and provide as much usable graft length as possible. A transverse incision is made in the forearm just distal

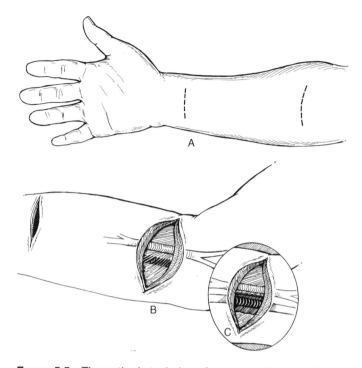

FIGURE 5.5 The author's technique for construction of a forearm loop bridge AV graft. Transverse incisions are made in the antecubital fossa and distal forearm. B. Exposure of the antecubital cephalic and or basilic veins is accomplished in the subcutaneous plane. C. The biceps aponeurosis is opened carefully, sparing trauma to the superficial branch of the radial and median nerves to expose the brachial artery. This artery is often surrounded by venae comitantes. D. A curved tunneller is used to tunnel the 6-mm graft in the subcutaneous space into a loop configuration. E. A long beveled venous anastomosis and slightly beveled or square arterial anastomosis is performed.

to the antecubital crease (Figure 5.5a). This placement prevents kinking of the anastomotic limbs by avoidance of the flexion crease. We try to keep this incision as small as possible to include the brachial artery and the chosen outflow vein. Care is taken not to injure the vein, which is often immediately under the dermis in the antecubital fossa. Enough vein is exposed on its anterior and lateral surfaces to construct an adequate venous anastomosis, since tourniquet occlusion is used for vascular control (Figure 5.5b). When vascular clamps are utilized, enough vein must be mobilized to permit application of loops or clamps. Once the vein segment is exposed, the bicipital aponeurosis is incised to gain exposure of the

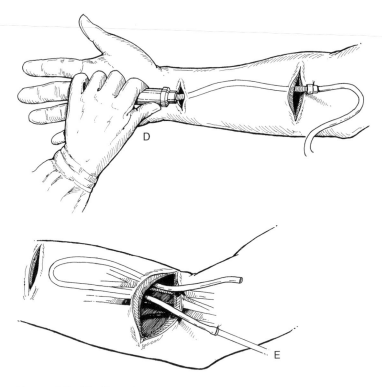

FIGURE 5.5 Continued.

brachial artery (Figure 5.5c). Care must be exercised to avoid injury to the median nerve, which lies close to the brachial artery. Because of its deep location, circumferential dissection of the brachial artery and control with Silastic loops is accomplished even if tourniquet occlusion will be utilized for vascular control. This maneuver permits elevation of the artery out of the depths of the wound to facilitate completion of the anstomosis. A transverse counterincision is made on the volar surface of the forearm 15 to 20 cm distal to the antecubital incision. A subcutaneous pocket is created on the proximal aspect of this incision to accomodate the apex of the loop graft such that it is not positioned directly under the skin incision.

We use the short, curved Kelly-Wick tunneler with a 6-mm head to tunnel the graft by first passing the tunneler from the counterincision to the site for the venous anastomosis (Figure 5.5d). The graft is then secured to the tunneler head with a suture and pulled through the tunnel, leaving enough graft to perform the venous anastomosis plus a few centimeters extra. The attached graft and 6-mm head are removed, a second 6-mm head is applied, and the tunneler is subsequently passed from the antecubital incision, distally to the counterincision. Reattachment of the graft/tunneler head assembly is followed by pulling the graft from the counterincision proximally to the antecubital incision, which completes graft placement. During these maneuvers, sterile towels are used to avoid any contact of the graft material with the skin. At the level of the antecubital incision, the graft should be tunneled just beneath the subcutaneous fascia, which is an important layer to close at the completion of the procedure. In the forearm proper, the graft should lie just beneath the dermis to permit easy access. Care must be taken in patients with delicate, thin skin to tunnel the graft just above the muscle fascia, thus avoiding skin breakdown and graft exposure. This technique adequately accommodates a 40- to 50-cm length of graft, maximizing the usable length of the loop for access and minimizing the waste and cost associated with longer lengths of prosthetic material.

With the graft properly tunneled and confirmed to be free of kinks or twists, we apply a sterile pneumatic tourniquet and cast padding to the above elbow position. Limb exsanguination is accomplished with a 4-in. Esmarch bandage and the tourniquet is inflated to 250 mmHg. We usually begin with the venous anastomosis, since this is the more critical connection in regard to long-term patency and may require exposure of a secondary venous site if unsuspected pathology is encountered upon opening the chosen vein. It is unusual to find pathology in the brachial artery that would alter the conduct of the procedure, so this anastomosis is reserved for later. A venotomy approximately 2 cm in length is made on the selected vein. Serial Garret coronary dilators are passed up the vein their full length to a maximal 4-mm diameter to confirm unobstructed venous patency. Even with a pneumatic tourniquet in place, passage of the dilators is usually possible in the absence of venous pathology. Occasionally the selected venous segment is patent at the antecubital fossa but occluded more proximally. Determination of this finding at this juncture permits exposure of a different venous outflow site at the elbow without significantly disrupting the progress of the operation. This may require extension of the antecubital incision medially or laterally to expose the basilic or cephalic veins, respectively. The graft is cut on a bevel using a curved hemostat and a scalpel and an end-to-side anstomosis is performed. The critical portion of the anstomosis is the toe on the outflow vein. Suture bites on the vein should be small and evenly placed to avoid narrowing the outflow channel. Wide patency of the toe of the anastomosis is confirmed by passage of a 4-mm dilator prior to completing the final suturing. Once the venous anastomosis is completed, an arteriotomy approximately 8 to 10 mm in length is made on the brachial artery. It is possible to use either the proximal radial or ulnar arteries if they are of adequate size (4 mm); if the brachial artery has a high bifurcation, this is sometimes necessary in order to avoid placing the arterial anastomosis accross the flexion crease. The arterial limb of the graft is gently beveled and sewn to the artery in an end-to-side configuration. With digital pressure occluding the brachial artery above the elbow, the tourniquet is released, allowing backbleeding of the venous and arterial anastomoses. This confirms patency of the distal artery and venous outflow. Depending on the proximity of a venous valve to the anastomosis, there may not be much backbleeding from the venous limb. Digital pressure is released and a flush is given to the arterial anastomosis prior to securing the anastomotic suture. Both the venous and arterial anastomotic sutures are securely tied as flow is established in the AV graft.

Various and sundry modifications of this technique exist, as discussed under "General Principles," above. No specific method has been demonstrated to provide superior results in terms of long-term primary and secondary patency; therefore individual surgeon preferences usually take precedence.

Of equal importance to the construction of the fistula is an immediate assessment of flow in the graft. When the pneumatic tourniquet is utilized, it is imperative to remove the tourniquet and the cast padding prior to assessing fistula function as even their passive compression can impede venous outflow enough to distort graft assessment. Successful fistula construction is usually manifest as a faint thrill palpable over the arterial limb of the graft. An assessment of hand perfusion in the absence of palpable radial and ulnar pulses is required as well to assure that early ischemia will not compromise the distal extremity. A sterile continuous-wave Doppler probe with sterile acoustic gel is used to interrogate the fistula and the hand. Insonation over the outflow vein should reveal a pulsatile audible flow signal that maintains flow through diastole. This should disappear completely when the fistula is compressed at its apex. Insonation over the arterial limb should reveal a similarly turbulent signal, which converts to a thump with fistula compression. Because of the large amount of air present within the interstices of ePTFE prosthetic grafts, which functions as an acoustic barrier to sound transmission, flow may not be detected by the Doppler when it is placed directly over graft material. This requires insonation over the anstomoses or outflow vein to assess flow. With time, the air becomes displaced from the graft (a process know as denucleation) as the graft heals into the subcutaneous tissue, permitting successful Doppler assessment over the graft material. Doppler interrogation of the radial, ulnar, and palmar arch arteries should also take place with and without fistula compression to document adequacy of the distal circulation and determine any effects the fistula may have on arterial flow in the hand. The absence of Doppler flow at the wrist, which returns when the fistula is compressed, is a worrisome sign of hand ischemia, which will require further assessment or intervention, including fistula ligation to prevent loss of the distal extremity (see Chapter 12).

Closure of the two incisions is individualized to the integrity of the skin. Healthy skin is closed with a running subcutaneous layer of an absorbable suture followed by a running subcuticular closure of a monofilament absorbable suture.

When the skin is thin and attenuated, closure of the subcutaneous layer with absorbable suture is attempted, followed by closure of the dermis with either interrupted or running, widely spaced sutures of monofilament nylon. The counter-incision in the distal forearm is usually closed with a two-layer closure using absorbable suture.

Straight Forearm Fistula

This fistula is usually constructed between the radial artery at the wrist and one of the antecubital veins at the elbow. For many surgeons, this is the first choice for a prosthetic access graft. These grafts can be effectively constructed using local, regional, or general anesthesia. They can be made using all of the available graft materials. In general, a 6-mm graft is chosen to accomodate the small size of the radial artery yet still provide enough flow through the graft for effective dialysis. In patients with very small radial arteries, size mismatch can be overcome by using one of the available 4- to 7-mm taper grafts. As with all access procedures, a careful assessment of extremity blood pressure and distal flow is necessary to minimize ischemic complications and early failure from inadequate arterial inflow. The presence of a strong radial pulse and a negative Allen's test are prerequisites for use of this access configuration.

Exposure of the radial artery is obtained at the wrist through a longitudinal incision. A superficial branch of the radial nerve is commonly encountered and should be protected from trauma (Figure 5.6). Circumferential exposure and control of the artery is not necessary if tourniquet ischemia will be used, otherwise, the artery is dissected and controlled with vessel loops. The selected outflow vein is then exposed in the forearm just distal to the antecubital crease, usually through a transversly oriented incision. Either the median antecubital, cephalic, or basilic vein is selected, based upon preoperative assessment with a tourniquet in place. In patients with generous subcutaneous fatty tissue, palpation with a tourniquet in place may be limited in delineating the size and patency of these veins. In these circumstances, duplex imaging and mapping preoperatively may be useful. The remaining conduct of the procedure is open to variation. The selected graft is tunneled between these two sites, concentrating the bulk of the graft on the radial aspect of the arm. This point is important, since most patients cannot hold the arm comfortably in supination during a dialysis session, which is necessary if the graft is positioned largely on the ulnar aspect of the forearm. Arterial and venous anatomoses are constructed as described above. Whether vascular clamps or a pneumatic tourniquet is used for control, it is important to flush the vessels and anastomoses adequately prior to establishing flow in the graft. Once flow is established through the graft, a palpable thrill should be appreciable at the arterial end of the graft. A sterile Doppler probe should be available to interrogate flow in the outflow vein as well as arterial circulation in the hand prior to exiting the operating suite.

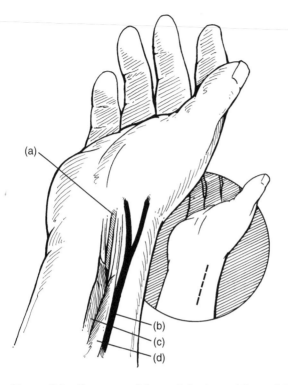

FIGURE 5.6 Exposure of the radial artery at the wrist for placement of a straight forearm bridge AV graft. The superficial branch of the radial nerve is the first structure encountered and should be spared any trauma to avoid paresthesias to the thumb and index finger. The artery lies deep to the nerve between the flexor carpi radialis tendon medially and the brachioradialis tendon laterally. (a) Superficial branch of the radial nerve, (b) radial artery, (c) palmaris longus tendon, (d) flexor carpi radialis tendon.

Upper Arm Bridge AV Grafts

Upper arm AV grafts are often secondary sites of access when forearm sites are exhausted. Occasionally, a patient may not have adequate arterial inflow or venous outflow at the antecubital level to permit construction of a forearm bridge fistula; therefore an upper arm graft becomes the primary access site. Because of durable primary and secondary patency rates, upper arm grafts have been recommended as preferential sites for primary access by some authors (47,48).

Upper arm AV grafts use the brachial artery just proximal to the antecubital crease as a source of arterial inflow (Figure 5.7). The venous outflow is usually

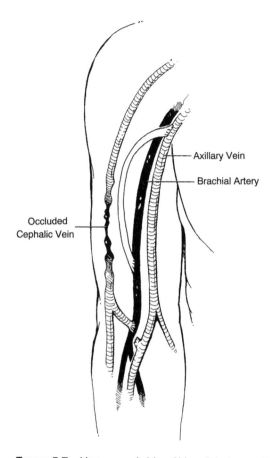

Axillary Vein

Brachial Artery

Occluded
Cephalic Vein

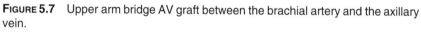

FIGURE 5.7   Upper arm bridge AV graft between the brachial artery and the axillary vein.

placed on the basilic, brachial, or axillary vein through an upper arm or axillary incision. Occasionally, the proximal cephalic vein in the deltopectoral groove is patent and of adequate caliber to provide venous outflow. Initial use of the cephalic vein reserves the axillary vein for fistula revision when failure at the venous anastomosis is encountered.

Upper arm fistula procedures can be performed using local, regional, or general anesthesia. Local and regional techniques are less common in this location because of the difficulty in obtaining adequate anesthesia in the axilla. Exposure is gained through a longitudinal incision made in the upper arm up to the anterior axillary line (Figure 5.8). The basilic and brachial veins are exposed as

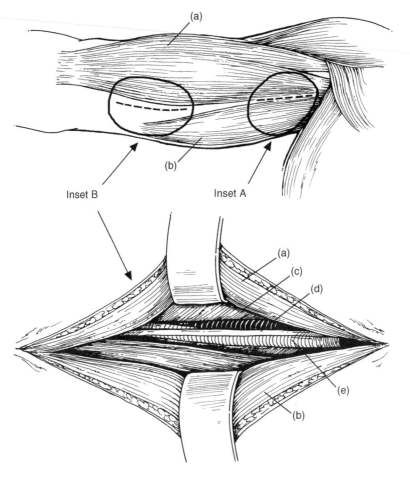

Figure 5.8 Incisions and anatomical exposure of the brachial artery (inset A) and the basilic/axillary veins (inset B) for placement of an upper arm bridge AV graft. (a) Biceps muscle (b) triceps muscle, (c) brachial artery, (d) median nerve, (e) median antebrachial nerve, (f) brachial vein, (g) ulnar nerve, (h) basilic vein, (i) pectoral muscle, (j) triceps muscle.

they transition into the axillary vein in the groove between the biceps and triceps muscles (Figure 5.8a). In dissecting out the venous structures, care must be exercised to avoid injury to the median, ulnar, and medial antebrachial cutaneous nerves, which surround the brachial artery at this level. If an adequate sized basilic or brachial vein is available, we reserve extension of the incision and subse-

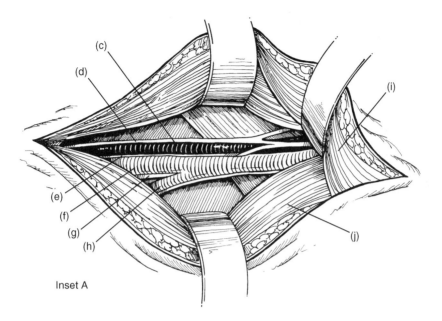

(c)
(d)
(i)
(e)
(f)
(g)
(h)
(j)

Inset A

FIGURE 5.8   Continued.

quent exposure of the axillary vein for a secondary procedure. Circumferential control of the venous outflow vein is accomplished with Silastic loops. Small branches can be ligated and divided to facilitate the mobilization and avoid traumatic tearing of these delicate vessels. The brachial artery is exposed and circumferentially dissected in the distal upper arm through a longitudinal incision similarly placed in the groove between the biceps and triceps muscle bellies (Figure 5.8b). A 6-mm graft is tunneled in a curvilinear fashion over the lateral aspect of the biceps muscle belly in the subcutaneous space toward the proximal incision. With the advent of the Kelly-Wick tunneler, this can often be accomplished without the need for a counterincision. A critical step in the construction is coursing the graft in a gently oblique fashion over the biceps muscle belly and into the proximal upper arm or axillary dissection (Figure 5.9). It is important to avoid an acute angulation of the graft over the muscle and into the vein, which often results in a kink in the graft when the incision is closed (Figure 5.10).

The venous and arterial anastomoses are completed as previously described. For these anastomoses, vascular control can be obtained through the use of fine vascular clamps, silastic vessel loops, or combinations of these methods. Passage of a 4-mm Garret dilator through the partially completed venous anastomosis confirms an adequate lumen without narrowing of the outflow. As with

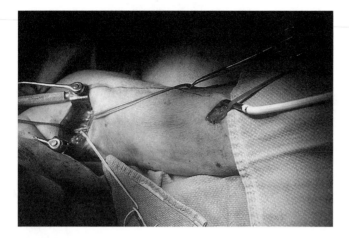

FIGURE 5.9 Tunneling of an upper arm AV bridge graft. The availability of curved tunnelers eliminates the need for counterincisions.

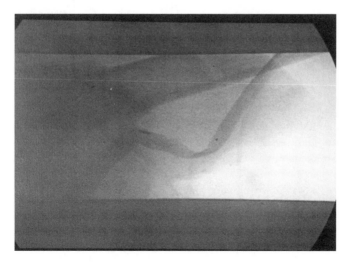

FIGURE 5.10 The venous limb of this upper arm AV graft has a kink caused by the acute angulation of the graft over the medial border of the bicep muscle and into the venous outflow at almost a right angle.

other AV grafts, backbleeding and flushing maneuvers should be performed before establishing flow in the graft. Assessment of graft patency by palpation and Doppler insonation is completed once flow is established in the graft, along with an assessment of distal circulation in the hand and wrist.

If the cephalic, basilic, or brachial vein is chosen as the venous outflow for the initial upper arm AV graft, the axillary vein provides a secondary site for revision of the venous anastomosis, which can be exposed by extension of the incision into the axilla and mobilizing the lateral border of the pectoralis major and minor muscles. Extension of the venous limb into the axillary vein avoids placing the graft across the shoulder joint. By contrast, further revision of an upper arm graft venous limb may require exposure of the axillosubclavian vein through an infraclavicular incision. When an extension of the venous limb to this level is necessary, the author chooses to use an externally supported ePTFE graft for the portion of the fistula that crosses the shoulder joint.

Lower Extremity Bridge AV Grafts

Once both upper extremities have been exhausted for placement of chronic AV access grafts, it is often necessary to move to the lower extremities for continued hemodialysis access. Fortunately, this route is inevitable in only a small percentage of dialysis patients. The lower extremity is a less desirable site for access construction for a number of reasons. The proximity of the access site to the chronic bacterial contamination of the perineum, associated with the digestive and genitourinary systems, raises concern for access site infection in the groin. Moreover, atherosclerotic occlusive disease is more likely to be present in the femoral arterial branches, precluding their use for arterial inflow for access construction. Preexisting femoral or iliac vein stenosis from prior catheterization may limit available sites for venous outflow in lower extremity AV grafts. Finally, complications related to the venous outflow of a lower extremity fistula may extend to involve the iliac veins, thereby compromising sites for renal transplantation if the patient is a suitable candidate. Despite these limitations, lower extremity access grafts provide another route for the maintenance of chronic access in patients who are no longer candidates for upper extremity grafts.

The general principles for access graft construction discussed above are similarly applicable in placing lower extremity AV grafts. All routes of anesthesia have been applied; however, either regional spinal/epidural or general techniques are most commonly utilized. Preoperative assessment includes a careful examination of the femoral, popliteal, and pedal pulses of both lower extremities. An ankle-brachial index should be calculated using the highest of the two arm systolic blood pressures as the denominator and the highest ankle pressure from each leg as the numerator. An index of greater than 0.80 implies adequate circulation to support a fistula without compromising distal perfusion. If any question exists as to the adequacy of arterial inflow for fistula construction based upon clinical and Doppler examinations, arteriography should be performed to assess the anatomical distribution of occlusive lesions. If prior femoral venous cannulation with large-bore catheters was performed for interim access, color-flow Doppler examination of each groin should be used to assess venous patency.

Prosthetic AV grafts placed in the lower extremity can have either the distal superficial femoral or common femoral arteries as their arterial inflow vessels (Figure 5.11). Similarly, either the saphenous or common femoral vein may be utilized for venous outflow. Exposure of the common femoral artery and vein is accomplished through a vertical groin incision made in the femoral triangle (Fig-

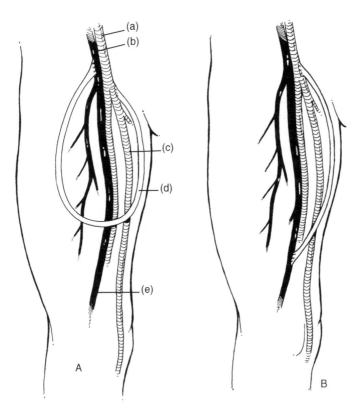

FIGURE 5.11   Lower extremity bridge AV grafts may originate from either the common femoral artery (A), or the distal superficial femoral artery (B). (a) Common femoral vein, (b) common femoral artery, (c) greater saphenous vein, (d) graft, (e) popliteal artery.

ure 5.12a). If the distal superficial femoral artery is chosen for the arterial inflow site, exposure is obtained through an incision in the medial thigh over the subsartorial canal (Figure 5.12b). Circumferential dissection and control of the selected arterial and venous structures is accomplished. The technical procedure of the graft placement is similar to those discussed above. The selected graft is tunneled in a loop or semilunar configuration in the subcutaneous tissue, usually routed toward the lateral aspect of the thigh to permit easy cannulation of the fistula without the need for uncomfortable external rotation of the hip. A counterincision may or may not be necessary to facilitate graft tunneling. As with AV fistulas in the upper extremity, a 6-mm graft will usually suffice, with no clear advantage achieved by the use of either the taper graft or larger sizes. When the saphenous vein is chosen as the site for the venous anastomosis, the distal vein is ligated to prevent venous hypertension in the saphenous system.

As in the case of upper extremity prosthetic access grafts, the usual cause of failure of lower extremity AV grafts is often narrowing at the venous anastomosis due to intimal hyperplasia. This can be treated by balloon angioplasty. Repeated failures require surgical revision, which may necessitate extension in the iliac venous system for adequate venous outflow. Since lower extremity prosthetic AV grafts are often placed as a last resort, little if any data exist to provide a measure of primary or secondary patency for this type of bridge fistula. As survival of patients on dialysis increases, this particular approach to chronic access will likely find increased application. As a consequence, better definitions of its durability will be obtained.

UNUSUAL SITES FOR AV GRAFT CONSTRUCTION

Site selection for placement of prosthetic AV grafts is limited only by the surgeon's imagination and the availability of adequate arterial inflow and venous outflow. The practical factors affecting site selection are accessibility of the graft for cannulation by the dialysis personnel and the morbidity due to either the placement procedure or operations to deal with potential complications related to the graft. Most patients are maintained throughout their dialysis lifetime with the upper extremity access grafts previously described. Infrequently, either lower extremity or unusual upper body access procedures are necessary to maintain uninterrupted access. The axilloaxillary, axillofemoral, and brachiojugular bridge fistulas are described briefly below.

Axilloaxillary Bridge Grafts

When anatomical or infectious factors preclude the use of the upper or lower extremity for access for hemodialysis, the axillary arteries and veins provide a suitable alternative. The exact configuration depends upon the individual patient

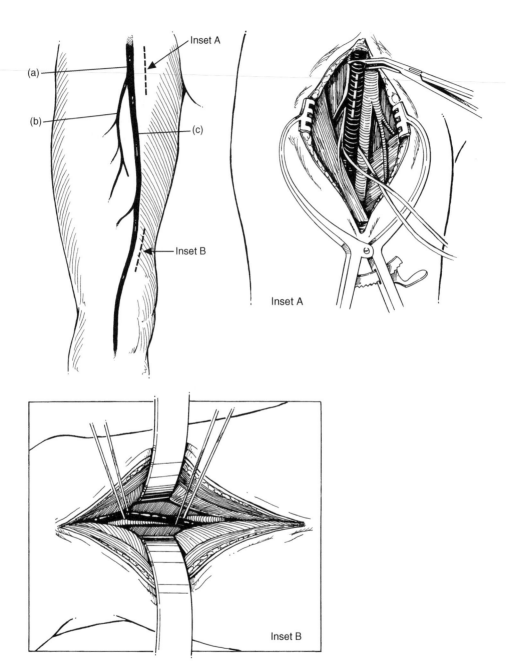

Figure 5.12 Exposure for construction of a lower leg bridge AV graft taking origin from the common femoral artery (inset A) or the distal superficial femoral artery (inset B). (a) Common femoral artery, (b) profundus femoral artery, (c) superficial femoral artery.

factors, but either axillary artery to contralateral axillary vein (straight or "necklace" fistula) or axillary artery to ipsilateral axillary vein (loop) grafts can be created (Figure 5.13).

The axillary artery and vein are exposed through an infraclavicular incision made between the sternal and clavicular portions of the pectoralis major muscle (Figure 5.14). It is possible to accomplish this exposure under local anesthesia if mandated by the patient's comorbid conditions. For the straight graft configuration, bilateral infraclavicular incisions are made and the graft is tunneled across the chest in the subcuticular plane with a minimal curve. For the loop arrangement, a single infraclavicular exposure is utilized and the graft is tunneled in the subcutaneous tissue over the pectoralis major muscle with the loop apex inferior to the ipsilateral nipple.

The overall experience reported with axilloaxillary AV grafts is limited. These grafts are usually reserved for end-stage access; however, the limited experience reported in the literature compares these grafts favorably with access grafts placed in more traditional positions (49,50). Owing to their proximal positioning on the axillary artery and vein of these access grafts, complications such as thrombosis or infection may have a more severe impact on the patient, related to surgical reexposure of the axillary artery and vein. Scarring around the brachial plexus and the difficulty of obtaining vascular control proximal to the thoracic outlet through the scarred infraclavicular dissection can conceivably require application of more complex and morbid exposures, such as median sternotomy or clavicular resection, to achieve the required vascular control. These considerations account for the practice of reserving these access grafts for end-stage patients.

Axillofemoral (Femoroaxillary) Bridge Grafts

These grafts represent another anatomic alternative for the patient in whom access is difficult. They may be configured as axillary artery to femoral vein or femoral artery to axillary vein, as mandated by the specific patient circumstance. These grafts can provide a route for dialysis access in the patient with adequate arterial inflow from the axillary artery but inadequate venous outflow due to occlusion of the axillosubclavian venous systems. When used to replace a functioning upper arm graft complicated by venous hypertension, resolution of the hypertension usually follows ligation of the old access graft. Similarly, the femoroaxillary route can be used for patients with adequate central venous patency in the axillosubclavian system but inadequate arterial inflow to support an AV graft.

The large size of the femoral and axillary vessels permits use of a 6- or 8-mm graft with high flow rates and ease of cannulation. Although no large series are reported, the use of externally supported ePTFE, as recommended for axillofemoral arterial bypass grafts, does not seem necessary and would make cannulation difficult. The limited reports on this graft configuration suggest satisfactory maintenance of access with few major complications (51).

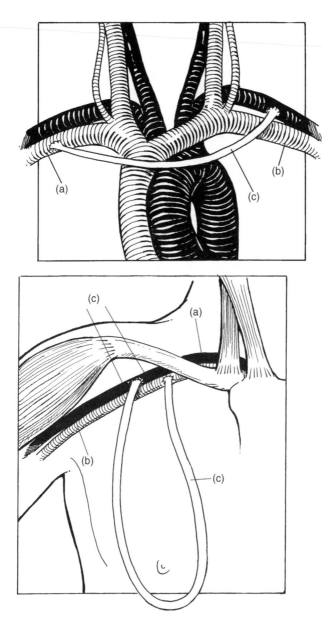

FIGURE 5.13   Configuration of axilloaxillary bridge AV grafts (a) axillary artery, (b) axillary vein, (c) axillary artery graft.

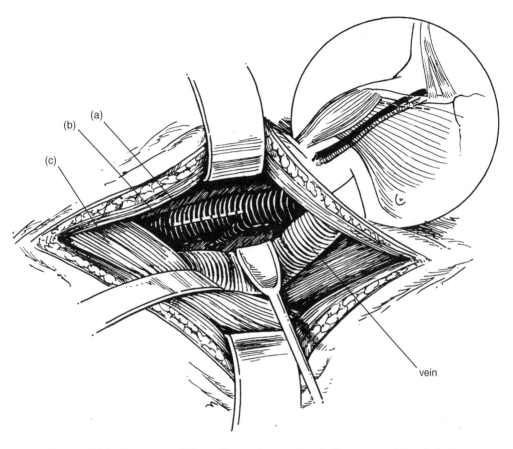

Figure 5.14   Exposure of the axillary artery and vein through an infraclavicular incision for placement of an axilloaxillary bridge AV graft (a) axillary artery, (b) axillary vein, (c) pectoralis major M.

Brachiojugular Bridge AV Graft

The brachiojugular bridge graft represents a method to salvage upper extremity access grafts that are failing or have failed due to venous obstruction at the axillo-subclavian level. If the ipsilateral jugular vein is patent, the venous limb of the graft can be extended to the base of the neck. Given the frequency of placement of temporary jugular catheters in dialysis patients to provide interval access when their primary fistula is dysfunctional, confirmation of patency of the jugular veins with duplex imaging and venography is requisite before placement of the jugular limb.

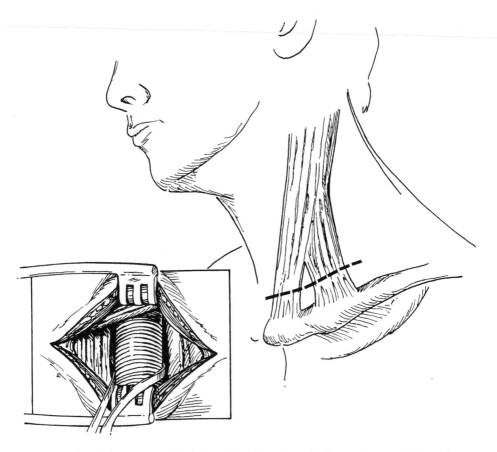

FIGURE 5.15 Exposure of the internal jugular vein at the base of the neck through the triangle formed by the sternal and clavicular heads of the sternocleidomastoid muscle.

The internal jugular vein is exposed through a transverse incision at the base of the neck over the triangle formed by the sternal and clavicular heads of the sternocleidomastoid muscle (Figure 5.15). The selected graft is tunneled between this site and the lateral aspect of the upper arm, where a smooth, straight transition to the venous limb of the graft can be achieved. Because the graft must traverse the shoulder joint, this section of the graft should be externally supported. Placement of a brachiojugular graft can be performed under local anesthesia if necessary. This approach can successfully alleviate venous hypertension due to a functioning fistula and subclavian vein stenosis or occlusion while providing an acceptable route to maintain dialysis access. As with the other end-stage access procedures, reported experience from any one center is limited, but small series have achieved acceptable results in this difficult population (52,53). In one of the largest series of this graft configuration reported, Polo et al. (54) achieved 24-month actuarial secondary patency of 70% in 16 of the original 40 patients. In their series, 20 patients had placement of the venous anastomosis on the external jugular vein. Two of these patients developed venous hypertension of the face, which resolved with ligation of the distal vein.

GRAFT SELECTION

As mentioned earlier in this chapter, ePTFE has become the most common prosthetic material employed for construction of AV grafts. A number of new prosthetic materials have recently been introduced for AV fistula construction and deserve mention.

One of the earliest modifications of ePTFE was the tapered graft configuration. This graft comprised a gentle taper from 4 mm at the arterial end to 7 mm at the venous end in an effort to limit flow through the graft and reduce the incidence of ischemic complications due to arterial steal (55). A secondary consequence of reducing flow through the graft may be a reduction in turbulence mediated intimal hyperplasia at the venous anastomosis (56). Because the incidence of clinically significant arterial steal that requires intervention is low, it has been difficult to verify that the taper or step-graft has substantially affected the occurrence of this problem (57,58). Moreover, there has been no documented advantage in primary or secondary patency provided by the use of the taper graft compared with standard 6-mm alternatives (57,58). In practice, the taper graft does provide an alternative prosthetic selection for patients with small (<4 mm) arteries who may be at higher risk for ischemic complications while maintaining adequate flow for effective hemodialysis.

With specific regard to the basic construction of ePTFE grafts, a number of modifications have appeared on the dialysis graft market in recent years. Each attempts to address the shortcomings of the original ePTFE (14). From its original appearance in 1976 up to the early 1990s, ePTFE access grafts were predominantly available as the Gore-Tex (W.L. Gore and Associates, Flagstaff, AZ) and Impra (Impra, Inc., Tempe, AZ) constructs. The fundamental difference between these two prostheses is the presence of an outer wrap on the Gore-Tex graft. Cannulation of these access grafts within the first 2 weeks after placement appears to be associated with the complications of seroma and hematoma formation. Although the use of new tunneling devices has addressed this concern to some degree, wide application of the practice of early cannulation had not been adopted with standard ePTFE grafts (41). The significance of this approach rests in the need to place a temporary jugular catheter for interim access during the 2-week period while the ePTFE graft incorporates sufficiently for safe cannulation.

A number of prostheses that incorporate modifications to the basic ePTFE structure have been produced to address this specific limitation. The plasma PTFE graft (pl-TFE, Medtronics, Inc., Minneapolis, MN) combines the hemostatic properties of the base polymer of Dacron—i.e., polyethylene terephthalate (PET)—with the low thrombogenicity of PTFE. The pl-TFE graft consists of an ultrathin woven PET prosthesis coated with PTFE using a glow-discharge methodology and external support with a helical polypropylene wrap (59). The early clinical experience with the pl-TFE graft confirmed the ability to accomplish early cannulation without excessive bleeding complications (60). However, a more recent study demonstrated significant difficulties in thrombectomizing the pl-TFE prosthesis, no apparent difference in patency, and a suggestion that a more exuberant hyperplastic response at the venous anastomosis may be related to the base material of the graft (61). Combined with recent reports documenting the safe early use of standard ePTFE prostheses, the pl-TFE graft has had limited clinical success (42).

An alternative to the pl-TFE graft that addresses the same issue of early cannulation is the Perma-Seal (Possis Medical, Inc., Minneapolis, MN) prosthesis. Rather than a modification of an ePTFE prosthesis, the Perma-Seal graft comprises a silicone-base polymer graft formed on a mandril, which is reinforced with polyester filaments within the external wall (25). The silicone graft is effectively impervious, with an internal porosity of zero. The addition of the polyester filaments in the outer layer produces a microporous lattice to enhance tissue ingrowth. The major advantage of the graft as claimed by the manufacturer is the self-sealing property of the silicone-base polymer. This occurs independent of graft healing and allows for immediate cannulation after implantation. At the time of this writing, the Perma-Seal graft was in clinical trials, with no data available on its performance in humans.

Two recent modifications of Gore-Tex ePTFE access grafts have been introduced by Gore. The first was an alteration in the extrusion process for producing ePTFE, which resulted in a graft possessing inherent longitudinal stretch due to the formation of microcrimps. The initial advantage of this graft over standard ePTFE was perceived to be the ease of handling and conformity provided by the longitudinal stretch. A secondary finding of the clinical experience in using the stretch ePTFE prosthesis for hemodialysis access grafts was the ability to safely cannulate new fistulas within 2 weeks of placement without significant sequelae (27,62,63). Initially, this attribute was ascribed to the microcrimping of the ePTFE. However, when the graft is stretched to the appropriate length at implantation, as recommended by the manufacturer, the ultrastructure as assessed by electron microscopy is identical to that of standard ePTFE. The successful early cannulation of the stretch graft is more likely a phenomenon of placement of the graft within a snug subcutaneous tunnel, as initially recommended by Taucher, and less likely related to the structure of the ePTFE (41). As more clinical experience was gained using the stretch ePTFE graft for chronic access, improvements in primary and secondary patency compared with standard ePTFE emerged as a consistent result (63–66).

To further address the issue of early cannulation, Gore, in 1994, began producing the Diastat ePTFE graft for dialysis access (67). The fundamental structure of this prosthesis is a basic 6-mm graft to a section of which an outer wrap of standard-thickness ePTFE has been added for cannulation. The cannulation segment is secured by a thin, perforated outer PTFE cover. The resultant graft has an outside diameter in the cannulation segment of 8 mm. The principle guiding this structure is a baffle effect provided by the outer layer over needle holes, which facilitates sealing and makes the graft amenable to early cannulation prior to graft incorporation. Impressive marketing demonstrations showing zero porosity to water after needle puncture of the cannulation segment were used to announce the commercial availability of this graft. However, clinical experience is limited to the study published by Bartlett et al. (26). Their report of 48 Diastat grafts demonstrated the ease with which hemostasis could be accomplished after cannulation even in the early postoperative period. Primary and secondary patency rates of the Diastat graft were not different from those reported for other ePTFE prostheses. Though anecdotal, our own experience with Diastat grafts has been disappointing, with a subjectively high incidence of graft infections experienced by our own centers as well as others (67). This finding is somewhat intuitive, given the marked increase in the volume of prosthetic material associated with the Diastat graft. Furthermore, these grafts are deprived of the protective effect of tissue incorporation by virtue of their early usage. It is clear that more clinical experience with the Diastat graft is required to determine its role in the construction of chronic access.

Another entry into the dialysis access graft arena is the carbon-PTFE prosthesis (Impra, Inc., Tempe, AZ). This modification of standard ePTFE was designed with an internal lumen composed of ePTFE and carbon in an effort to take advantage of the lower thrombogenicity of the negatively charged carbon (68). In the only clinical study of this experimental graft, performance of the carbon-PTFE AV fistula was equivocal to standard PTFE in regard to primary patency. A recent addition to the carbon lining is a built-in hood at the venous end. This construct of the carbon-coated AV graft, known as the Venaflo (Impra Inc., Tempe, AZ), was designed to alter shear stress at the venous anastomosis and thereby reduce intimal hyperplasia. Escobar et al., in their single-center study, demonstrated improved primary and secondary patency of the hooded graft compared with conventional ePTFE AV grafts (69).

A further modification in the basic ePTFE vascular graft was introduced as the Atrium Hybrid PTFE (Atrium Medical Corp., Hollis, NH). The structure of this graft is intended to optimize graft healing by providing low porosity, 20-μm internodal distance on the lumen surface, and 60-μm internodal distance porosity on the adventitial surface (24). This construct theoretically will allow capillary ingrowth from the adventitial surface into the graft wall and enhancement of pseudointimal growth. Early results from a multicenter trial of the Atrium Hybrid ePTFE graft for AV access have shown comparable primary and secondary patency rates compared with standard ePTFE grafts (personal communication) (Figure 5.16). More prolonged experience with this graft will determine if the altered microstructure will change graft healing in a way that affects long-term AV access.

A recent addition to the expanding family of prosthetic grafts for AV access is the polyurethane graft manufactured by Thoratek. At the time of this publication, there was no published experience with this device for adequate comparison with standard materials.

No discussion of prosthetic AV grafts would be complete without mention of adjunctive vein cuffs and patches. As in the case of lower extremity arterial bypass grafts, various configurations of vein cuffs and patches have been added to the venous anatomoses of AV grafts in an effort to prolong patency (70–72). No study to date has demonstrated superior patency with these adjunctive techniques. The study by Gagne et al. actually demonstrated a higher incidence

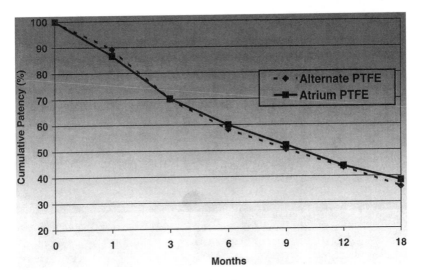

FIGURE 5.16   Multicenter trial of PTFE graft.

of hyperplasia at the venous anastomosis of Tyrell patches than at conventional grafts (71). The role of vein patches in prosthetic AV grafts remains ill defined.

CONCLUSION

Despite emerging vascular graft technologies, the basic autogenous AV fistula described by Brescia and Cimino (1) remains the first choice for chronic access for hemodialysis (1). Once autogenous options have been exhausted, prosthetic fistulae become the mainstay of maintenance hemodialysis access alternatives. Placement should begin in the nondominant upper extremity at the most distal site possible to achieve durable functioning. Grafts constructed of ePTFE provide the most consistent uninterrupted performance, have low rates of infectious and aneurysmal complications, and are easy to thrombectomize when thrombosis occurs. At the present time, there is no clear advantage provided by one specific brand or type of ePTFE prosthesis; therefore economic issues may guide individual selection in this regard without significant differences in overall performance.

REFERENCES

1. Brescia MJ, Cimino JE, Appel K, Hurwich BJ. Chronic hemodialysis using venipuncture and a surgically created arteriovenous fistula. N Engl J Med 275:1089–1092, 1966.
2. NKF-DOQI Clinical Practice Guidelines for Vascular Access. New York: National Kidney Foundation; 1997:17–78.
3. Hinsdale JG, Lipkowitz GS, Hoover EL. Vascular access for hemodialysis in the elderly: Results and perspectives in a geriatric population. Dial Transplant 14:560–565, 1985.
4. Kaufman JL. The decline of the autogenous hemodialysis access site. Semin Dial 8:59–61, 1995.
5. Connolly JE et al. Complications of renal dialysis access procedures. Arch Surg 119:1325, 1984.
6. Burger H et al. A survey of vascular access for hemodialysis in the Netherlands. Nephrol Dial Transplant 6:5, 1991.
7. Churchill DN, Taylor DW, Cook RJ, et al. Canadian hemodialysis morbidity study. Am J Kidney Dis 19:214–234, 1992.
8. Kolff WJ, Berk HTJ, ter-Welle M, et al. The artificial kidney: A dialyzer with a great area. Acta Med Scand 117:121–134, 1944.
9. Quinton W, Dillard D, Scribner BH. Cannulation of blood vessels for prolonged hemodialysis. Trans Am Soc Artif Intern Organs 6:104–113, 1960.
10. Rajagopalan PR, Fitts CT. Use of Allen-Brown shunt between profunda femoris artery and long saphenous vein for hemodialysis access. Ann Surg 44:226–228, 1978.

11. Thomas GI. A large-vessel applique A-V shunt for hemodialysis. Trans Am Soc Artif Intern Organs 15:288–292, 1969.

12. Buselmeier TJ, Kjellstrand CM, Rattazzi LC, et al. A new subcutaneous prosthetic A-V shunt: advantages over the Quinton-Scribner shunt and A-V fistula. Proc Clin Dial Transplant Forum 2:67–75, 1972.

13. Butt KMH, Rao TKS, Maki T, et al. Bovine heterograft as a preferential hemodialysis access. Trans Am Soc Artif Intern Organs 20:339–342, 1974.

14. Baker LD, Johnson JM, Goldfarb D. Expanded polytetrafluoroethylene (PTFE) subcutaneous arteriovenous conduit: An improved vascular access for hemodialysis. Trans Am Soc Artif Intern Organs 22:382–385, 1976.

15. Dunn I, Frumkin E, Forte R. Dacron velour vascular prosthesis for hemodialysis. Proc Clin Dial Transplant Forum 2:85, 1972.

16. Dardik H, Ibrahim IM, Dardik I. Arteriovenous fistula constructed with modified human umbilical cord vein graft. Arch Surg 111:60, 1976.

17. Lilly L, Ngheim D, Mendez-Picon G, Lee HM. Comparison between bovine heterograft and expanded PTFE grafts for dialysis access. Am Surg 46:694–696, 1980.

18. Doyle DL, Fry PD. Polytetrafluoroethylene and bovine grafts for vascular access in patients on long-term hemodialysis. Can J Surg 25:379–382, 1982.

19. Reese JC, Esterl R, Lindsey L, et al. A prospective randomized comparison of bovine heterografts versus Impra grafts for chronic hemodialysis. In Henry ML, Ferguson RM, eds. Vascular Access for Hemodialysis III. Chicago: Gore; 1993: 157–163.

20. Hurt AV et al. Bovine carotid artery heterografts versus polytetrafluoroethylene grafts—A prospective randomized study. Am J Surg 146:844–847, 1983.

21. Butler HG, Baker LD, Johnson JM. Vascular access for hemodialysis: Polytetrafluoroethylene (PTFE) versus bovine heterografts. Am J Surg 134:791–793, 1977.

22. Reed WP, Sadler JH. Experience with a needless vascular access device (Hemasite) for hemodialysis. South Med J 77:1501, 1984.

23. Golding AL, Nissenson AR, Raible D. Carbon transcutaneous access device (CTAD). Proc Clin Dial Transplant Forum 9:242–246, 1979.

24. Martakos P, Karwoski T. Healing characteristics of hybrid and conventional polytetrafluoroethylene vascular grafts. ASAIO J 41:735–741, 1995.

25. Drasler WJ, Wilson GJ, Stenoien MD, et al. A spun elastomeric graft for dialysis access. ASAIO J 39:114–119, 1993.

26. Bartlett ST, Schweitzer EJ, Roberts JE, et al. Early experience with a new ePTFE vascular prosthesis for hemodialysis. Am J Surg 170:118–122, 1995.

27. Dawidson I, Melone D. Preliminary experience with a new PTFE graft for vascular access. In Henry ML, Ferguson RM, eds. Vascular Access for Hemodialysis III. Chicago: Gore; 1993:133–136.

28. Machold C, Gideon T, Berman SS. Use of tunneled hemodialysis catheters and autogenous arteriovenous fistulas in patients who need acute and chronic dialysis access. In Henry ML, ed. Vascular access for hemodialysis VI. Chicago: Gore Precept Press; 1999:347–353.

29. Comeaux ME, Bryant PS, Harkrider WW. Preoperative evaluation of the renal access patient with color Doppler imaging. J Vasc Tech 17:247–250, 1993.

30. Didlake R, Curry E, Rigdon EE, et al. Outpatient vascular access surgery: Impact of a dialysis unit-based surgical facility. Am J Kidney Dis 19:39–44, 1992.

31. Taylor B, Sigley RD, May KJ. Fate of infected and eroded hemodialysis grafts and autogenous fistulas. Am J Surg 165:632, 1993.

32. Yu VL et al. Staphylococcus aureus nasal carriage and infection in patients on hemodialysis. N Engl J Med 315:91, 1986.

33. Kaiser AB, Clayson KR, Mulherin JL. Antibiotic prophylaxis in vascular surgery. Ann Surg 188:283–289, 1978.

34. Kaiser A, Petracek M, Lea J IV. Efficacy of cephazolin, cefamandole, and gentamicin as prophylactic agents in vascular surgery. Ann Surg 206:791–797, 1987.

35. Law MM, Gelabert HA. Antibiotic prophylaxis of vascular graft infection. In Moore WS, ed. Vascular Surgery: A Comprehensive Review. Philadelphia: Saunders; 1993: 350–369.

36. Charvat J, Kestlerova M, Jarosova H, Mlejnkova M. Correlation between the blood coagulation status in hemodialyzed patients and arteriovenous fistula thrombosis—A prospective study. Cas Lek Cesk 133:242–244, 1994.

37. Dal Ponte DB, Berman SS, Patula VB, et al. Anastomotic tissue response associated with expanded polytetraflouroethylene access grafts constructed using non-penetrating clips. J Vasc Surg 30:325–333, 1999.

38. Moore WM, Bunt TJ, Hermann GD, Fogarty TJ. Assessment of transmural force during application of vascular occlusive devices. J Vasc Surg 8:422–427, 1988.

39. Pabst TS, Flanigan DP, Buchbinder D. Reduced intimal injury to canine arteries with controlled application of vessel loops. J Surg Res 47:235–241, 1989.

40. Berman SS, Lopez J. Use of a pneumatic tourniquet for vascular control in the management of vascular access for hemodialysis. In Henry ML, Ferguson RM, eds. Vascular Access for Hemodialysis V. Chicago: Gore; 1997:307–315.

41. Taucher L. Immediate, safe hemodialysis into arteriovenous fistulas created with a new tunneler: An eleven year experience. Am J Surg 150:212–215, 1985.

42. Haag BW, Paramesh V, Roberts T, Taber T. Early use of polytetrafluoroethylene grafts for hemodialysis access. In Sommer BG, Henry ML, eds. Vascular Access for Hemodialysis II. Chicago: Gore; 1991:173–178.

43. Schmidt SP, Field FI. Forearm vascular access: Loop versus staright polytetrafluoroethylene grafts. In Sommer BG, Henry ML, eds. Vascular access for hemodialysis II. Chicago: Gore; 1991:179–185.

44. Mehta S. Statistical summary of clinical results of vascular access procedures for hemodialysis. In Sommer BG, Henry ML, eds. Vascular Access for Hemodialysis II. Chicago: Gore; 1991:145–157.

45. Schuman ES, Gross GF, Hayes JF, Standage BA. Long-term patency of polytetrafluoroethylene graft fistulas. Am J Surg 155:644–646, 1988.

46. Raju S. PTFE grafts for hemodialysis access: Techniques for insertion and management of complications. Ann Surg 206:666–673, 1987.

47. Berman J, Celoria G, Garb J. Upper arm arteriovenous bridge grafts for hemodialysis. Vasc Surg 26:85–92, 1992.

48. Bittner HB, Weaver JP. The brachioaxillary interposition graft as a successful tertiary vascular access procedure for hemodialysis. Am J Surg 176:615, 1994.

49. Haimov M. Vascular access for hemodialysis—New modifications for the difficult patient. Surgery 92:109–110, 1982.
50. Garcia-Rinaldi R, Von Koch L. The axillary artery to axillary vein bovine graft for circulatory access. Am J Surg 135:265–268, 1978.
51. Rueckmann I, Ouriel K, Berry C, Hoffart N. The synthetic axillofemoral graft for hemodialysis access. ANNA J 18:567–571, 1991.
52. Posner MP, McNeil P, Lee HM, et al. Salvage of hemoaccess in the presence of symptomatic subclavian vein stenosis/occlusion. Transplant Proc 19:137–145, 1987.
53. Campistol JM, Abad C, Torras A, Revert L. Salvage of upper arm access graft in the presence of symptomatic subclavian vein thrombosis. Nephron 51:551–552, 1989.
54. Polo JR, Sanabia J, Calleja J. Brachial-jugular expanded PTFE grafts for dialysis. In Henry ML, Ferguson RM, eds. Vascular Access for Hemodialysis IV. Chicago: Gore; 1995:203–209.
55. Rosental JJ, Bell DD, Gaspar MR, et al. Prevention of high flow problems of arteriovenous grafts. Am J Surg 140:231–233, 1980.
56. Fillinger MF, Resetarits DE, Brendenberg CE. Graft geometry and venous intimal medial hyperplasia in arteriovenous loop grafts. J Vasc Surg 16:556–566, 1990.
57. Hines LH, Turner GR, King WS, et al. 4–7 mm tapered expanded PTFE access grafts: Techniques of construction and preservation of graft life. In Henry ML, Ferguson RM, eds. Vascular Access for Hemodialysis III. Chicago: Gore; 1993:175–185.
58. Sabanayagam P. 15-Year experience with tapered (4–7 mm) and straight (6 mm) PTFE angio-access in the ESRD patient. In Henry ML, Ferguson RM, eds. Vascular Access for Hemodialysis IV. Chicago: Gore; 1995:159–169.
59. Garfinkle AM, Hoffman AS, Ratner BD, et al. Effects of tetrafluoroethylene glow discharge on patency of small diameter Dacron vascular grafts. Trans Am Soc Artif Intern Organs 30:432–439, 1984.
60. Jendrisak M, Bander S, Windus D, Delmez J. Early cannulation of plasma tetrafluoroethylene (Plasma-TFE) grafts for dialysis. Kidney Int 37:303, 1990.
61. Didlake R, Curry E, Rigdon E, et al. Dialysis access using PTFE-coated woven grafts. In Henry ML, Ferguson RM, eds. Vascular Access for Hemodialysis III. Chicago: Gore; 1993:146–156.
62. Simoni EJ, Jain KM, Munn JS. Use of 6 mm stretch PTFE grafts for early use in hemodialysis. In Henry ML, Ferguson RM, eds. Vascular Access for Hemodialysis III. Chicago: Gore; 1993:142–145.
63. Pärsson H, Jundzill W, Hallberg E, et al. Acute thrombogenicity and 4 weeks healing properties of a new stretch-ePTFE graft. Eur J Vasc Surg 7:63–70, 1993.
64. Colonna JO II, Swanson SJ, Shaver TR. Successful early use of the stretch PTFE graft. In Henry ML, Ferguson RM, eds. Vascular Access for Hemodialysis IV. Chicago: Gore; 1995:273–276.
65. Tordoir JHM, Hofstra L, Bergmans DCJJ, et al. Stretch versus standard ePTFE grafts for hemodialysis access. In Henry ML, Ferguson RM, eds. Vascular Access for Hemodialysis IV. Chicago: Gore, 1995:277–285.
66. Derenoncourt FJ. PTFE for A-V access: Six years experience with 310 reinforced

and stretch grafts. In Henry ML, Ferguson RM, eds. Vascular Access for Hemodialysis IV. Chicago: Gore; 1995:286–291.

67. Lohr JM, James KV, Heam A, Ogden SA. Lessons learned from the DIASTAT vascular access graft. Am J Surg 172:205–209, 1996.

68. Bourquelot P, Stolba J, Cheret P, et al. Carbon-PTFE versus standard PTFE A-V bridge grafts for chronic hemodialysis. In Henry ML, Ferguson RM, eds. Vascular Access for Hemodialysis IV. Chicago: Gore; 1995:303–307.

69. Escobar FS, Schwartz SA, Abouljoud M, et al. Comparison of a new "hooded" graft with a conventional ePTFE graft: A preliminary study. In Henry ML, ed. Vascular Access for Hemodialysis VI. Chicago: Precept Press; 1999:205–211.

70. Lemson MS, Tordoir JH, van Det RJ, et al. Effects of a venous cuff at the venous anastomosis of polytetrafluoroethylene grafts for hemodialysis vascular access. J Vasc Surg 32:1155–1163, 2000.

71. Gentile AT, Mills JL, Gooden MA, et al. Vein patching reduces neointimal thickening associated with prosthetic graft implantation. Am J Surg 176:601–607, 1998.

72. Gagne PJ, Martinez J, DeMassi R, et al. The effect of a venous anastomosis Tyrell vein collar on the primary patency of arteriovenous grafts in patients undergoing hemodialysis. J Vasc Surg 32:1149–1154, 2000.

73. Pipinos II, Escobar FS, Anagnostopoulos PV, et al. Early experience with Taylor and notched vein patching in the construction of arteriovenous hemodialysis access procedures: Results of a prospective study. In Henry ML, ed. Vascular Access for Hemodialysis–VI. Chicago: Precept Press, 1999:213–222.

74. Dal Ponte DB, Berman SS, Patula VB, et al. Anastomotic tissue response associated with expanded polytetrafluorethylene access grafts constructed by using nonpenetrating clips. J Vasc Surg 30:325–333, 1999.

6

Postoperative Surveillance of Dialysis Access

Joseph L. Mills
The University of Arizona Health Sciences Center,
Tucson, Arizona

Scott S. Berman
The University of Arizona, Carondelet St. Mary's Hospital, and The
Southern Arizona Vascular Institute, Tucson, Arizona

It is estimated that nearly 300,000 U.S. citizens suffer from end-stage renal disease (ESRD), a majority of whom require lifetime hemodialysis (1). In 1990, approximately 17,000 new permanent vascular accesses were placed in established chronic hemodialysis patients in the Medicare ESRD program (2). The most frequently performed procedure in the United States for establishing chronic hemodialysis is a prosthetic fistula, which accounts for over 80% of primary access operations (2). The major cause of hospitalization for chronic renal failure patients is failure of dialysis access. This single problem accounts for the majority of hospital days for ESRD patients. It would thus seem of critical importance to establish a protocol for the identification and correction of significant fistula abnormalities prior to fistula thrombosis. Unfortunately, such a protocol is not uniformly applied at the national level (3).

The vast majority of reoperative fistula procedures are performed after the access has already thrombosed. This causes a great deal of inconvenience for the patient as well as for the dialysis care team. Patients often need to have their dialysis rescheduled or postponed, or they may undergo emergency placement of a temporary central venous dialysis catheter to obtain access for dialysis until the fistula can be repaired or a new fistula placed. Reliance upon clinical means to diagnose failing fistulae prior to thrombosis has been a dismal failure. Fortunately, recent data document improved fistula lifespan when a protocol of surveillance is initiated and prophylactic intervention is undertaken to correct high-grade stenoses. In fact, two recent reports document with high statistical significance that, compared with interventions, prophylactic balloon angioplasty or revision of stenotic arteriovenous (AV) fistulae prolongs patency once access thrombosis has occurred (4,5).

Any useful method of access surveillance should be sensitive in the detection of venous outflow stenosis, since it is the most common cause of access failure. The problem of distal anastomotic myointimal hyperplasia is well recognized. It is estimated that 60 to 90% of access fistulae fail because of venous outflow stenosis (6,7). Surveillance methods should also be able to detect more proximal venous outflow problems, given the significant incidence of subclavian vein stenosis due to the previous placement of a line for subclavian dialysis access (8). Unfortunately, surveillance of dialysis grafts has not yet gained widespread acceptance. This chapter outlines the clinical markers of impending access failure as well as methods of surveillance that can readily be performed either in the hemodialysis facility or the outpatient noninvasive vascular laboratory (Tables 6.1 and 6.2).

CLINICAL INDICATIONS OF IMPENDING DIALYSIS ACCESS FAILURE

There are several important clinical indications of impending fistula failure. These signs are often noted by attentive personnel in the dialysis facility and should not be ignored. Prolonged bleeding after needle removal is a subtle sign of venous outflow obstruction either at the venous anastomosis or in the proximal subclavian vein. Significant arm edema, occasionally with noted development of prominent chest wall venous collaterals, is also an important clinical sign of central vein stenosis or occlusion. This problem should be pursued aggressively with fistulography and venography. Good results with salvage of failing fistulae have been reported with balloon angioplasty and stent placement for proximal subclavian vein stenosis (8–10).

Routine palpation of the fistula or access can also provide useful clinical information (11,12). If palpation of the fistula reveals that flow has become pulsatile, this is a strong clinical sign of venous outflow obstruction. In addition, the character of the thrill is important. With a low-flow fistula, either due to venous outflow problems or an arterial inflow stenosis, the thrill is often decreased. Moreover, as venous outflow stenosis progresses, the thrill over the venous anastomosis will often increase in severity and be associated with a harsh bruit. Such physical findings should lead to further evaluation of the access, as outlined be-

TABLE 6.1 Monitoring Dialysis AV Grafts for Stenosis

1. Physical examination of an access graft should be performed weekly and should include but not be limited to inspection and palpation for pulse and thrill at the arterial, mid-, and venous sections of the graft.
2. Dialysis AV graft accesses should be monitored for hemodynamically significant stenosis. The Work Group recommends an organized monitoring approach with regular assessment of clinical parameters of the AV access and dialysis adequacy. Data from the monitoring tests, clinical assessment, and dialysis adequacy measurements should be collected and maintained for each patient's access and made available to all staff. The data should be tabulated and tracked within each dialysis center as part of a Quality Assurance/Continuous Quality Improvement (QA/CQI) program.
3. Prospective monitoring of AV grafts for hemodynamically significant stenosis, when combined with correction, improves patency and decreases the incidence of thrombosis. Techniques, not mutually exclusive, that can be used to monitor for stenosis in AV grafts include (a) intra-access flow, (b) static venous pressure, and (c) dynamic venous pressures.
4. Other studies or information that can be useful in detecting AV graft stenosis include (a) measurement of access recirculation using urea concentrations; (b) measurement of recirculation using dilution techniques (non-urea-based); (c) unexplained decreases in the measured amount of hemodialysis delivered (URR, Kt/V); (d) physical findings of persistent swelling of the arm, clotting of the graft, prolonged bleeding after needle withdrawal, or altered characteristics of pulse or thrill in a graft; (e) elevated negative arterial prepump pressures that prevent increasing to acceptable blood flow; and (f) Doppler ultrasound.
5. Persistent abnormalities in any of these parameters should prompt referral for venography.

Source: Modified Ref. 3, Guideline 10.

TABLE 6.2 Monitoring Primary AV Fistulae for Stenosis

1. Primary AV fistulae should be monitored as outlined for dialysis AV grafts.
2. Direct flow measurements, if available, are preferable to more indirect measures.
3. Methods appropriate for monitoring stenosis in grafts (e.g., static and dynamic venous pressures) are not as accurate for monitoring in primary AV fistulae. Recirculation and Doppler analysis are of potential benefit.

Source: Modified from Ref. 3, Guideline 11.

low. Finally, difficulty in accessing the fistula and increased intragraft pressures when the fistula is first accessed are important signs of impending fistula failure, which can be identified in the dialysis center.

ACCESS SURVEILLANCE TECHNIQUES

Methods of AV access surveillance fall into two broad categories. The first includes measurements performed at the time of hemodialysis. Such measurements should be obtained and recorded on a regular basis to establish baseline values for each individual's access site and to detect serial changes in access function. These measurements include the following:

1. Intragraft pressure measurement
2. Venous pressure measurement
3. Recirculation time
4. Efficiency of dialysis by kinetic modeling (Kt/V)

The second broad category of surveillance techniques involves the application of Doppler technology based duplex scanning. Duplex surveillance has revolutionized the management of lower extremity bypass grafts. It has been generally accepted that a regular protocol of duplex-based surveillance for such grafts greatly improves outcome following lower extremity infrainguinal vein graft reconstructions (13,14). Repair of high-grade infrainguinal vein graft stenoses detected by duplex surveillance significantly improves patency rates (15). Reliable criteria have been developed for lower extremity vein grafts, which include the detection of peak systolic velocities greater than 300 cm/s within the conduit itself and velocity ratios across the stenosis exceeding 3.5 (16,17). While the use of duplex surveillance for AV access grafts lags far behind the widespread clinical application of infrainguinal vein graft surveillance, criteria have been developed for the detection of significant stenosis in AV grafts and native fistulae.

Intragraft Pressure

In addition to the clinical findings noted above, several fairly simple measurements can be made at the time of hemodialysis access, which may result in the identification of impending access failure. In patients with AV grafts, a pressure greater than 50 mmHg recorded in the venous needle prior to initiating blood flow suggests venous outflow stenosis (18). When such a stenosis is suspected, complete duplex scanning of the access should be performed to identify the site of the stenosis. If no stenosis is evident in the graft or the venous outflow site, fistulography should be performed to include views of the proximal subclavian vein, as this might be the site of stenosis and a cause of increased intragraft pressure.

Venous Pressure

Measurement of venous pressures during dialysis has been shown to be an accurate method for the identification of impending fistula failure. Schwab et al. (8) have performed detailed studies using the measurement of venous pressures at the initiation of hemodialysis. It is important to note that the venous pressure measurement is blood flow–dependent. In many modern dialysis access facilities, blood flow rates exceeding 400 mL/min are now used in order to increase the efficiency of dialysis and decrease the time required for the dialysis session. Measurement of venous pressures at such high flow rates has not proven to be accurate. However, the measurement of venous pressures exceeding 150 mmHg at blood flow rates of 200 to 225 mL/min is associated with a failing fistula and usually a greater than 50% stenosis within the fistula itself (8,19,20). Choudhury et al. (6) confirmed this observation by measuring venous pressures in a series of 46 patients who subsequently underwent formal venography. Choudhury's group also confirmed that venous pressures were blood flow–dependent. Like the method in widespread use, their technique measures the pressure at the dialyzer's blood outlet line (the venous outlet pressure) during the first 5 min of dialysis at a blood flow of 200 mL/min. With the use of a 16-gauge needle, the venous pressure will usually average approximately 75 $\pm$ 30 mmHg (SD). A venous pressure measured in this fashion during the first portion of dialysis greater than 145 to 150 mmHg is abnormal and suggests a greater then 50% stenosis in the fistula. When blood flow rates are increased to 300 mL/min, a venous pressure of greater than 170 mmHg is considered abnormal (6). At standard high blood flow rates of greater than 400 mL/min, which are currently obtained with high-flow dialysis, measurement of venous pressures is unreliable (6,21). Venous pressures should thus be measured at the beginning of dialysis and at flow rates of 200 to 225 mL/min. When such a protocol is used regularly in the dialysis treatment center and two or three successive venous pressure measurements are elevated, the fistula should be further evaluated by duplex ultrasound and/or fistulography.

In our experience, we have had difficulty achieving compliance among the staff at a large dialysis unit for strict adherence to the protocol for venous pressure measurement. As an alternative, we have tracked venous pressure measurements during every dialysis run and have found good correlation between a consistently elevated venous pressure greater than 300 mmHg and an elevation in recirculation percentage and/or a decline in Kt/V or urea reduction ratio (URR). With this random venous pressure threshold, confirmatory fistulograms have consistently demonstrated significant obstructive lesions within the fistula (unpublished data) (Table 6.3).

Urea Recirculation

Calculation of urea recirculation has also been useful for detecting impending fistula failure (22) (Table 6.4). It is somewhat more cumbersome than simple

TABLE 6.3 Dynamic Venous Dialysis Pressure Monitoring Protocol

- Establish a baseline by initiating measurements when the access is first used.
- Measure venous dialysis pressure from the hemodialysis machine at Qb 200 mL/min during the first 2 to 5 min of hemodialysis at every hemodialysis session.
- Use 15-gauge needles (or establish own protocol for different needle size).
- Assure that the venous needle is in the lumen of the vessel and not partially occluded by the vessel wall.
- Pressure must exceed the threshold three times in succession to be significant.
- Assess at same level relative to hemodialysis machine for all measurements.
- Interpretation of Result: Three measurements in succession above the threshold are required to eliminate the effect of variation caused by needle placement. Hemodialysis machines measure pressure with different monitors and tubing types and lengths. These variables, as well as needle size, influence venous dialysis pressure. The most important variable affecting the dynamic pressure at a blood flow of 200 mL/min is the needle gauge. It is essential to set thresholds for action based on machine manufacturer, tubing type, and needle gauge.

  Using 15-gauge needles, the threshold that indicates elevated pressure (and therefore the likely presence of a hemodynamically significant venous outlet stenosis) for Cobe Centry 3 machines is a pressure of 125 mmHg, whereas the threshold for Gambro AK 10 machines is a pressure of 150 mmHg. Data for Baxter, Fresenius, Althin, and other dialysis machines are not available but are likely to be similar to those of the Cobe Centry 3 if the same gauge venous needle is used. Trial and error at each institution will determine each unit's threshold pressure.

  Trend analysis is more important than any single measurement. Upward trends in hemodialysis pressure over time are more predictive than absolute values. Each unit should establish its own venous pressure threshold values.

  Patients with progressively increasing pressures or those who exceed the threshold on three consecutive hemodialysis treatment should be referred for venography.

Source: Modified from Ref. 3, Table III-3.

venous pressure measurement and no data exist to suggest that it is more accurate. Nevertheless, it can be readily performed in the dialysis center and is usually done monthly during the first hour of hemodialysis. The suggested method involves a two-needle technique in which blood urea nitrogen (BUN) samples are drawn from both the arterial and the venous lines. The methodology is summarized in Table 6.5.

TABLE 6.4 Recirculation Methodology, Limits, Evaluation, and Follow-up

1. Recirculation should be measured using a non-urea-based dilutional method or by using the two-needle urea-based method. The three-needle method of measuring recirculation using a peripheral vein should not be employed.
2. Any access recirculation is abnormal. Recirculation exceeding 10% using the recommended two-needle urea-based method, or 5% using a nonurea-based dilutional method, should prompt investigation of its cause.
3. If access recirculation values exceed 20%, correct placement of needles should be confirmed before further studies are conducted.
4. Elevated levels of access recirculation should be investigated using angiography (fistulography) to determine whether stenotic lesions are impairing access blood flow.

Source: Modified from Ref. 3, Guideline 12.

It is important to note that as blood flow rates are increased, the urea circulation also increases. For this reason, determination of urea recirculation is less accurate at higher blood flow rates. Data suggest that if the urea recirculation is greater than 10%, there is a 79% likelihood of detecting a venous stenosis by fistulography (22). It is also important to note that urea recirculation is dependent on the location of the fistula, with higher-flow proximal fistulae and loop fistulae having greater baseline urea recirculation values than distally placed or low-flow fistulae. Measurement of urea recirculation can also be evaluated following fistula revision. If the fistula revision is successful, the urea recirculation should return

TABLE 6.5 Protocol for Urea-Based Measurement of Recirculation

Perform test after approximately 30 min of treatment and after turning off ultrafiltration.
1. Draw arterial (A) and venous (V) line samples.
2. Immediately reduce blood flow rate (BFR) to 120 mL/min.
3. Turn blood pump off exactly 10 s after reducing BFR.
4. Clamp arterial line immediately above sampling port.
5. Draw systemic arterial sample (S) from arterial line port.
6. Unclamp line and resume dialysis.
7. Measure BUN in A, V, and S samples and calculate percent recirculation (R).
Recirculation formula:

$$R = \frac{S - A}{S - V} \times 100$$

Source: Modified from Ref. 3, Table III-5.

to normal (less than 10%). Urea recirculation calculations are not expensive, and newer dialysis machines are incorporating the technology to provide continuous biochemical feedback during the dialysis session.

MEASURING THE EFFICIENCY OF DIALYSIS

The management of the dialysis prescription for ESRD patients is often guided by modeling equations of urea kinetics. As such, access graft and fistula problems may be suggested by deterioration in urea clearance, as represented by the value for Kt/V. A detailed discussion of urea kinetic modeling is beyond the scope of this chapter; interested readers are referred to the excellent summary by Daugirdas (23). Briefly, the efficiency of dialysis may be calculated using Kt/V, where K = mass transfer coefficient specific to the dialyzer kidney; t = time of the dialysis session; and V = urea distribution volume.

The actual calculation of Kt/V is based upon measurement of urea removal and the urea reduction ration (URR), UN refers to urea nitrogen:

$$URR = \frac{postplasma\ UN}{preplasma\ UN}$$

The lower the URR, the greater the amount of urea cleared during the session. Effective dialysis and low morbidity are associated with URR values <0.32. The subsequent value for Kt/V is derived from a number of formulae relating the URR to the ultrafiltrate volume removed and the patient's postdialysis weight through either linear or logarithmic equations. Depending upon the specific relationship chosen, acceptable values for Kt/V range from 0.9 to 1.3.

It is important to note that these calculated values may be affected by numerous variables such as the methodology of the blood draw, the underlying renal function of the patient, and the patient's protein intake. The importance of both the Kt/V and URR in regard to access surveillance lies not only in their absolute values but with their trends in serial measurements. Falling values of Kt/V or rising values for the URR may be attributed to poor access function related to anatomical lesions. Since these biochemical measures are a routine part of managing the dialysis prescription for ESRD patients, careful attention to their trends provides a means for selecting patients for investigation of their AV access with either duplex scanning or fistulography if deterioration in dialysis efficiency is demonstrated.

It would appear the combination of regular venous pressure determinations combined with interval measurements of urea recirculation, Kt/V, and URR would be a reasonable way to monitor AV access grafts and fistulae in the dialysis center. When either acute changes or suspicious trends are noted, investigation of the access site is warranted once other factors have been eliminated to explain the changes in these parameters. Further evaluation of the access can be carried out with duplex scanning or fistulography. The cost-effectiveness of this approach has not been studied in a controlled manner and is the basis of an ongoing prospective study at our institution.

DUPLEX ULTRASOUND DETECTION OF AV FISTULA STENOSES

The impact of duplex surveillance on infrainguinal arterial bypass grafting has been substantial, with nearly all revisions of autogenous vein bypasses being performed on patent grafts with stenotic segments discovered by surveillance. With this approach, long-term patencies are excellent (13–17). The converse is true when discussing hemodialysis access, with nearly all interventions performed after fistula thrombosis has already occurred. This problem can be corrected only when serial surveillance of AV fistulae is performed and prophylactic intervention carried out when significant anatomic lesions are identified. Duplex ultrasound detection of AV fistula stenoses is a theoretically attractive technique. The studies are noninvasive, can be repeated serially, and are accurate in the localization of fistula stenoses. Since AV fistulae and access grafts are subcutaneous, the inflow artery, the proximal anastomosis, the entire AV graft, the distal anastomosis, and the outflow vein can all be easily examined. Several interesting techniques have been described for evaluating fistula dysfunction (24–29).

The simplest technique is examination of the inflow arterial waveform (29). It is important to remember that the diastolic component of an arterial waveform reflects the resistance of the vascular bed being perfused. For example, normal peripheral arterial waveforms exhibit no forward flow in diastole or even reversal of flow in diastole because of the elastic recoil of high-resistance peripheral arteries. Normal peripheral arterial waveforms are thus triphasic. An example of a normal triphasic Doppler waveform in the brachial artery is shown in Figure 6.1. In contrast, in circulatory beds with low resistance, there will be significant forward flow in diastole. Examples include both the cerebral and the renal circulations. Cerebral blood flow is subject to autoregulation and maintained at constant levels between pressures of 60 and 150 mmHg. The renal circulation is also of low resistance. Similar flow patterns are exhibited by AV fistulae because they perfuse low-resistance venous outflow beds and therefore display significant forward flow in diastole.

Harkrider and Comeaux (29) have devised a unique technique for monitoring arteriovenous fistulae by examining the native arterial waveform proximal to the fistula. For example, the brachial artery supplying a forearm loop fistula is examined proximal to the arterial anastomosis. A normally functioning AV fistula has significant diastolic flow (Figure 6.2), and the ratio of the Doppler-derived velocity in peak diastole divided by the velocity in peak systole makes

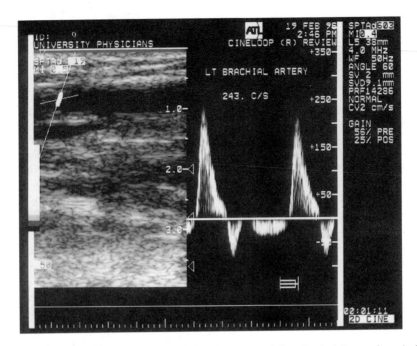

FIGURE 6.1 Normal high-resistance triphasic peripheral arterial waveform in brachial artery.

it possible to determine a flow ratio (Vd/Vs). With measurements made at a Doppler angle of 60 degrees, Harkrider and Comeaux (29) determined that a normally functioning fistula without significant outflow problems has a Vd/Vs ratio >0.4. With significant stenosis in the fistula or outflow tract, the diastolic flow component decreases, resulting in a Vd/Vs ratio <0.3. This becomes a very easy, indirect method to detect problems with the access site by interrogation of the proximal arterial waveform in the feeding artery. Thus, when the flow pattern reverts from a low-resistance, normal fistula pattern to a high-resistance peripheral arterial waveform, the presence of a graft or outflow stenosis can be inferred. This technique is, by virtue of its design, an indirect method, as it does not examine the fistula itself.

Ermers et al. (30) have performed detailed duplex surveillance of AV fistulae and reported that a greater than 50% stenosis could be detected in 70 to 80% within the first month following implantation. However, this group was unable to document an improvement in patency rate by intervention in fistulae with these early stenoses. Tordoir et al. (7) developed specific criteria for the determination of fistula stenosis as outlined in Table 6.6. For Brescia-Cimino or forearm autoge-

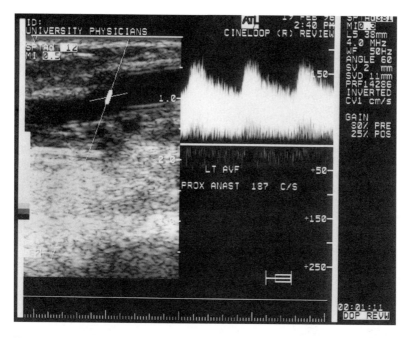

FIGURE 6.2 Biphasic low-resistance flow pattern in prosthetic AV fistula with Vd/Vs ratio of 0.6.

TABLE 6.6 Threshold Values for Access Evaluation and Prophylactic Intervention to Prevent Thrombosis

Parameters Measured at Dialysis Facility	
Intragraft pressure	>50 mmHg
Venous pressure	>150 mmHg at flow rate of 200–225 mL/min
Recirculation percent	>15–20%
Urea kinetics	Kt/V < 1.2
	URR > 0.32
	(Both are dependent on dialysis unit variables)
Duplex Surveillance in the Vascular Laboratory	
Vd/Vs	≤0.3
PSF	
Autogenous fistula	>12 kHz
Prosthetic fistula	>10 kHz or F ratio > 3.5
Efferent vein	>8 kHz
Volume flow (prosthetic fistulae)	<450 mL/min

nous fistulae, a peak systolic frequency of greater than 12 kHz is indicative of greater than 50% stenosis. For 6-mm prosthetic polytetrafluoroethylene (PTFE) AV grafts, the presence of a peak systolic frequency greater than 10 kHz is indicative of stenosis. Figure 6.3 illustrates an example of a high-grade venous outflow stenosis detected by duplex surveillance with a peak systolic frequency (PSF) of 19.6 kHz.

In addition, for prosthetic fistulae, a PSF ratio greater than 3.5 was indicative of graft stenosis in the study by Tordoir et al. (7). To measure this ratio, the PSF obtained at the site of stenosis is divided by the PSF in the inflow artery several centimeters proximal to the anastomosis. This yields a velocity ratio analogous to that obtained in peripheral arterial graft surveillance. In determining criteria for infrainguinal vein grafts, multiple authors have determined that a PSF or velocity ratio greater than 3.5 correlates with a failing bypass graft (13,14). It is extremely interesting to note that very similar threshold criteria have been derived for AV access stenosis. Similar velocity or frequency ratio data are not available for autogenous fistulae. Finally, a PSF greater than 8 kHz in the efferent vein has also been shown to correlate highly with the presence of a stenosis (7).

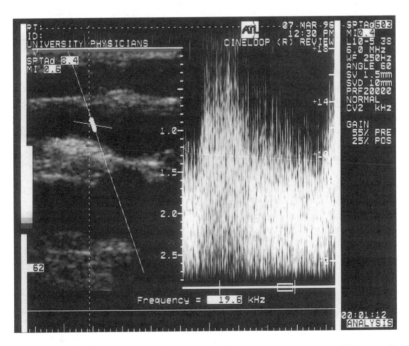

FIGURE 6.3 High-grade stenosis of distal venous anastomosis of forearm loop AV fistula identified by duplex surveillance. The peak systolic frequency is 19.6 kHz (abnormal > 10 kHz).

Volume flow has been used by some investigators to evaluate fistula function. According to Rittgers et al. (31), the average 6 mm PTFE fistula has a volume flow of 750 ± 383 mL/min. This group measured the velocity at least 10 cm downstream from the proximal artery to the graft anastomosis to diminish the effects of turbulence near the anastomosis. All grafts in which a volume flow <450 mL/min was measured by duplex scanning occluded within 2 weeks. Similar findings were reported by Shackleton et al. (32), who achieved a sensitivity of 83% and specificity of 75% for predicting interval thrombosis when a flow rate of 450 mL/min was selected as a low-flow threshold. It would thus appear that any prosthetic 6-mm PTFE access with a volume flow of less than 500 mL/ min should be further examined for the presence of a lesion that might predispose the graft to failure.

To perform duplex surveillance, the entire fistula or graft should be examined, including the inflow artery, the proximal anastomosis, the graft/fistula itself, the distal anastomosis, and the outflow vein. The peak systolic frequencies or velocities are then recorded and ratios determined by comparing the frequency at the site of the stenosis with the baseline frequency in the inflow artery proximal to the anastomosis. Color-flow Doppler can assist in identifying anatomic areas of stenosis for further interrogation with velocity or frequency measurements. Once velocity data are obtained, volume flow can be determined in areas of uniform diameter by using calculations incorporated in most imaging systems.

RESULTS

Until recently, there were no convincing data to demonstrate that prophylactic intervention in failing fistulae was superior to thrombectomy and revision once fistula failure had occurred. Kirkman (33) points out that the most failures occur at the venous outflow site, so a simple surgical approach to cut down on the venous outflow stenosis, patch or extend the graft to a more central vein, and thrombectomize the inflow appears to be adequate to restore patency to the majority of failed AV access fistulae. In Kirkman's view, a large proportion of acutely thrombosed grafts can be salvaged, so there may be little harm to this approach other than the time constraints involved in scheduling emergency thrombectomy and graft revision. However, it is certainly much easier to perform elective revision, either with balloon angioplasty or surgery, when a stenosis is identified prior to graft occlusion. This allows the procedure to be done on an outpatient basis and permits dialysis to continue without interruption. It also obviates the need for emergency placement of temporary central venous dialysis catheters, with their attendant morbidity, to continue dialysis until the fistula patency can be restored.

There are two recent papers that strongly support prophylactic revision of fistulae with impending failure. Sands et al. (4), using a duplex surveillance protocol and elective balloon angioplasty for identified access stenoses of greater than

50%, noted extensively prolonged survival of the access in patients who underwent elective revision as compared with those who had primary clotting and emergency revision. Duplex surveillance and elective revision resulted in a mean of 1222.7 days of access patency, compared with only 689 days for the emergency thrombectomy and revision group—a difference that was statistically significant ($p = 0.013$).

Moreover, Katz and Kohl (5) convincingly demonstrated that elective balloon angioplasty for failing PTFE AV grafts resulted in a marked improvement in secondary patency compared with the results of cases of identified stenoses treated with thrombolytic therapy and angioplasty after the graft had already occluded. In their experience, grafts not requiring thrombolysis had significantly higher patency rates than those that were thrombosed ($p < 0.0001$) (5). In addition, the patency of grafts undergoing angioplasty at sites remote from the venous anastomosis, such as the subclavian vein, had a significantly higher patency rate than those that underwent venous anastomotic balloon angioplasty. Nevertheless, in a very well controlled series, their results conclusively demonstrated that graft surveillance with prophylactic intervention when significant stenoses were identified was superior to thrombolytic therapy and angioplasty.

IN-LINE DILUTIONAL METHODS OF ACCESS FLOW MEASUREMENT

An emerging technology that allows measurement of access flow during the dialysis treatment revolves around the use of ultrasound flow measurements and indicator dilution (34–36). These devices are incorporated into the dialysis system and provide a simple method to monitor access function. Experience with these technologies is accumulating, with measurements of access flow being correlated with duplex and angiographic findings (37). These in-line measurements of access flow may offer a more convenient method to screen access for significant lesions that may compromise function and lead to access thrombosis. In a study comparing multiple techniques of access surveillance—including pressures, urea recirculation, duplex ultrasound, and access blood flow by dilutional methods—May et al. demonstrated that access flow measured by either Doppler ultrasound or dilutional methods was the best predictor of subsequent thrombosis (38).

CONCLUSION

The determination of whether to proceed with balloon angioplasty or elective surgical revision of a failing AV fistula is beyond the scope of this chapter. Nonetheless, when significant graft or outflow stenoses are corrected, the flow characteristics of the fistula return to normal and there is no question that the lifespan of these fistulae is thereby prolonged. It would thus appear undeniable that surveillance has a significant role to play in extremity access surgery. Practicing nephrologists and surgeons should no longer be content to remain the proverbial ostriches, burying their collective heads in the sand until fistula thrombosis has occurred. It is unquestionably more difficult to resurrect a failed access than to perform a prophylactic revision of a failing access that is still patent. Proactive protocols must be instituted at each dialysis center in order to permit the recognition of impending access failure. It would seem reasonable to combine hemodialysis access measurements, such as venous pressures and urea kinetic measurements, with duplex surveillance. In-line measurements of access flow during dialysis treatments may also have a role in this schema. The frequency and specific combination of surveillance options will need careful assessment in the current climate of cost containment in health care. However, once significant flow abnormalities are detected, prophylactic intervention should be undertaken. With this approach, the significant drain on the health care system and on the dialysis patient resulting from an access thrombosis could be obviated.

REFERENCES

1. US Renal Data System. Excerpts from the United States Renal Data System 1998 Annual Data Report. Incidence and Prevalence of ESRD. Am J Kidney Dis 32(suppl I):S38–S49, 1998.
2. Windus DW. Permanent vascular access: A nephrologist's view. Am J Kidney Dis 21:457–471, 1993.
3. NKF-DOQI. Clinical Practice Guidelines for Vascular Access. New York: National Kidney Foundation; 1997:34–42.
4. Sands JJ, Jabyac PA, Miranda CL, Kapsick BJ. Intervention based on monthly monitoring decreases hemodialysis access thrombosis. ASAIO J 45:147–50, 1999.
5. Katz SG, Kohl RD. The percutaneous treatment of angio access graft complications. Am J Surg 170:238–242, 1995.
6. Choudhury D, Lee J, Elivera HS, et al. Correlation of venography, venous pressure, and hemoaccess function. Am J Kidney Dis 25:269–275, 1995.
7. Tordoir JH, de Bruin HG, Hoeneveld H, et al. Duplex ultrasound scanning in the assessment of arteriovenous fistulas created for hemodialysis access: Comparison with digital subtraction angiography. J Vasc Surg 10:122–128, 1989.
8. Schwab SJ, Raymond JR, Saeed M, et al. Prevention of hemodialysis fistula thrombosis. Early detection of venous stenosis. Kidney Int 36:707–711, 1989.
9. Beathard GA. Percutaneous transvenous angioplasty in the treatment of vascular access stenosis. Kidney Int 42:1390–1397, 1992.
10. Kanterman RY, Veseley TM, Pilgram TK, et al. Dialysis access grafts: Anatomic location of venous stenosis and results of angioplasty. Radiology 195:135–139, 1995.
11. Trerotola SO, Scheel PJ, Powe N. Physical examination vs. color flow Doppler US for detecting impending vascular graft failure (abstr). J Vasc Intervent Radiol 5:39, 1994.

12. Beathard GA. Physical examination of AV grafts. Semin Dial 5:74, 1992.
13. Bandyk DF, Schmitt DD, Seabrook GR, et al. Monitoring functional patency of in situ saphenous vein bypasses: The impact of a surveillance protocol and elective revision. J Vasc Surg 9:286–296, 1989.
14. Mills JL, Harris EJ, Taylor LM Jr, et al. The importance of routine surveillance of distal bypass grafts with duplex scanning: A study of 379 reverse vein grafts. J Vasc Surg 12:379–394, 1990.
15. Bergamini TM, George SM, Massey HT, et al. Intensive surveillance of femoro-popliteal-tibial autogenous vein graft bypasses improves long-term patency and limb salvage. Ann Surg 221:507–518, 1995.
16. Gahtan V, Payne LP, Roper LD, et al. Duplex criteria for predicting progression of vein graft lesions: Which stenoses can be followed? J Vasc Tech 19:211–215, 1995.
17. Sladen JG, Reid JDS, Cooperberg PL, et al. Color flow duplex screening of infrainguinal grafts combining low- and high-velocity criteria. Am J Surg 158:107–112, 1989.
18. Besarab A, Sullivan KL, Ross RP, Moritz MJ. Utility of intra-access pressure monitoring in detecting and correcting venous outlet stenoses prior to thrombosis. Kidney Int 47:1364–1373, 1995.
19. Besarab A, Dorrell S, Moritz M, et al. Determinants of measured dialysis venous pressure and its relationship to true intra-access venous pressure. Trans Am Soc Artif Intern Organs 37:270–271, 1991.
20. Besarab A, Moritz M, Sullivan K, et al. Venous access pressures and the detection of intra-access stenosis. Trans Am Soc Artif Intern Organs 38:519–523, 1992.
21. Collins DM, Lambert MB, Middleton JP, et al. Fistula dysfunction: Effect on rapid hemodialysis. Kidney Int 41:1292–1296, 1992.
22. Sherman RA, Kapoian T. Recirculation, urea disequilibrium and dialysis efficiency: Peripheral artereiovenous versus central venovenous vascular access. Am J Kidney Dis 29:479–489, 1997.
23. Daugirdas JT. Chronic hemodialysis prescription: A urea kinetic approach. In Daugirdas JT, Ing TS, eds. Handbook of Dialysis, 2nd ed. Boston: Little Brown; 1994: 92–109.
24. Villemarette PY, Hower JF. Evaluation of functional longevity of dialysis access grafts using color flow Doppler imaging. J Vasc Tech 16:183–188, 1992.
25. Martin SP. Routine color Doppler evaluation of dialysis access grafts should be performed. Semin Dial 6:206–207, 1993.
26. Walters GK, Jones CE. Color duplex evaluation of arteriovenous access for hemodialysis. J Vasc Tech 18:295–298, 1994.
27. Tordoir JH, Hoeneveld H, Eikelboom BC, Kitslaar P. The correlation between clinical and duplex ultrasound parameters and the development of complications in arteriovenous fistulae for hemodialysis. Eur J Vasc Surg 4:179–184, 1990.
28. Strauch BS, O'Connell RS, Geoly KL, et al. Forecasting thrombosis of vascular access with Doppler color flow imaging. Am J Kidney Dis 19:554–557, 1992.
29. Harkrider WW, Comeaux ME. Proximal arterial waveform as an indicator functional significance in color Doppler imaging of the AV fistula for hemodialysis. In Henry ML, Ferguson RM, eds. Vascular Access for Hemodialysis IV. Chicago: Gore, 1995: 169–174.

30. Ermers EJM, Langeveld APM, Penders RPA, et al. Duplex ultrasound detection of stenoses in newly created hemodialysis AV fistulas: Its significance in relation to fistula complications. J Vasc Tech 16:295–297, 1992.

31. Rittgers SE, Garcia-Valdez C, McCormick MS, Posner MP. Noninvasive blood flow measurements in expanded polytetrafluoroethylene grafts for hemodialysis. J Vasc Surg 3:635–642, 1986.

32. Shackleton CR, Taylor DC, Buckley AR, et al. Predicting failure in polytetrafluoroethylene vascular access grafts for hemodialysis: A pilot study. Can J Surg 30:442–444, 1987.

33. Kirkman RL. Can diagnostic testing help prolong access function? A prophylactic approach to graft thrombosis is not yet justifiable. Semin Dial 6:203–208, 1993.

34. Krivitski NM. Novel method to measure access flow during hemodialysis by ultrasound velocity dilution technique. ASAIO J 41:741–745, 1995.

35. Dener TA. Hemodialysis access—The role of monitoring. In-line methods. ASAIO J 44:38–9, 1998.

36. Lindsay RM, Rothera C, Blake PG. A comparison of methods for the measurement of hemodialysis access recirculation: an update. ASAIO J 44:191–193, 1998.

37. Sands J, Glidden D, Miranda C. Hemodialysis access flow measurements. Comparison of ultrasound dilution and duplex ultrasonography. ASAIO J 42:899–901, 1996.

38. May RE, Himmelfarb J, Yenicesu M, et al. Predictive measures of vascular access thrombosis: A prospective study. Kidney Int 52:1656–1662, 1997.

7

Revisional Surgery for Failed Dialysis Access

Alex Westerband

Southern Arizona Veterans Affairs Health Care Systems and The University of Arizona Health Sciences Center, Tucson, Arizona

Bruce E. Jarrell

The University of Maryland School of Medicine, Baltimore, Maryland

Scott S. Berman

The University of Arizona, Carondelet St. Mary's Hospital, and The Southern Arizona Vascular Institute, Tucson, Arizona

The 1994 report of the U.S. Renal Data System (USRDS) has shown a progressive annual increase in the number of newly treated end-stage renal disease (ESRD) patients in this country, with an 8.76% annual growth since 1982 (1). Among the three main treatment modalities—hemodialysis, renal transplantation, and peritoneal dialysis—hemodialysis is instituted in approximately two-thirds of these patients. For the 200,000 hemodialysis patients in the United States, it is imperative to establish an effective arteriovenous (AV) fistula with a reasonable long-term patency rate, even with the required three-time weekly needle punctures at the access site. In spite of our best efforts, most if not all of these vascular accesses will eventually thrombose and require either a revision or the creation of a new fistula or graft at a different site. Over the course of an ESRD patient's dialysis lifetime, complications related to the establishment or

125

maintenance of vascular access is the most common reason for admission to a health care facility (2). The limited number of easily accessible sites and the good results obtained after revision of failed dialysis access grafts have led vascular access surgeons to attempt revision prior to constructing a new AV fistula elsewhere. For autogenous fistulae, Kinnaert et al. (3) and Rohr et al. (4) report secondary patency rates of 88 and 65% at 1 year and 88 and 55% at 2 years, respectively. For prosthetic arteriovenous grafts, similar secondary patency rates of 75 and 95% at 1 year and 61 and 81% at 2 years have been achieved in the respective series reported by Kherlakian et al. (5) and Puckett and Lindsay (6). Moreover, Palder et al. (7) have shown that successfully revised fistulae, either autogenous or prosthetic, maintain a patency survival similar to that of unrevised fistulae. The purpose of this chapter is to review the surgical approaches to throm-

TABLE 7.1 Treatment of Thrombosis and Associated Stenosis in Dialysis AV Grafts

Thrombosis of an AV graft should be corrected with surgical thrombectomy or with pharmacomechanical or mechanical thrombolysis. The choice of technique to treat thrombosis should be based on the expertise of the center. However, it is essential that:

1. Treatment be performed rapidly following detection of thrombosis so as to minimize the need for temporary access. No more than one and preferably no femoral vein catheterization should be required (opinion).
2. The access be evaluated by fistulogram for residual stenosis postprocedure (evidence).
3. Residual stenosis be corrected by angioplasty or surgical correction. Outflow venous stenoses are present in >85% of instances of thrombosis; the need for PTA or surgical revision is expected in most instances (evidence).
4. The procedure be performed on an outpatient basis under local anesthesia. Access revision may require up to a 24-h observation to evaluate swelling and steal (opinion).
5. Monitoring tests used to screen for venous obstruction should return to normal following intervention (evidence).
6. Centers should monitor outcome results on the basis of patency. Minimum reasonable goals (for the center as a whole) of percutaneous thrombolysis and surgical revision thrombectomy should be (a) Percutaneous thrombolysis with PTA—40% unassisted patency and functionality at 3 months; (b) Surgical thrombectomy and revision—50% unassisted patency and functionality at 6 months and 40% unassisted patency and functionality at 1 year (opinion); (c) For both techniques—immediate patency, defined as patency to the next dialysis session, of 85%.

Source: Modified from Ref. 8, Guideline 21.

TABLE **7.2** Treatment of Thrombosis in Primary AV Fistulae

Thrombosis of an AV fistula is difficult to treat. Neither percutaneous nor surgical techniques offer good results. Each institution should attempt to resolve thrombosis with the technique that is preferred at the institution (opinion).

Source: Modified from Ref. 8, Guideline 22.

bectomy and revision for the most commonly encountered failures of AV dialysis access (Tables 7.1 and 7.2) (8).

CLINICAL ASSESSMENT

The ESRD patient is typically referred to the surgeon by the dialysis center staff, either before or after a dialysis session, when the fistula or graft is clotted. Occasionally, the patient will note the disappearance of a thrill and notify the dialysis staff prior to a scheduled dialysis session. With the success of percutaneous procedures for salvaging thrombosed access fistulae (see Chapter 8), a third pathway for the patient to return to the access surgeon is after repeated procedures on the same access site by interventional radiologists.

When the patient with a thrombosed access presents to the surgeon, important aspects of the patient's history are ascertained, which help guide the surgical intervention as follows:

The age of the fistula
Time interval to thrombosis from last intervention
Prior episodes of thrombosis and selected intervention
Recent fistula performance on dialysis, such as increased venous pressure or long recirculation times
Contributing factors for thrombosis, such as hypotension during dialysis or improper digital pressure on the fistula after needle removal

The patient must be carefully examined prior to any treatment. The physical examination may provide clues to the cause of thrombosis, such as graft aneurysms or anastomotic pseudoaneurysms. Documentation of the arterial circulation distal to the fistula is imperative to establish a baseline for comparison after fistula thrombectomy. If a good pulse is found at the arterial anastomosis upon palpation of the graft, the problem is likely to be on the venous side. Conversely, absence of a pulse in the arterial limb of the graft with a paucity of thrombus in the body of the graft implies a problem at the arterial anatomosis. Equally important to the treatment of the patient is a careful review of previous operative reports and fistulograms. Operative reports may comment on the integrity of alternative venous outflows should revision of the venous anastomosis become necessary. Previously preformed fistulograms, particularly during percutaneous interventions, may demonstrate the cause of the most recent thrombosis and show patency of alternative sites for venous outflow. Moreover, prior fistulograms should confirm patency of the surgically inaccessible central venous outflow in the brachiocephalic and subclavian systems, which is imperative for successful revision and salvage of the extremity as an access site.

On occasion, an autogenous fistula that has remained patent but has failed to adequately ''arterialize'' must be evaluated for revision or replacement. Preoperative fistulography is necessary to determine whether revision of the autogenous access will be possible. If an anatomic lesion—stenosis in either the inflow artery, outflow vein, or at the anastomosis—is not demonstrated, revision is not possible and replacement to a prosthetic graft will be necessary.

SURGICAL METHODS FOR REVISION

The general principles for perioperative management do not differ whether a new vascular access or a thrombectomy/revision is contemplated. For patients who are medically unstable, with florid fluid overload or severe electrolyte disturbances, a temporary jugular or femoral dual lumen dialysis catheter is placed and the patient is dialyzed before proceeding with any intervention to treat the thrombosed fistula. Perioperative antibiotic prophylaxis with high activity against *Staphylococcus aureus* is recommended any time prosthetic materials are used (9). Anesthetic technique is individualized based upon the usual selection factors, such as the patient's comorbid condition and planned extent of surgical intervention. Whereas local anesthesia generally suffices in creating a native arteriovenous fistula at the wrist, the presence of scarred tissues makes a local anesthetic less effective for fistula revision. For that reason, a regional anesthesia such as an axillary block is preferred. General anesthesia may be safely applied and is sometimes necessary when extension of an upper extremity graft into the axilla or infraclavicular region is anticipated. For lower extremity AV grafts, regional anesthesia using spinal or epidural techniques may be adequate to accomplish thrombectomy/revision.

Whenever a surgical revision has been performed, the hemodialysis staff must be instructed to avoid cannulation of a new segment of fistula. A simple drawing added to the operative note clearly illustrating the procedure performed and demonstrating the direction of the blood flow will be particularly useful for proper and safe cannulation of the revised access.

Autogenous Fistulas

The autogenous radiocephalic fistula has remained unsurpassed since its introduction by Brescia et al. (10) in 1966, since it continues to provide better long-term patency rates (4,11,12) and a lower rate of complications (12,13) than other forms of angioaccess. Its superiority makes it the access of choice when it is technically feasible and vein maturation can be obtained. When fistula thrombosis occurs, a common approach today is to institute thrombolytic therapy by local infusion of a lytic agent to reopen the fistula. Kumpe and Cohen (14) achieved recanalization rates of 58 to 90%, even in the presence of late thrombosis, with this approach. When lytic therapy has been successful at reopening the fistula, defects identified by a fistulogram may be treated percutaneously or surgically. The initial success rate using percutaneous techniques such as balloon angioplasty for stenosis or stricture has been reported to be as high as 80 to 90%, but the patency rate dramatically decreases soon after (14–16). Surgical revision usually requires a vein patch angioplasty as directed by the fistulogram findings.

For the Cimino fistula that has remained patent but has failed to mature, the cephalic vein in the forearm may have a short-segment stenosis near the anastomosis (5). This may be treated with a venous patch or a simple interposition vein graft to salvage the fistula.

When the cephalic vein in the forearm has become thrombosed and unusable, there may be an adequate basilic forearm vein that can be transposed and anastomosed end-to-side with the radial artery. This eventuality is rather rare, and because it requires more dissection, this procedure is avoided by many, especially in patients with diabetes.

With a satisfactory arterial inflow at the wrist, a simple conversion to a straight bridge fistula between the radial artery and a large antecubital vein may be accomplished using expanded polytetrafluoroethylene (ePTFE) (Figure 7.1). On rare occasions, when the antecubital vein is of insufficient caliber, the venous outflow tract can be expanded using an antebrachial venoplasty (Figure 7.2) as described by Alexander (17).

Frequently, the distal forearm veins are no longer suitable for cannulation due to repeated venipunctures and subsequent thrombosis. However, the cephalic vein in the upper arm has already become arterialized and can be readily anastomosed to the brachial artery, creating an autogenous brachiocephalic fistula (Figure 7.3). This access fistula is often usable in 1 to 2 weeks, since the upper arm cephalic vein has served as the outflow for the more distally placed Cimino. Satisfactory and even superior results with elbow autogenous fistulas have been reported (18). When an adequate cephalic vein in the upper arm is available, this is our preferred secondary approach after the Cimino fistula has failed and cannot be revised without using a prosthetic graft.

Infrequently, a so-called reverse fistula can be constructed by anastomosing the basilic vein and the brachial artery side to side in the upper arm and plicating the vein above the anastomosis (19). To establish flow retrograde into the subcutaneous antecubital branches, however, requires a valvulotomy within the first few centimeters of the antecubital vein. On rare occasions a reverse fistula may

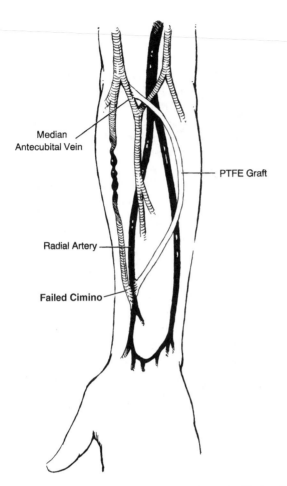

FIGURE 7.1 Conversion of a failed Brescia-Cimino fistula to a straight prosthetic bridge graft.

spontaneously develop secondary to outflow obstruction in an upper arm brachio-cephalic fistula. To maintain patency and adequate flow in this scenario requires only ligation of the cephalic vein in the mid-upper arm (Figure 7.4).

Prosthetic A-V Grafts

General Principles

Although different types of materials have been offered as arteriovenous conduits when an autogenous fistula cannot be constructed, the e-PTFE graft is considered

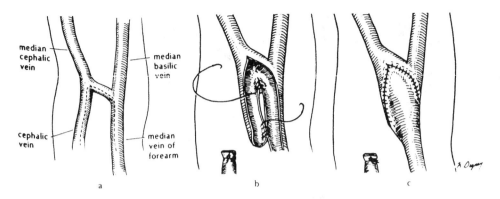

FIGURE 7.2 Technique of antebrachial venoplasty as described by Alexander. (From Ref. 17.)

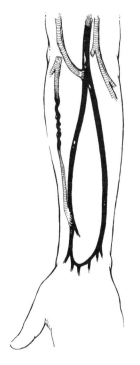

FIGURE 7.3 Treatment of a failed Brescia-Cimino fistula by conversion to an antecubital brachiocephalic fistula.

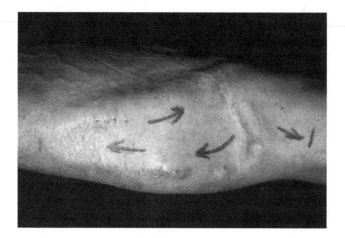

FIGURE 7.4 Spontaneous upper arm reverse fistula in a patient with outflow stenosis in a native upper arm brachiocephalic fistula.

superior based upon better patency rates, lower complication rates, and ease of thrombectomy compared to other biological or prosthetic materials (20,21). Reports of 1- and 2-year patency rates of 71 to 80%, and of 60 to 70%, respectively, appear in the literature (4,6,22).

When thrombosis develops in a prosthetic AV graft within the first 30 days after placement, technical failure at one of the anastomoses is often incriminated as the precipitating event. The traditional approach to this problem mandated immediate surgical exploration of both anastomoses. After thrombectomy is performed, fistulography is mandatory to determine the etiology of the thrombosis. More often than not, early thrombosis is caused by poor selection of the venous outflow. Not uncommonly, however, no anatomic reason for the graft failure is found, which portends a poor prognosis for long-term patency at that specific site. If adequate fistulograms are not obtainable in the operating suite, an alternative approach to early graft thrombosis uses the success of percutaneous thrombolysis and thrombectomy. These techniques are discussed in detail in the following chapter.

Even within the first 2 to 3 weeks after fistula placement, percutaneous methods can be applied to restore patency. The advantage of this approach is the ability to obtain detailed fistulograms to assess the anatomic arrangement of the graft and the proximal venous system. This information allows more focused surgical intervention to take place and on occasion spares the patient reoperation when no technical problem is discovered. In that circumstance, consideration must be given to nonsurgical causes for thrombosis, such as an underlying hypercoagulable state or poor circulatory hemodynamics. These conditions will require adjustments to the dialysis prescription to prevent recurrent problems with graft thrombosis.

For surgical revision, the patient should be adequately prepped and draped so as not to limit the possible options for revision. Routinely, we have the patient prepped from the axilla to the hand for upper extremity access work. If an upper arm access graft is already in place, the prep should be extended to include the infraclavicular region should revision to this level be necessary. It is equally important to include the wrist and hand in the prep so that the distal circulation can be assessed after the procedure for any evidence of embolization that would mandate immediate intervention.

The sequence of steps in performing thrombectomy depend upon the clinical situation. If graft revision is planned, thrombectomy is performed at the end of the operative procedure. Alternatively, if the etiology of graft thrombosis is unknown, thrombectomy is the initial step of the operation. With the advent of temporary jugular dialysis catheters, graft thrombectomy may be postponed until the patient is medically stable for surgery. We still prefer to intervene within 2 weeks of thrombosis because it becomes more difficult to perform a complete and satisfactory thrombectomy beyond that period.

We use systemic heparinization routinely for thrombectomy procedures. A dose between 3000 and 5000 U is given intravenously prior to the start of the procedure. One of the authors (SSB) uses a sterile pneumatic tourniquet for all forearm AV graft thrombectomy/revision procedures, which minimizes blood loss and minimizes the need for extensive dissection for circumferential control of the graft and anastomotic vessels. In addition, excellent views of the arterial anastomosis and arterial tree distal to the fistula may be obtained with the tourniquet in place during intraoperative fistulography. Most often a Fogarty balloon catheter is used to thrombectomize the fistula. Since most grafts are 6 mm in diameter, a No. 4 catheter is usually adequate to accomplish complete thrombectomy. Larger and smaller catheters are available but are unnecessary in most circumstances.

The venous limb of the arteriovenous fistula is declotted first; then the Fogarty catheter is advanced with great caution through the arterial anastomosis. Several passes may be necessary to achieve removal of the characteristic bullet-shaped plug of thrombus from the arterial anastomosis with its characteristic meniscus (Figure 7.5). Diligence in pursuing this plug must be applied to assure complete thrombectomy, since a strong pulsatile blood flow may be achieved despite persistence of this adherent plug at the arterial anastomosis. Failure to completely remove this dense plug will almost certainly result in recurrent thrombosis.

Two additional catheters which may be useful in AV graft thrombectomy are the Fogarty adherent clot catheter and the Fogarty graft thrombectomy cathe-

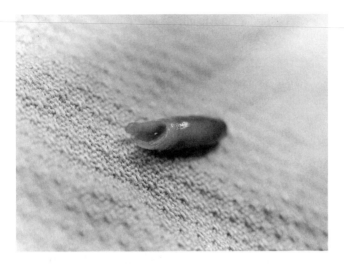

FIGURE 7.5   Characteristic dense thrombus plug with meniscus obtained from the arterial anastomosis of a successfully thrombectomized access graft.

ter (Figure 7.6). These devices employ a serpentine wire either covered or bare, respectively, which upon withdrawal engages the dense adherent clot and pseudointima which line prosthetic grafts allowing for a more complete thrombectomy. Often, restoration of the bare internal prosthetic surface is possible with these adjunctive maneuvers. The use of coronary dilators can help to determine the magnitude of a stenosis and to dislodge an organized thrombus if present. An intraoperative fistulogram is performed to verify the cause of the thrombosis. It is often difficult to adequately visualize the axillosubclavian and brachiocephalic venous systems with intraoperative fistulograms; therefore, if pathology in the central venous system is suspected, formal fistulograms are obtained in the radiology department after graft patency is restored. If a central vein stenosis is found to be responsible for the failure of the graft, balloon angioplasty with or without placement of an endovascular stent, can be accomplished with a cumulative patency rate as high as 93% being reported for stenting of subclavian and innominate venous stenosis and occlusions (23).

Graft curretage and angioscopy are adjunctive procedures to further assess and achieve complete graft thrombectomy (24,25). Though both techniques have their own proponents, the additional cost and time required for these procedures

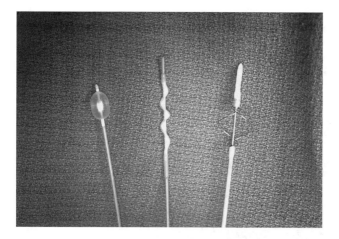

FIGURE 7.6 Catheters available for access graft thrombectomy (from left): Fogarty balloon catheter, Fogarty adherent clot catheter, Fogarty graft thrombectomy catheter.

has not yet been justified by consistently superior results when compared with intraoperative fistulography.

For late AV graft thrombosis, the problem usually occurs at the venous anastomosis due to the development of intimal hyperplasia. This problem is more frequently being managed by percutaneous interventions. In large centers, thrombolytic therapy in combination with balloon angioplasty is being used more frequently, with results equivalent or even superior to those obtained with surgical revision (26–28). Some reports, however, have shown a higher recurrence rate when stenoses are treated with percutaneous transluninal angioplasty (PTA) (14,16). The surgical approach for late fistula thrombosis in the absence of previous fistulography or interventions relies upon adequate thrombectomy and intraoperative fistulography to determine the etiology of thrombosis and guide therapy. For failing or failed AV grafts that have been previously treated by percutaneous interventions, review of previous treatment reports and fistulograms serves as a useful guide to focus surgical treatment.

Forearm Bridge AV Grafts

When the problem is suspected to be at the venous anastomosis, those failed dialysis accesses will generally be approached by reopening the incision just over the venous anastomosis. The hood of the graft is opened longitudinally, graft thrombectomy is performed, and if intimal hyperplasia is noted at the anastomo-

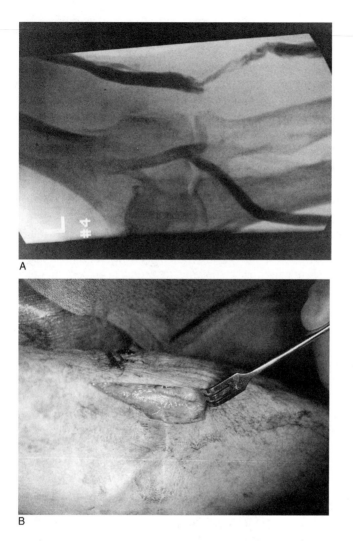

FIGURE 7.7 Venous anastomotic stenosis in a prosthetic bridge AV graft seen on fistulogram (A) and treated with a patch angioplasty (B).

sis, revision can be accomplished either by a patch angioplasty using a trimmed segment of ePTFE (Figure 7.7) or a jump graft bypassing the stenotic segment (Figure 7.8).

When the graft is configured as a forearm loop, it is sometimes difficult to accomplish complete thrombectomy of the arterial limb from access through

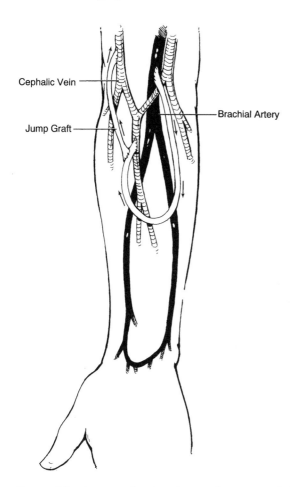

Cephalic Vein

Brachial Artery

Jump Graft

FIGURE 7.8 Jump graft extension on the venous limb of a prosthetic bridge AV graft.

the venous anastomosis. Sufficient forward force to drive the thrombectomy catheter through the thrombus may not be achieved due to the curvature in the apex of the graft before the catheter kinks and bends. As an alternative, thrombectomy may begin through a cutdown over the apex of the graft. This approach permits easy straight line access to both the arterial and venous anastomoses (Figure 7.9). Complete thrombectomy of each limb of the graft is easy to accomplish without the need for dissection over the anastomoses and through scar tissue, making this approach amenable to the use of local anesthesia. Following thrombectomy,

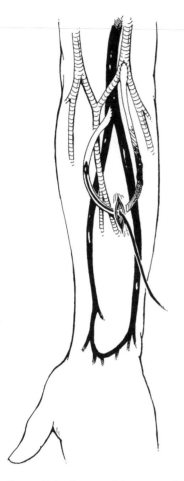

FIGURE 7.9 Approach to access thrombectomy through the apex of a forearm loop bridge graft. This technique provides access to both the venous and arterial limbs of the access and proves useful when the suspected course of access thrombosis is not well delineated prior to surgery.

fistulograms of each limb of the graft are obtained. Should venous outflow stenosis adjacent to or involving the venous anastomosis be demonstrated, intraoperative balloon angioplasty may be utilized for primary treatment with acceptable patency results (29).

A more complex situation occurs when the cephalic venous outflow tract is thrombosed to an extent where a jump graft to the cephalic vein would no longer be feasible. A jump graft to the basilic vein would be subject to kinking

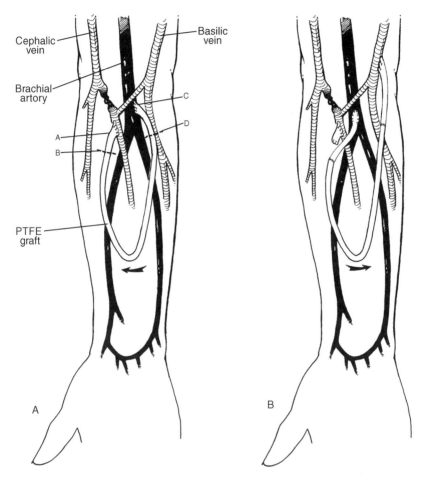

FIGURE 7.10 Revision of the venous limb of a forearm loop bridge graft from the antecubital veins to the basilic vein. (A) Segments A-B and C-D indicate the zones of transection. (B) Completion of the B-C anastomosis and the addition of a segment of graft at D reverses the original flow direction in the graft.

and subsequent thrombosis, due to its oblique position while crossing the elbow crease. In these particular circumstances, with cephalic vein outflow obstruction, Schulak et al. (30) have successfully accomplished a reversal of the direction of blood flow through the graft with subsequent venous anastomosis with the median basilic vein proximal to the elbow crease (Figure 7.10).

Not infrequently, a long-standing AV graft will have multiple areas of intra-

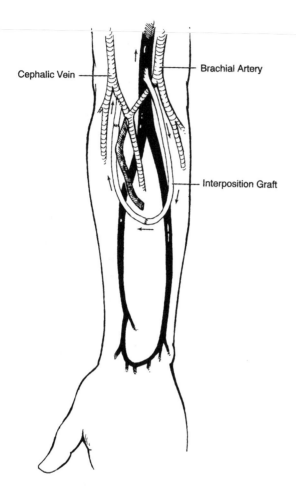

Cephalic Vein

Brachial Artery

Interposition Graft

FIGURE 7.11   Replacement of a diffusely stenotic segment of a forearm loop bridge graft with an interposition graft.

graft stenosis with otherwise adequate arterial inflow and venous outflow. These problems occur in areas of repeated cannulation and usually require graft replacement. Segmental graft resection and replacement can be done when the diseased segment is short or an interposition graft can be used for a longer diseased segment (Figure 7.11) while the stenotic segment is excluded and left in place. However, midgraft stenosis may be due to organized thrombus, in which case a graft curettage may be effective in restoring an adequate lumen size (5), avoiding the

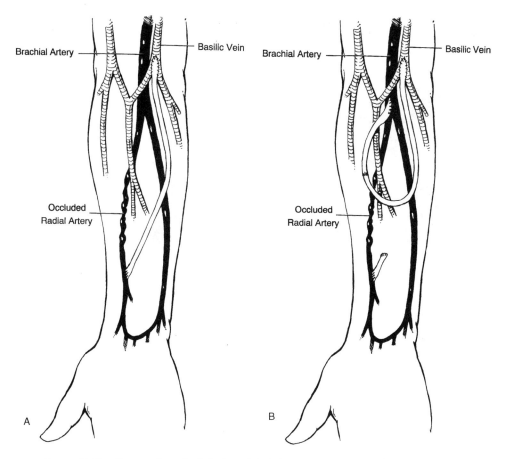

FIGURE 7.12 Conversion of a failed straight bridge graft (A) into a loop bridge graft (B) when arterial inflow is the source of failure.

need for graft replacement or interposition. Multiple incisions with their attendant risk of breakdown and infection, may be necessary to restore complete patency.

In the clinical situation in which a straight forearm bridge graft has failed because of arterial stenosis and poor inflow, conversion to a loop graft based upon the brachial artery is easily performed. Arterial stenosis is responsible for failure of vascular access in as many as 15 to 19% of clotted grafts (30,31). A new arterial limb is placed on the brachial artery and anastomosed to form a loop apex in the distal forearm to the old straight graft (Figure 7.12).

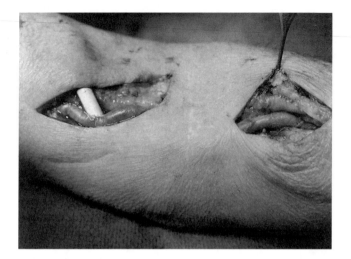

FIGURE 7.13   Salvage of an upper arm AV graft that failed due to occlusive disease in the brachial artery. Here the brachial artery is replaced with a segment of the greater saphenous vein from above the elbow to the forearm; a new segment of ePTFE is anastomosed to the vein graft to replace the arterial limb of the AV graft.

The most favorable method of managing a thrombosed forearm bridge graft is conversion to an autogenous fistula. When the cephalic vein in the upper arm has functioned as the primary outflow for the prosthetic bridge graft, it may become adequately arterialized to permit simple conversion to a native fistula when the bridge graft thromboses. By simply anastomosing the cephalic vein to the brachial artery in an end-to-side configuration, either in the antecubital fossa or just proximal to the antecubital crease, a durable native fistula is created that can often be cannulated within a few days (see Figure 4.8). These fistula achieve the long-term patency of other autogenous access routes.

Upper Arm Bridge AV Grafts

Thromboses of upper arm AV grafts are similarly related to venous outflow stenoses in the majority of cases. In those rare instances where progression of atherosclerosis in the inflow artery results in access failure, vascular reconstruction may provide inflow reestablishment and allow successful AV graft revision (Figure 7.13). The approach to surgical thrombectomy and revision does not deviate from that described for forearm bridge grafts with notable exceptions. General anesthesia is more commonly required, since revision may involve incision and dissection in the axilla and infraclavicular region. Tourniquet occlusion is limited to use only when the arterial anastomosis needs revision. Whereas stent placement after balloon angioplasty in the peripheral cephalic and basilic veins has not been effective, stent deployment in the axillary vein has provided patency rates equivalent to surgical revision in this region for venous stenosis (32). Rarely occlusive disease in the brachial artery may cause access failure. Correcting the arterial lesion requires either limited patch angioplasty, transposition of the access to a more proximal arterial site, or arterial reconstruction as depicted in Figure 7.13.

Alternative Bridge AV Grafts

Permanent vascular access in the lower extremity is usually considered only after all the technical possibilities and potential locations for placement have been exhausted in both upper extremities. Despite reports establishing a better patency rate for thigh grafts as compared to arm grafts (33), presumably due to a higher flow in larger vessels, there is a higher incidence of infection and ischemia with a greater risk of potential limb loss (12), which makes thigh AV grafts less desirable alternatives. Occasionally, other configurations are encountered. Examples include bridge AV graft between the axillary or subclavian artery on one side and the axillary or subclavian vein on the contralateral side (necklace fistula). As with bridge fistulas in other locations, the same principles of thrombectomy/revision apply. However, due to their anatomical locations and the morbidity associated with reoperative exposure in these locations, emphasis has been placed on angioplasty to maintain access graft patency.

CONCLUSION

The goal of thrombectomy and revision of access grafts and fistulae is to prolong the use of a specific access site before a new access construction is required. Traditionally this required surgical approaches. However, as techniques for percutaneous intervention evolve, combinations of these therapies will likely form the basis of treatment algorithms. Currently available surgical and nonsurgical methods are considered successful if patency is maintained for 6 to 12 months following treatment. The costs of surgical versus nonsurgical techniques are equivalent in many centers. If pharmaceutical thrombolysis becomes unnecessary, nonsurgical techniques will clearly be less costly. More and more emphasis is being placed on developing reliable methods to detect failing fistulae and to intervene prior to thrombosis (34–37). The savings in both cost and patient morbidity by avoiding the need for urgent interventions and for placement of temporary jugular catheters should support the application of these screening methods. With the expanding success of percutaneous treatment for failed and failing access fistulae and grafts, the role of the access surgeon will evolve to specific surgical repair of lesions as guided by prior percutaneous treatment and to construction of secondary access grafts and fistulae. Less emphasis will be placed upon surgical thrombectomy and revision as a primary pathway for treatment of thrombosed access sites.

REFERENCES

1. U.S. Renal Data System. USRDS 1994 Annual Data Report. Am J Kidney Dis 24 (suppl 2):548–556, 1994.
2. Lazarus JM, Huang WH, Lew NL, Lowrie EG. Contribution of vascular access–related disease to morbidity of hemodialysis patients. In Henry ML, Ferguson RM, eds. Vascular Access for Hemodialysis III. Chicago: Gore; 1993:3–13.
3. Kinnaert P, Veerstraeten P, Toussaint C, et al. Nine years' experience with internal arteriovenous fistulas for hemodialysis: A study of some factors influencing the results. Br J Surg 64:242–246, 1977.
4. Rohr MS, Brewder W, Frentz GD, et al. Arteriovenous fistulas for long-term dialysis. Arch Surg 113:153–155, 1978.
5. Kherlakian GH, Rodersheimer LR, Arbaugh JJ, et al. Comparison of autogenous fistula versus expanded polytetrafluoroethylene graft fistula for angioaccess in hemodialysis. Am J Surg 152:238–243, 1986.
6. Puckett J, Lindsay S. Midgraft curettage as a routine adjunct to salvage operation for thrombosed polytetraflueroethylene hemodialysis access grafts. Am J Surg 156:139–143, 1988.
7. Palder SB, Kirkman RL, Whittemore AD, et al. Vascular access for hemodialysis. Patency rates and results of revision. Ann Surg 202:235–239, 1985.
8. NKF-DOQI. Clinical Practice Guidelines for Vascular Access. New York: National Kidney Foundation; 1997.
9. Bennion RS, Hiatt JR, Williams RA, et al. A randomized, prospective study of perioperative antimicrobial prophylaxis for vascular access surgery. J Cardiovasc Surg 26:270–274, 1985.
10. Brescia M, Cimino J, Appel K, et al. Chronic hemodialysis using venipuncture and a surgically created arteriovenous fistula. N Engl J Med 275:1089, 1966.
11. Chazan, JA, London MR, Pond LM. Long-term survival of vascular accesses in a large chronic hemodialysis population. Nephron 69:228–233, 1995.
12. Zibari GB, Rohr MS, Landroneau MD, et al. Complications from permanent hemodialysis vascular access. Surgery 104:681–686, 1988.
13. Jenkins A, Buisk TAS, Glover SD. Medium-term follow-up of forty arteriovenous and forty PTFE grafts for dialysis access. Surgery 88:667–672, 1980.
14. Kumpe DA, Cohen MA. Angioplasty/thrombolytic treatment of failing and failed hemodialysis access sites: Comparison with surgical treatment. Prog Cardiovasc Dis 34:263, 1992.
15. Glanz S, Gordon DH, Butt KMH, et al. The role of percutaneous angioplasty in the management of chronic hemodialysis fistulas. Ann Surg 206:777, 1987.
16. Brooks JL, Sigley RD, May KJ, et al. Transluminal angioplasty versus surgical repair for stenosis of hemodialysis graft. Am J Surg 153:530–531, 1987.
17. Alexander JJ. Expansion of the venous outflow tract in arteriovenous grafts of the forearm using antebrachial venoplasty. Surg Gynecol Obstet 173:235–236, 1991.
18. Bender MHM, Bruyninckx CMA, Gerlag PGG. The brachiocephalic elbow fistula: A useful alternative angioaccess for permanent hemodialysis. J Vasc Surg 20:808–813, 1994.

19. Geis WP, Giacchino JL, Iwatsuki S, et al. The reverse fistula for vascular access. Surg Gynecol Obstet 145:901–904, 1977.
20. Haimov M, Burrows L, Schanzer H, et al. Experience with arterial substitutes in the construction of vascular access for hemodialysis. J Cardiovasc Surg 21:149, 1980.
21. Lilly L, Nigheim D, Mendez-Picon G, et al. Comparison between bovine heterograft and expanded PTFE grafts for dialysis access. Am Surg 46:694, 1980.
22. Rizzuti RP, Hale JC, Burkart TE. Extended patency of expanded polytetrafluoroethylene grafts for vascular access using optimal configurations and revisions. Surg Gynecol Obstet 166:23, 1988.
23. Shoenfeld R, Hermano H, Novick A, et al. Stenting of proximal venous obstructions to maintain hemodialysis access. J Vasc Surg 19:532–539, 1994.
24. Puckett JW, Lindsay SF. Graft curettage. In Henry ML, Ferguson RM, ed. Vascular Access for Hemodialysis III. Chicago: Gore; 1993:186–195.
25. Miller A, Maracaccio EJ, Goodman WS, Gottlieb MN. The role of angioscopy in vascular access surgery. In Henry ML, Ferguson RM, ed. Vascular Access for Hemodialysis III. Chicago: Gore; 1993:210–218.
26. Dapunt O, Feurstein H, Rendl K, et al. Transluminal angioplasty versus conventional operation in the treatment of hemodialysis fistula stenosis: Results from a 5-year study. Br J Surg 74:1004–1005, 1987.
27. Valjik K, Bookstein JJ, Roberts AC, et al. Pharmacomechanical thrombosis and angioplasty in the management of clotted hemodialysis grafts: Early and late clinical results. Radiology 178:243–247, 1991.
28. Hood DB, Yellin AE, Richman MF, et al. Hemodialysis graft salvage with endoluminal stents. Am Surg 60:733–737, 1994.
29. Romero A, Polo JR, Morato EG, et al. Salvage of angioaccess after late thrombosis of radiocephalic fistulas for hemodialysis. Int Surg 71:122–124, 1986.
30. Schulak JA, Lukens ML, Mayers JT. Salvage of thrombosed forearm polytetrafluoroethylene vascular access grafts by reversal of flow direction and venous bypass grafting. Am J Surg 161:485–489, 1991.
31. Raja S. PTFE grafts for hemodialysis access—Techniques for insertion and management of complications. Ann Surg 206:666–673, 1987.
32. Vorwerk D, Guenther RW, Bohndorf K, Gladziwa U, Kistler D. Self-expanding stents in peripheral and central veins used for arteriovenous shunts: Five years of experience. Radiology 189:174, 1993.
33. Owens ML, Stabile BE, Gahr MD et al. Vascular grafts for hemodialysis: An evaluation of sites and materials. Dial Transplant 8:521, 1979.
34. Schwab SJ, Raymond JR, Sared M, et al. Prevention of hemodialysis fistula thrombosis. Early detection of venous stenosis. Kidney Int 36:707, 1989.
35. Gani JS, Fowler PR, Steinberg AW, et al. Use of the fistula assessment monitor to detect stenosis in access fistulae. Am J Kidney Dis 3:303–306, 1991.
36. Strauch BS, O'Connel RS, Geoly KL, et al: Forecasting thrombosis of vascular access with Doppler color flow imaging. Am J Kidney Dis 6:554–557, 1992.
37. Berkoben M, Schwab SJ. Maintenance of permanent hemodialysis vascular access patency. ANNA J 22(1):17–24, 1995.

8

Nonsurgical Methods for Salvaging Failed Dialysis Access

Donald J. Roach
Radiology Limited, Tucson, Arizona

Thomas Stejskal
Carondelet St. Mary's Hospital and The Southern Arizona Vascular
Institute, Tucson, Arizona

Scott S. Berman
The University of Arizona, Carondelet St. Mary's Hospital, and The
Southern Arizona Vascular Institute, Tucson, Arizona

The preceding chapter reviews in detail the approach to surgical revision of a failing or failed dialysis access site. In this section we discuss nonsurgical methods for intervening in the failing or failed AV access, largely focusing on percutaneous techniques. Of critical importance in maintaining uninterrupted access for hemodialysis is the identification of AV fistulae and grafts at risk for failure prior to the onset of thrombosis (1). Accomplishing this goal relies heavily on a surveillance protocol that may incorporate one or a number of the methods described in Chapter 6.

TREATMENT OF THE FAILING ACCESS SITE

One of the primary goal of physicians involved in the care of patients on hemodialysis is the maintenance of uninterrupted access. Since the first description by Brescia and Cimino (2) of the native radiocephalic AV fistula at the wrist 30 years ago, no other form of chronic vascular access has achieved the same durable results. However, even native AV fistulae develop anatomic lesions which, if not corrected, will lead to thrombosis and failure. Whether the dialysis patient has a native fistula or a prosthetic AV graft, intervention to correct anatomical lesions prior to the onset of access thrombosis is a more cost-effective approach. It spares the patient the potential morbidity associated with temporary access catheters and spares the health care system the cost associated with treating access thrombosis. Adopting this philosophy depends on the availability of techniques to identify fistulae and grafts at risk. Currently available surveillance methods use measures of dialysis efficiency, venous pressure, and access flow to screen patients for anatomic lesions. Once an access site has been identified that may be at risk for thrombosis, further intervention is guided most commonly by contrast fistulography.

Fistulography

Fistulograms are usually performed by radiologists using modern angiographic equipment. If adequate image intensifiers and radiolucent tables are available in the operating suite, acceptable fistulograms can be obtained at the time of surgical placement or revision of fistulae or AV grafts, thereby providing a means for the identification of anatomical lesions and confirmation of technical results.

The most common cause of AV graft or fistula failure resides in stenosis at the venous anastomosis or in the venous outflow tract. Our approach to diagnostic fistulography, therefore, begins with cannulation of the venous limb of the graft or the dilated venous outflow of the fistula using the Seldinger over-the-wire technique with a simple 18-gauge angiocath. Digital subtraction techniques permit the acquisition of abundant information with small hand injections of contrast agents. Several injections utilizing multiple projections are usually required to adequately visualize the venous anastomosis and often complex collateral network of venous outflow channels (Figure 8.1). It is imperative to visualize the entire venous outflow, including the central venous system, to exclude the presence of occult occlusive disease. There is a significant incidence of subclavian vein stenosis in patient's who have previously undergone placement of subclavian dialysis catheters. Only visualization of the central venous system can exclude pathology at this site as the cause for access dysfunction. A qualitative appraisal of fistula flow is made during contrast injection. Flow through a patent, obstruction-free access site should be rapid and should not demonstrate any areas of stagnation.

By manipulating the diagnostic catheter under fluoroscopy toward the arterial limb of the graft or the AV anastomosis of the fistula, interrogation of the arterial inflow can be accomplished. A tourniquet or blood pressure cuff inflated above the elbow to a pressure exceeding systemic blood pressure will interrupt flow and allow contrast to reflux into the arterial limb of the graft, enabling visualization of the arterial anastomosis and arterial inflow. If needed, a guidewire followed by a diagnostic catheter can be advanced retrograde up the brachial

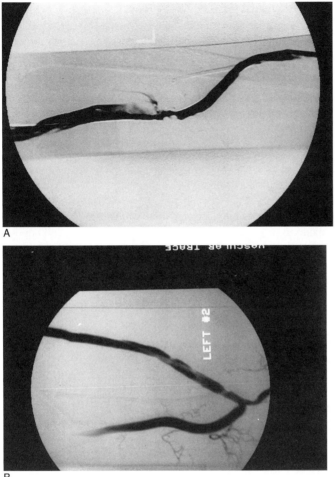

FIGURE 8.1 Diagnostic fistulogram obtained through the venous (A) and arterial (B) limbs of an arteriovenous graft.

artery to the takeoff of the subclavian artery to completely assess the arterial tree and exclude obstructive lesions of the arterial inflow as a cause of access dysfunction.

As an alternative, diagnostic fistulography can be performed through indwelling dialysis needles following a dialysis treatment. The needles are capped and secured by the dialysis staff after the run is completed and the patient is transported to the imaging suite. The indwelling dialysis needles provide a conduit for contrast injection without the need for additional cannulation of the access. If therapeutic intervention such as balloon angioplasty is subsequently indicated, guidewires may be introduced and the needles exchanged for appropriately sized sheaths.

Balloon Angioplasty

Stenosis involving the venous anastomosis or the venous outflow tract is the predominant reason for vascular access failure (3). Balloon angioplasty has emerged as a common method to treat stenotic lesions, particularly in the venous outflow, and thereby prolong access patency (4–8). One of the major presumed advantages of balloon angioplasty compared with surgical revision is the preservation of venous sites for future access revision. The initial effectiveness and long-term durability of balloon angioplasty for the treatment of AV access site stenosis are comparable to surgical revision. Moreover, intervention with balloon angioplasty prior to access thrombosis is less costly than surgical methods of access salvage (9).

Balloon angioplasty is readily accomplished at the time of diagnostic fistulography. An appropriately sized sheath is advanced over a guidewire into either the venous or arterial limb of the fistula or graft. Sheath size will be guided by the selection of balloon catheters and should always begin with the smallest diameter possible to accomplish the intervention. Generally, simple balloon angioplasty can be performed through a 6F sheath; however, sheaths ranging in size from 5F to 11F should be at hand. An appropriate selection of guidewires is necessary and should be available in a range of sizes (0.025 to 0.038 in.) and variable qualities (stiff, steerable, hydrophilic). Similarly, angioplasty catheters—which come in a number of different balloon diameters, balloon lengths, shaft sizes, and balloon materials—should be readily accessible. A representative assortment is required to overcome the pathology that can be encountered in managing AV fistula stenosis.

Performance of balloon angioplasty is straightforward when certain general principles are applied. One fundamental tenet is to maintain guidewire access across lesions and limit the advancement of diagnostic and therapeutic catheters to the over-the-wire technique. Adherence to this principle prevents having to ''recross'' stenotic areas, which can be difficult and time-consuming, particularly after angioplasty. With this in mind, a guidewire is advanced through the sheath and across the stenotic lesion. Once guidewire access is obtained, the balloon angioplasty catheter can be advanced across the lesion as well. Balloon inflation is performed using a dilute solution of contrast and a syringe with pressure monitoring capabilities. Each type of balloon has its own unique burst pressure, which should not be exceeded during balloon inflation. For simple angioplasty, this detail is usually not that critical, as balloon rupture is usually of no consequence and it may be necessary to exceed burst pressure by 25 to 50% to dilate resistant lesions. Selection of the appropriately sized balloon is important to successful angioplasty. This aspect is somewhat dependent upon knowledge surrounding the anatomical details of the fistula or graft and the size and location of the stenosis.

Our own experience over the last 5 years has revealed that overdilation, particularly of venous lesions, is crucial for long-term success. For example, most prosthetic AV grafts are constructed of 6-mm polytetrafluoroethylene, with a slight bevel cut in the graft at the venous anastomosis resulting in an anastomostic opening of 1 to 2 cm. To adequately dilate a stenosis at the venous anastomosis requires balloon diameters of at least 8 or 9 mm (Figure 8.2). We have found most consistent success when 9-mm balloons are used on venous lesions in the periphery and 9- to 12-mm balloons for angioplasty of central venous lesions. For arterial anatomostic lesions, however, balloons on the order of 5 or 6 mm are usually adequate to dilate arterial or arterial anastomotic stenoses. Finally, for intragraft lesions, 7- or 8-mm balloons usually suffice.

At the conclusion of the angioplasty procedure, completion fistulography should confirm a widely patent access with brisk flow throughout if the intervention was successful. The measurement of pressure gradients across lesions in AV access grafts provides another method to assess the effectiveness of angioplasty. Focal gradients should be virtually eliminated with effective angioplasty; however, an inherent pressure drop across the length of the graft of 75 to 80% of systemic pressure should be expected (10). Any residual focal pressure gradient should prompt repeat angioplasty with upsizing of the balloon by 1 mm (Table 8.1).

The principal debate in the field of dialysis access management revolves around the most effective method for treating a failing access site: percutaneous angioplasty versus surgical revision. The superiority of either approach over the other can be rationalized by reviewing the available literature from different perspectives. In reality, the two procedures should be considered complementary and not exclusionary. The method chosen often depends upon factors specific to the dialysis practice, such as caseload and local expertise with the available treatment options. Cumulative primary patency following percutaneous angioplasty of failing AV grafts at 6 months is on the order of 60% (4–9,12). Failures are largely due to recurrence of the stenosis at the site of angioplasty, which is often amenable to retreatment. Secondary patency rates for balloon angioplasty of access-site stenoses on the order of 80% at 12 months have been achieved (13). The main advantages of simple balloon angioplasty alone of failing access sites are the preservation of venous positions for future fistulae or grafts and the ability to prolong access patency with a simple outpatient procedure. These specific

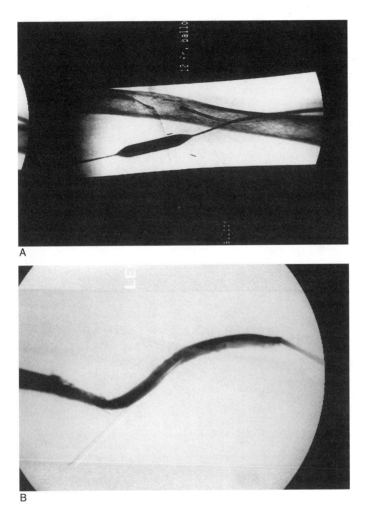

FIGURE 8.2 A and B. Balloon angioplasty of venous stenosis seen in Figure 8.1 with 9-mm balloon.

benefits are difficult to glean from the available literature and are largely recognized based upon the authors' experience with over 1500 treatments. These benefits may be negated in the setting of access-site thrombosis or when more complicated interventions, such as endovascular stents, are required to salvage the access site, as discussed in later sections of this chapter.

TABLE 8.1 Treatment of Stenosis Without Thrombosis in Dialysis AV Grafts and Primary AV Fistulae

---

Stenosis Treatment

1. Stenoses that occur in a dialysis AV graft or primary AV fistula (venous outflow or arterial inflow) should be treated with percutaneous transluminal angioplasty or surgical revision if the stenosis is >50% of the lumen diameter and is associated with the following clinical/physiological abnormalities: (a) Previous thrombosis in the access, (b) Elevated venous dialysis pressure, (c) Abnormal urea or other recirculation measurements, (d) Abnormal physical findings, (e) Unexplained decrease in measurement of dialysis dose, and (f) Decreasing access flow.
2. Each dialysis center should determine which procedure (angioplasty versus surgical revision) is best for the patient based on the expertise at that center.
3. Stenosis, as well as the clinical parameters used to detect it, should return to acceptable limits following intervention.

Stenosis Treatment Outcomes

1. Centers should monitor stenosis treatment outcomes on the basis of patency. Reasonable patency goals (for the center as a whole) for PTA and surgical revision in the absence of thrombosis are (a) PTA—50% unassisted patency[a] at 6 months, no more than 30% residual stenosis postprocedure, and resolution of physical indicator(s) of stenosis and (b) surgical revision—50% unassisted patency at 1 year.
2. If angioplasty is required more than two times within 3 months, the patient should be referred for surgical revision if such an option is available and if the patient is a good surgical candidate.
3. Stents are useful in selected instances (e.g., limited residual access sites, surgically inaccessible lesions, contraindication to surgery) when PTA fails.

---

[a] Unassisted patency is defined as patency until either thrombosis or access failure occurs or an intervention to prevent thrombosis is performed.
Source: Modified from Ref. 11, Guideline 19.

TREATMENT OF THROMBOSED ACCESS SITES

Once a dialysis access site has failed and progressed to thrombosis, salvage of the fistula becomes more difficult. Patients who are medically unstable and in need of dialysis must undergo placement of a jugular catheter, with its attendant risks, to accomplish temporary dialysis until permanent access can be reestablished. Percutaneous methods to treat thrombosed fistulae and grafts incorporate the balloon angioplasty techniques previously discussed. In addition, thrombectomy of the graft or fistula must be achieved, either with mechanical or pharmaceutical techniques or combinations of these modalities (pharmacomechanical approaches) (Table 8.2).

TABLE 8.2   Treatment of Thrombosis and Associated Stenosis in Dialysis AV
Grafts

Thrombosis of an AV graft should be corrected with surgical thrombectomy or
with pharmacomechanical or mechanical thrombolysis. The choice of technique
to treat thrombosis should be based on the expertise of the center. However, it
is essential that:
1.   Treatment be performed rapidly following detection of thrombosis so as to
     minimized the need for temporary access. (No more than one and prefera-
     bly no femoral vein catheterization should be required.)
2.   The access be evaluated by fistulogram for residual stenosis postproce-
     dure.
3.   Residual stenosis be corrected be angioplasty or surgical correction. Out-
     flow venous stenoses are present in >85% of instances of thrombosis; the
     need for PTA or surgical revision is expected in most instances.
4.   The procedure be performed on an outpatient basis under local anesthesia.
     Access revision may require up to a 24-h observation to evaluate swelling
     and steal.
5.   Monitoring tests used to screen for venous obstruction should return to nor-
     mal following intervention.
6.   Centers should monitor outcome results on the basis of patency. Minimum
     reasonable goals (for the center as a whole) for percutaneous thrombolysis
     and surgical revision thrombectomy should be (a) Percutaneous thromboly-
     sis with PTA—40% unassisted patency and functionality at 3 months, (b)
     Surgical thrombectomy and revision—50% unassisted patency and function-
     ality at 6 months and 40% unassisted patency and functionality at 1 year,
     (c) For both techniques—immediate patency, defined as patency to the
     next dialysis session, of 85%.

Source: Modified from Ref. 11, Guideline 21.

Pharmaceutical Thrombectomy

Infusion Thrombolysis

Dissolution of occluding thrombus in AV access grafts and fistulae using thrombolytic agents was first described in the mid-1980s. Streptokinase was the agent
utilized in the early reports from Klimas et al. (14) and Young et al. (15). These
previous reports combined direct infusion of the lytic agent with external massage
of the access site and, not surprisingly, had relatively poor success rates around
50%. As in the scenario of arterial thrombosis, urokinase has now become the
lytic agent of choice for managing dialysis access thrombosis. In comparison to
streptokinase, urokinase has a shorter half-life, lacks antigenicity, and is associated with significantly fewer systemic hemorrhagic complications. Repeated
treatments can be given with no fear of anaphylaxis. Difficulty arises in compar-

ing series of thrombosed fistulae treated with thrombolysis because of the various techniques use to deliver the lytic agent.

Early experience with thrombolysis of AV fistulae relied upon infusion techniques to deliver the lytic agent. This methodology was the purest form of pharmaceutical thrombectomy, as no mechanical manipulation of the thrombus took place. Infusions of urokinase ranging from 60,000 to 500,000 U/h resulted in successful lysis in up to 93% of cases. However, this often required prolonged overnight infusions and observation in an intensive care setting. Thus, the infusion technique was associated with considerable cost both for the amount of urokinase required for successful lysis and the associated hospitalization (16,17). Any perceived benefit of the percutaneous technique was negated by these factors in studies comparing thrombolysis to surgical thrombectomy.

Pulse-Spray Thrombolysis

The drawbacks of the infusion technique—namely, costs for the lytic agent and time required for successful lysis—stimulated the evolution of the pulse-spray method of thrombolysis (18). Various permutations of the pulse-spray technique account for the most common method of percutaneous thrombectomy of dialysis grafts practiced today.

The basic premise of the pulse-spray technique is to rapidly deliver a high concentration of lytic agent throughout the entire length of the clot burden. This is accomplished using the crossed-catheter technique. Briefly, one catheter is placed in the arterial limb of the graft and directed toward the venous outflow while the other is placed in the venous limb of the graft and directed toward the arterial inflow (Figure 8.3). If balloon angioplasty or mechanical manipulation is contemplated, appropriately sized sheaths should be placed (arterial 5F, venous 7F). Care must be taken not to forcibly dislodge clot from the arterial limb into the native arterial tree with either catheter manipulation or contrast "test" injections into the thrombosed graft. Catheters with multiple side holes, such as the Mewisson (Meditech Inc., Watertown, MA) or the Cook multiside-hole infusion catheter (Cook Inc., Bloomington, IN), are used to assure drug delivery throughout the length of the thrombus. Once flow is reestablished through the fistula, resolution of residual thrombus is hastened by either massaging the fistula or performing "balloon angioplasty" of residual areas of thrombus (Figure 8.4). These mechanical techniques further disrupt adherent clot, exposing more thrombus to the lytic agent and thereby facilitating complete lysis. At the conclusion of the thrombolytic session, residual areas of graft, anastomotic, or venous stenosis are subsequently treated with balloon angioplasty, as previously described.

The combination of a lytic agent, pulse-spray delivery techniques, and clot maceration, either manually or with balloon catheters, results in a pharmacomechanical system to effectively declot access fistulae (19). Unlike the simple infusion technique, pharmacomechanical thrombectomy is rapid and uses much less lytic

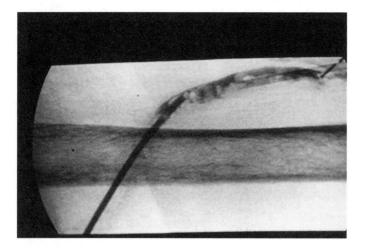

FIGURE 8.3 Crossed-catheter technique for pulse-spray thrombolysis of an occluded arteriovenous graft.

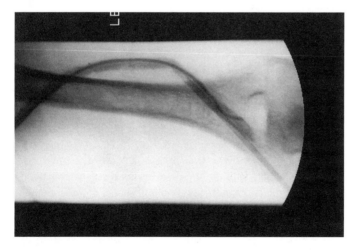

FIGURE 8.4 Successful pharmacomechanical treatment of a thrombosed arteriovenous access graft.

agent. Most patients are successfully treated on an outpatient basis with a procedure time of 30 to 90 min. In contrast to lytic infusion alone, pulse-spray techniques attain more reliable success rates that parallel surgical thrombectomy. Initial clinical success rates on the order of 80 to 95% have been reported using the crossed-catheter technique with pulse-spray delivery of urokinase in the series reported by Brunner et al. (20), Roberts et al. (21), and Cohen et al. (22). Moreover, pharmacomechanical thrombolysis combined with balloon angioplasty of uncovered stenotic lesions has been shown to be less costly yet equally effective in prolonging access function as compared with surgical thrombectomy/revision in the series reported by Sands et al. (23) and Schwartz et al. (24). In a retrospective review of 71 thrombolysis procedures and 75 surgical thrombectomies, Sands et al. (23) demonstrated equivalent technical success and 6-month patency in each group. Total cost for the surgery group exceeded that for the thrombosis group by a significant amount ($12,740 vs. $6802, $p = 0.018$). Unfortunately, meager results have been obtained in native AV fistulas with the pulse-spray technique. Clinical success ranging from 48 to 59% has been reported in limited series by Gmelin et al. (13) and Kumpe et al. (25).

The recent withdrawal of urokinase from the United States market by Abbott Laboratories has forced physicians who manage thrombosed access sites to rely on either mechanical means to declot grafts or the selective use of tissue plasminogen activator (TPA) or a related compound as a substitute lytic agent. Too few series using this agent have been reported to adequately assess efficacy for this application (26).

Percutaneous Mechanical Thrombectomy

A further effort to increase the overall effectiveness of percutaneous interventions for thrombosed AV grafts resulted in the development of the percutaneous mechanical thrombectomy technique for clotted AV grafts (3,27,28). This technique achieves rapid resolution of occluding thrombus without the expense of thrombolytic agents.

Percutaneous mechanical thrombectomy is accomplished using the crossed-catheter technique previously described. The procedure begins by placing a balloon catheter through the sheath inserted into the arterial limb of the graft. Both balloon angioplasty catheters and Fogarty embolectomy catheters can be utilized. With the catheter in place in the venous limb, the balloon is inflated and the catheter advanced through the venous limb and into the venous outflow. This maneuver effectively pushes the occlusive thrombus through the venous outflow and into the central venous circulation. Once the venous limb is clear of thrombus and any uncovered stenotic lesions have been treated with balloon angioplasty, attention is turned to declotting the arterial limb. A balloon catheter is advanced from the sheath placed into the venous limb retrograde through the arterial anastomosis. The balloon is inflated and pulled back across the arterial anastomosis, thereby dislodging the thrombus plug characteristic of this site. As the catheter is withdrawn across the arterial anastomosis, flow is reestablished in the graft and any residual loose debris is carried out the venous outflow.

Published experience with percutaneous mechanical thrombectomy is somewhat limited to date. Trerotola et al. (27), authors of one of the earliest reports, achieved an initial clinical success in 84% of the 34 clotted grafts treated in this fashion. Middlebrook et al. (28) compared percutaneous mechanical thrombectomy to pulse-spray thrombolysis. There was no significant difference in the initial clinical success (88 vs. 90%), patency at 3 months (30 vs. 40%), or patency at 12 months (8 vs. 13%) for 33 clotted ePTFE AV grafts treated with percutaneous mechanical thrombectomy compared with 30 grafts treated with pulse-spray thrombolysis, respectively. Beathard et al. (3) combined mechanical thrombectomy with pulse-spray thrombolysis in their series of 103 patients with clotted AV grafts. An initial clinical success rate of 93% was reported in that study, in which 55 grafts were pretreated with heparinized saline and 58 were pretreated with urokinase and heparin prior to mechanical thrombectomy. No significant difference was demonstrated between the urokinase group and the heparinized saline group, implying that use of a lytic agent was unnecessary in accomplishing effective graft declotting. The exact role that percutaneous mechanical thrombectomy will play in access graft management remains to be defined. The obvious concern with respect to creating iatrogenic pulmonary emboli is addressed in the subsequent section.

Recently, a number of new catheters have been introduced that macerate the clot through either a vortex of fluid or mechanical means and permit evacuation of the material, thereby avoiding embolization of large volumes of thrombus (29). None of the available devices addresses the dense plug of thrombus usually seen at the arterial anastomosis of a thrombosed AV access. If treated exclusively through percutaneous means, the plug is still addressed with balloon dislodgement and embolization into the venous circulation.

COMPLICATIONS OF PERCUTANEOUS THROMBOLYSIS

As one might expect, the most common complication associated with the use of lytic agents for fistula declotting is extravasation and hematoma at the access site. This can occur either around the diagnostic and therapeutic catheterization position or, more commonly, at needle puncture sites from recent hemodialysis (21,22). Local bleeding problems were more likely to be seen with prolonged infusion techniques. However, the rapidity of clot clearing seen with pulse-spray techniques has minimized the probability of this complication. Simple tamponade with manual pressure usually suffices to prevent an expanding hematoma from forming while the procedure is completed. Patients are observed at the conclusion of any percutaneous procedures for hemostasis to assure that no significant bleeding occurs at the access site prior to discharge.

Significant bleeding remote from the site of intervention—gastrointestinal, intracranial, or retroperitoneal—is rare particularly when the pulse-spray methodology is applied (15,21). Though not indicated for therapeutic intervention for fresh grafts that thrombose within the first few weeks, thrombolysis can be safely performed to define the precipitating lesion and the venous outflow anatomy without significant bleeding complications. Complications related to balloon angioplasty of AV access sites are similarly infrequent, with most series reporting less than a 5% incidence (12,13,30,31). Disruption of either an anastomosis or a native artery or vein is the most commonly reported complication (Figure 8.5). Anastomotic disruption generally requires surgical revision. Disruption of an outflow vein can often be treated with compression. Once fistula patency is reestablished, extravasation from the vein disruption ceases without requiring further intervention.

With the evolution of percutaneous mechanical thrombectomy techniques, embolization into both the arterial and central venous/pulmonary circulations has become a primary concern. Embolization into the arterial runoff distal to an AV fistula occurs in less than 3% of treatments and is usually detected at the time of completion fistulography. These emboli are usually amenable to treatment with direct intraarterial infusion of a thrombolytic agent (19). Long-term ischemic complications related to repeated percutaneous treatment of thrombosed AV access sites are unusual.

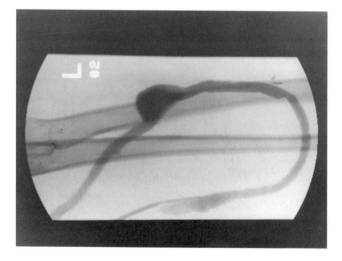

FIGURE 8.5   False aneurysm of a venous anastomosis resulting from balloon angioplasty of a stenosis.

Significant concern has been expressed over the creation of iatrogenic pulmonary emboli with percutaneous mechanical thrombectomy techniques (32,33). The creation of a pulmonary embolus is prerequisite for successful percutaneous graft thrombectomy. The clinical significance of these iatrogenic emboli is poorly understood. The incidence of clinically apparent pulmonary embolism in the available literature is low. In the series by Middlebrook et al. (28) comparing mechanical thrombectomy to pulse-spray thrombolysis, no clinically apparent episodes of pulmonary embolization occurred. They argued that the actual volume of clot occupying an AV graft is low (8 to 11 mL) and would not be expected to cause significant cardiopulmonary compromise. The only other published experience with pure percutaneous mechanical thrombectomy, by Trerotola et al. (27), failed to identify clinical pulmonary emboli in any of the 34 patients treated. However, both studies relied only upon clinical factors to identify patients with pulmonary embolism.

Our own experience with 43 clotted AV access grafts provides some further insight into this problem (33). Despite clinical success of restoring access patency in 95% of 43 patients, 2 patients succumbed to pulmonary embolization. Post-treatment perfusion lung scans were obtained in 22 patients and demonstrated findings consistent with pulmonary embolism in 59%. Our technique was not purely mechanical, but combined pulse-spray thrombolysis with balloon thrombectomy. Clearly, percutaneous mechanical thrombectomy is contraindicated in patients with severe underlying cardiopulmonary disease. Along with the selection/exclusion criteria for this treatment modality, the impact of repeated pulmonary embolization in these patients, who often require multiple treatments over their dialysis lifetime, remains ill defined.

ENDOVASCULAR STENTS IN DIALYSIS ACCESS SALVAGE

The first description of an endovascular stent that could be inserted from a site remote from its final location appeared in 1969 by Dotter (34). Stents are designed to function as an endoskeleton and provide supportive expansion to diseased vessels. The wide success realized by the Palmaz stent (Johnson & Johnson) in the iliac arteries, either following or in combination with balloon angioplasty, has equaled the results of surgical intervention in this vascular bed (35). The use of stents in treating AV access pathology has not achieved a similar level of success.

One of the earliest reports describing the placement of commercially available endovascular stents in dialysis access patients was that of Gross et al. (36). They placed stainless steel Gianturco stents in 13 dialysis patients, 8 with central vein stenosis and 5 with peripheral vein stenosis. Of 13 procedures, 11 were initially successful and remained patent for a mean of 8 months. By far the largest experience with endovascular stents in dialysis patients involves the use of the

Wallstent (Schneider, Minneapolis, MN) (37–40). The experience of Hood and associates is representative of the prevailing prejudice. They placed 19 Wallstents and 1 Palmaz stent in 14 access sites: 9 peripheral venous outflow, 7 venous anastomosis, 3 central venous outflow, and 1 intragraft. Mean patency of the stented segments was on the order of 6 months. Central venous sites (7.3 months) did better than either peripheral venous (5 months) or venous anastomoses (1.8 months). Restenosis occurred in 25% of the peripheral venous or venous anastomosis stents and in none of the subclavian vein stents during the follow-up period.

Our own experience with endovascular stents for fistula salvage parallels that in the literature. We have used Wallstents to treat refractory stenoses in 18 patients (unpublished data). The majority of these stents were placed at the venous anastomosis bridging the axillobrachial venous segment in 15 patients with upper arm AV grafts (Figure 8.6). Follow-up was available for 9 of 15 patients, with a mean patency of 5 months. An additional 3 patients with forearm loop grafts had stents placed in either the basilic vein outflow (1), the cephalic vein outflow (1), or at the venous anastomosis with the antecubital-cephalic vein (1). Mean stent patency in this small subgroup was 3.75 months. One patient with an upper arm graft in place underwent multiple angioplasties and stent placements resulting in the complete lining of the graft with Wallstents (Figure 8.7). This patient continued to receive dialysis through the stented portion of the access for 12 months.

The poor overall results obtained with endovascular stenting of dialysis access stenoses are not surprising when one considers the pathology. Venous anastomotic and outflow stenoses resulting from a patent AV fistula or graft comprise the most resilient forms of neointimal hyperplasia (41). This somewhat accounts for the theoretical benefit of stent placement to provide an endoskeletal support against the elastic recoil of the stenotic lesion. However, in the small-diameter peripheral veins and at sites of anastomosis, recurrent stenosis within the stented segment has evolved as the limiting factor. Retreatment with balloon angioplasty provides a means to maintain patency of these peripheral segments, though cumulative assisted rates vary between 20 and 70% (39,42). Because of the larger size of the central veins, more tolerance exists to the development of hyperplasia before a hemodynamically significant stenosis results. This may explain the improved results of endovascular stenting of central lesions compared with peripheral lesions (39,40). Furthermore, options for treating central lesions are limited, with significant morbidity associated with surgical approaches. Rather than abandoning the extremity as an access site, stenting of central venous stenoses may prolong the useful life of the access.

The available endovascular stents are not without their own inherent design characteristics, which favors one over the other in the specific application of dialysis access stenoses. The Palmaz stent requires a balloon to expand and deploy it within the vessel. It has no inherent recoil; therefore it is susceptible to

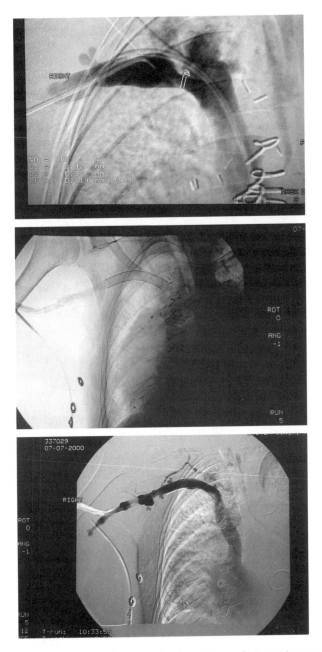

FIGURE 8.6   A to C. Wallstent placement in the axillary vein to treat venous anastomotic stenosis.

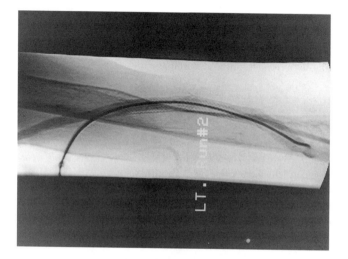

FIGURE 8.7   Upper arm graft with near completely lining of Wallstents. This patient continued to have dialysis for 12 months through this access site.

crushing when exposed to extrinsic compression and may migrate without intrinsic vessel pathology to fixate against (43,44). Its rigidity also makes it unsuitable for locations that require flexibility. These specific attributes, which are paramount in dealing with venous stenoses, are addressed nicely by the self-expanding Wallstent and argue for its preeminent role in vascular access applications today. However, the Wallstent has less hoop strength and, in stenotic lesions that demonstrate a large amount of elastic recoil, the stent's lumen may be compromised.

Precise indications for the placement of an endovascular stent within the vasculature of an AV access graft are not yet available. No study to date has compared primary stenting with balloon angioplasty in the treatment of venous outflow lesions. In the periphery, where surgical revision is associated with little morbidity other than consumption of venous "real estate," poor results with

TABLE 8.3   Treatment of Central Vein Stenosis

1. Percutaneous intervention with transluminal angioplasty is the preferred treatment for central vein stenosis.
2. Stent placement combined with angioplasty is indicated in elastic central vein stenosis or if a stenosis recurs within a 3-month period.

Source: Modified from Ref. 11, Guideline 20.

stenting do not justify the present cost of nearly $1000 per device. This is in contrast to the circumstance of central venous stenosis, where more favorable results with angioplasty and stenting justify the added expense in light of the limitations of the available options to otherwise manage these lesions (Table 8.3).

REFERENCES

1. Windus DW. Permanent vascular access: A nephrologist's view. Am J Kidney Dis 21:457–471, 1993.
2. Brescia MJ, Cimino JE, Appel K, Hurwish BJ. Chronic hemodialysis using venipuncture and a surgically created arteriovenous fistula. N Engl J Med 275:1089–1092, 1966.
3. Beathard GA. Mechanical versus pharmacomechanical thrombolysis for the treatment of thrombosed dialysis access grafts. Kidney Int 45:1401–1406, 1994.
4. Beathard GA. Percutaneous transvenous angioplasty in the treatment of vascular access stenosis. Kidney Int 42:1390–1397, 1992.
5. Brooks JL, Sigley RD, May KJ Jr, Mack RM. Transluminal angioplasty versus surgical repair for stenosis of hemodialysis grafts: A randomized study. Am J Surg 153:530–531, 1987.
6. Daput O, Feurstein M, Rendl KH, Prenner K. Transluminal angioplasty versus conventional operation in the treatment of hemodialysis fistula stenosis: Results from a 5-year study. Br J Surg 74:1004–1005, 1987.
7. Kanterman RY, Vesely TM, Pilgram TK, et al. Dialysis access grafts: Anatomic location of venous stenosis and results of angioplasty. Radiology 195:135–139, 1995.
8. Schwab SJ, Raymond JR, Saeed M, et al. Prevention of hemodialysis fistula thrombosis. Early detection of venous stenosis. Kidney Int 36:707–711, 1989.
9. Sands JJ, Young S, Miranda CL. The effect of Doppler flow screening studies and elective revision on dialysis access failure. ASAIOJ 38:M524–M527, 1992.
10. Sullivan KL, Besarab A, Bonn J, et al. Hemodynamics of failing dialysis grafts. Radiology 186:867–872, 1993.
11. NKF-DOQI. Clinical Practice Guidelines for Vascular Access. New York: National Kidney Foundation; 1997.
12. Saeed M, Newman GE, McCann RL, et al. Stenoses in dialysis fistulas: Treatment with percutaneous angioplasty. Radiology 164:693–697, 1987.
13. Gmelin E, Winterhoff R, Rinast E. Insufficient hemodialysis access fistulas: Late results of treatment with percutaneous balloon angioplasty. Radiology 171:657, 1989.
14. Klimas VA, Denny KM, Paganini EP, et al. Low dose streptokinase therapy for thrombosed arteriovenous fistulas. Trans Am Soc Artif Intern Organs 30:511, 1984.
15. Young AT, Hunter DW, Castaneda-Zuniga WR, et al. Thrombosed synthetic hemodialysis access fistulas: Failure of fibrolytic therapy. Radiology 154:639–642, 1985.
16. Schuman E, Quinn S, Standage B, Gross G. Thrombolysis versus thrombectomy for occluded hemodialysis grafts. Am J Surg 167:473–476, 1994.

17. Summers S, Drazan K, Gomes A, Freischlag J. Urokinase therapy for thrombosed hemodialysis access grafts. Surg Gynecol Obstet 176:534–538, 1993.
18. Bookstein JJ, Saldinger E. Accelerated thrombolysis: In vitro evaluation of agents and methods of administration. Invest Radiol 20:7331, 1985.
19. Valji K, Bookstein JJ, Roberts AC, Davis GB. Pharmacomechanical thrombolysis and angioplasty in the management of clotted hemodialysis grafts: Early and late clinical results. Radiology 178:243–247, 1991.
20. Brunner MC, Matalon TA, Patel SK, Ultrarapid urokinase in hemodialysis access occlusion. J Vasc Intervent Radiol 2:503–506, 1991.
21. Roberts AC, Valji K, Bookstein JJ, Hye RJ. Pulse-spray pharmacomechanical thrombolysis for treatment of thrombosed dialysis access grafts. Am J Surg 166:221–225, 1993.
22. Cohen MAH et al. Improved treatment of thrombosed hemodialysis access sites with thrombolysis and angioplasty. Kidney Int 46:1375, 1994.
23. Sands JJ, Patel S, Plaviak DJ, Miranda CL. Pharmacomechanical thrombolysis with urokinase for treatment of thrombosed hemodialysis access grafts: A comparison with surgical thrombectomy. ASAIO J 40:M886–M888, 1994.
24. Schwartz CI, McBrayer CV, Sloan JH. Thrombosed dialysis grafts: Comparison of treatment with transluminal angioplasty and surgical revision. Radiology 194:337–341, 1995.
25. Kumpe DA, Durham JD, Mann DJ. Thrombolysis and percutaneous transluminal angioplasty. In Wilson SE, ed. Vascular Access. Principles and Practice, 3rd ed. St. Louis: Mosby–Year Book, 1996:239–261.
26. Andriani M, Drago G, Bernardi AM, et al. Recombinant tissue plasminogen activator (rt-PA) as first-line therapy for declotting of haemodialysis access. Nephrol Dial Transplant 1995; 10:1714–1719.
27. Trerotola SO, Lund GB, Scheel PJ Jr, et al. Thrombosed dialysis access grafts: Percutaneous mechanical declotting without urokinase. Radiology 191:721–726, 1994.
28. Middlebrook MR, Amygdalos MA, Soulen MC, et al. Thrombosed hemodialysis grafts: Percutaneous mechanical balloon declotting versus thrombolysis. Radiology 196:73–77, 1995.
29. Lazzaro CR, Trerotola SO, Shah H, et al. Modified use of the Arrow-Trerotola percutaneous thrombolytic device for the treatment of thrombosed hemodialysis access grafts. J Vasc Intervent Radiol 10:1025–1031, 1999.
30. Glanz S, Gordon DH, Butt KMH, et al. The role of percutaneous angioplasty in the management of chronic hemodialysis fistulas. Ann Surg 206:777–781, 1987.
31. Hunter DW, So SK, Castaneda-Zuniga WR, et al. Failing or thrombosed Brescia-Cimino arteriovenous dialysis fistulas: Angiographic evaluation and percutaneous transluminal angioplasty. Radiology 149:105–109, 1983.
32. Dolmatch BL, Gray RJ, Horton KM. Will iatrogenic pulmonary embolization be our pulmonary embarrassment? Radiology 191:615–617, 1994.
33. Swan TL, Smyth SH, Ruffenach SJ, et al. Pulmonary embolism following hemodialysis access thrombolysis/thrombectomy. J Vasc Intervent Rad 6:683–686, 1995.
34. Dotter CT. Transluminally placed coilspring endarterial tube grafts. Long-term patency in canine popliteal artery. Invest Radiol 4:329–332, 1969.
35. Palmaz JC, Laborde JC, Rivera FJ, et al. Stenting of the iliac arteries with the Palmaz

stent: Experience from a multicenter trial. Cardiovasc Intervent Radiol 15:291–297, 1992.

36. Gross GF, Quinn SF, Standage BA, et al. Endovascular stents in hemodialysis patients. In Sommer BG, Henry ML, eds. Vascular Access for Hemodialysis-II. Chicago: Gore; 1991:209–211.

37. Hood DB, Yellin AE, Richman MF, et al. Hemodialysis graft salvage with endoluminal stents. Am Surg 60:733–737, 1994.

38. Gray RJ, Horton KM, Dolmatch BL, et al. Use of Wallstents foe hemodialysis access-related venous stenoses and occlusions untreatable with balloon angioplasty. Radiology 195:479–484, 1995.

39. Quinn SF, Schuman ES, Hall L, et al. Venous stenoses in patients who undergo hemodialysis: Treatment with self-expandable endovascular stents. Radiology 183:499–504, 1992.

40. Vorwerk D, Guenther RW, Mann H, et al. Venous stenosis and occlusion in hemodialysis shunts: Follow-up results of stent placement in 65 patients. Radiology 195:140–146, 1995.

41. Swedberg SH, Brown BG, Sigley RT, et al. Intimal fibromuscular hyperplasia at the venous anastomosis of PTFE grafts in hemodialysis patients. Circulation 80:1726–1736, 1989.

42. Beathard GA. Gianturco self-expanding stent in the treatment of stenosis in dialysis access grafts. Kidney Int 43:872–877, 1993.

43. Gray RJ, Dolmatch BL, Horton KM, et al. Migration of Palmaz stents following deployment for venous stenoses related to hemodialysis access. J Vasc Intervent Radiol 5:117–120, 1994.

44. Bjarnason H, Hunter DW, Crain MR, et al. Collapse of a Palmaz stent in the subclavian vein. Am J Roentgenol 160:1123–1124, 1993.

II

Dialysis Access Complications

9

Current Concepts in Dialysis Access Failure

Stuart K. Williams
The University of Arizona, Tucson, Arizona

Bruce E. Jarrell
The University of Maryland, Baltimore, Maryland

The creation of acceptable vascular access conduits does not always result in permanent access availability because of numerous complications. Difficulties in maintaining vascular access are often called the Achilles' heel of dialysis. A full understanding of the etiology of access failure requires an evaluation of numerous factors, including patient demographics, fistula type, and patient compliance with fistula care. The cost of failed access grafts is staggering, both in regard to patient morbidity (dialysis access complications are generally believed to be the cause of at least 25% of the hospitalizations of dialysis patients) and cost (1,2). The annual cost of revising failed or failing vascular access in the United States is in excess of $500 million (3). Before discussing the mechanisms underlying the failure of vascular access grafts an evaluation of the extent of failure through review of patency rates is enlightening.

PATENCY RATES IN DIALYSIS ACCESS

A large number of studies from numerous institutions around the world have now been published that provide information on the observed patency of both AV fistulas and AV grafts (4–27). This information must be evaluated cautiously, since significant differences in studies are inherent, including the definition of patency, patient demographics, anatomic site, and type of access, to name a few. The optimal analysis of access failure would be an evaluation of the intervention-free period with correction for life expectancy of the patient population (28). Unfortunately, few reports provide adequate information to complete a totally unambiguous analysis of access patency. Not all investigators reporting primary and secondary patency rates conform to the same standards of definition of a failed dialysis fistula or graft. For this reason the expected primary and secondary patency rates for fistulae and grafts can only be estimated within a range established by complete review of the literature. Nevertheless, general conclusions have been drawn regarding the initial and long-term patency that can be expected from different access methods. Moreover, these patency data have provided benchmarks for comparison to evaluate quality control in dialysis clinics and provide criteria for access selection based upon comorbidities such as diabetes and age. The National Kidney Fondation Dialysis Outcomes Quality Initiatives (DOQI) provide standards for early patency but appropriately do not establish guidelines for cumulative long-term patency.

Early Primary Patency (30 Days)

The primary AV fistula, constructed using the cephalic vein, historically provides the lowest incidence of early failure. One-month patency for Cimino fistulae has been reported to be between 97 (29) and 87% (30). One-month patency for synthetic grafts is generally in a similar range when reported (8). DOQI standards have been recommended for 1-month patency of AV grafts, based on placement site, ranging from 95% for upper arm grafts and 90% for forearm loop grafts to 85% for forearm straight grafts. As discussed above, DOQI guidelines are not stated for primary AV fistulae.

Based simply on patency considerations, the 1-month results appear equivocal. However, time to maturation is a major factor distinguishing native AV fistulae from AV grafts. Native fistulae show a site-specific difference in failure due to lack of maturation, with the highest incidence of failure to mature in primary radiocephalic AV fistulae. Nonmaturation rates for radiocephalic AV fistulae have been reported to be as high as 70% (31). In general, it can be estimated that 20 to 25% of native fistulae will fail due to inability to mature. Porous synthetic grafts, while not requiring a maturation period, do require a period for tissue ingrowth and stabilization of the graft material before first cannulation. The choice of synthetic over native fistulae should not be made on the basis of maturation alone due to the observed superiority of native fistulae with respect to long-term patency.

Long-Term Primary Patency

Numerous studies have now been completed comparing a variety of synthetic and native fistulae during long-term follow-up. Specific patency rates to be expected for different access types cannot be established due to differences in patient populations and technical expertise at various dialysis centers. A range of expected patency can be established based on findings from numerous groups (4–31). Cumulative primary patency rates for AV fistulae range from 60 to 75% at 1 year. Cumulative primary patency for ePTFE grafts at 1 year range from 60 to 85%. Two-year primary patency for these different access types are estimated to be 50 to 65% for native fistulae and 50 to 75% for synthetic grafts. While these numbers appear somewhat similar, it is critical to realize that native fistula failure includes the 20 to 25% of constructed fistulae that fail to mature. Correction for non-maturation provides evidence of the superior long-term patency of native fistulae.

Secondary Patency Rates

Failure of access devices is commonplace, with 0.5 to 0.8 episodes of access failure per patient-year on dialysis (32). Repair of the access to restore appropriate blood flow designates the beginning of a phase of secondary patency. Quite often investigators suggest that this phase be designated as assisted primary patency; however, this label is incorrect and misleading. Secondary patency is most accurately defined as beginning at the time a fistula or graft is subjected to intervention to correct a defect, leading to restoration of maximal blood flow. Secondary patency rates for repaired AV fistulae range from 60 to 90% at 1 year to 45 to 80% at 3 years. Secondary patency of ePTFE AV grafts ranges from 65 to 95% at 1 year to 40 to 75% at 3 years. No significant differences in secondary patency have been established between native fistulae and synthetic grafts.

MECHANISMS OF ACCESS FAILURE

The mechanisms underlying the failure of dialysis accesses are extensive (Table 9.1). This list indicates the multitude of problems that can befall access devices and that call for some form of intervention. By far the most common mechanism of access failure is reported as thrombosis; however, the mechanism underlying this may involve one or more of the mechanisms listed in Table 9.1. Multiple dialysis center–based trials have been conducted to assess the mechanisms responsible for the loss of access availability. Again, it is reiterated that failure of an access site is not equivalent to loss of blood flow, since many access sites defined as failed continue to exhibit flow but at rates that do not support dialysis.

The list of mechanisms underlying access failure, illustrated in Table 9.1, can be organized into the three general categories of thrombosis, infection, and aneurysms. The relative incidence of these complications in native fistulae as compared with synthetic grafts is presented in Table 9.2. As is evident from this table and has previously been discussed, primary fistulae are subject to early failure due to nonmaturation and early thrombosis, while synthetic grafts are more prone to late failure due to cellular stenosis.

TABLE 9.1 Mechanisms Associated with the Failure of Vascular Access

Thrombosis	Graft erosion
Stenoses	Venous hypertension
Infection	Hypotension
Intimal hyperplasia/thickening	Operative complication
Turbulence	Insufficient wound healing response
Increased hematocrit	Physical constriction of graft
Fistula compression during sleep or following dialysis	Arterial steal necessitating revision
	Premature fistula cannulation
Prothrombogenic surface lack of or dysfunctional endothelium	Poor fistula cannulation technique
	Compliance mismatch
Aneurysm/pseudoaneurysm	Extremity edema
Intravascular volume depletion	Prolonged puncture bleeding
Coagulopathy	Prolonged/inappropriate pressure to control puncture bleeding

Risk Factors for Access Failure

Numerous risk factors have been evaluated to determine patient populations that may be predisposed to access failure. The possible risk factors and current results of clinical trials evaluating these factors and their association with failure are provided in Table 9.3. A caveat in this analysis is the occurrence of conflicting data in the analysis of many risk factors. Therefore the predictive values stated in this table are based on currently available data; the in-depth evaluation of these risk factors in large clinical trials is still necessary. In spite of these uncertainties, some relatively noncontroversial conclusions can be drawn. First, it is generally agreed that diabetic patients with dialysis access are more prone to hospitalization to reestablish access (33). Second, the nonwhite dialysis population is also at higher risk for hospitalization to repair dialysis access. Age at time of primary access placement indicates that patients <40 years old exhibit increased risk for

TABLE 9.2 Relative Incidence of Access Complications—Comparison Between Native Vessel Fistulas and Prosthetic Grafts

Failure to mature	Fistula > graft
Early thrombosis	Fistula > graft
Long-term stenosis	Graft > fistula
Infection	Graft > fistula
Aneurysm	Graft > fistula

TABLE 9.3 Risk Factors Studied for Effect on Primary
Access Patency—Predictive (PR) or Nonpredictive (NP)

Risk	Fistula	Graft
Age	NP	PR ($<$40 years)
Diabetes	NP/PR	PR
Race		PR
Peripheral vascular disease	PR	PR
Previously failed ePTFE	PR	PR
Congestive heart failure	NP	NP
Erythropoeitin use	NP	NP
Aspirin use	NP	NP
Platelet disorders	NP	NP
Graft blood flow	NP	$<$500 mL/min
Age and diabetes	PR	PR

prosthetic graft failure, suggesting the preferred use of native AV fistulae in younger patients. Finally, the concomitant risk factors of age ($>$65 years) and diabetes appear to be unequivocally associated with increased risk of access failure in both native fistulae and synthetic grafts (34). The remaining risk factors included in Table 9.3 but not firmly associated with access failure should still be considered in assessing possible mechanisms of failure and choice of access (35–37).

Thrombosis and Stenosis

The relationship between stenosis and thrombosis in identifying failure modes of vascular access devices is best described with respect to the time following access creation. Access failure during the first month after creation is almost universally considered to be technical in nature, blamed either on premature or incorrect use of the fistula or graft or technical errors in creation of the access. While technical errors are most often the cause of early access failure, certain patients are predisposed to early access failure. The etiology of this early failure remains elusive but is generally considered to be related to either a platelet, leukocyte, or coagulation disorder or a combination of these.

After the first month of maturation, the causes of graft thrombosis shift significantly toward the occurrence of narrowing of the vessel lumen, defined as stenosis. Complications due to technical errors during dialysis remain, as well as patient-related complications such as compression of the fistula or graft during rest. However, the most significant complication to appear progressively with time is the occurrence of intimal lesions, both within the fistulae and grafts as well as within the arterial and venous segments associated with synthetic grafts. The terminology for this anatomical stenosis is often confusing, utilizing many terms including *restenosis, intimal hyperplasia, intimal thickening, neointima formation, extracellular hypertrophy*, and *arterialization*. All these terms describe the same general series of cellular and extracellular events, which occur following the establishment of an access site. The corresponding native vessels undergo a response to injury, which in a significant number of patients results in an anatomical stenosis. The site of this stenosis is different in fistulae and grafts and is described separately. A common mechanism to describe the process of intimal thickening and thus providing a pharmacological target has not been universally accepted.

AV Graft Stenosis

Following implantation of a synthetic AV graft, numerous cellular responses are initiated at several sites including the (a) arterial anastomosis, (b) graft-tissue interface, (c) graft-blood interface, (d) venous anastomosis, and (e) vein segment distal to the anastomosis. The progressive nature of these cellular and extracellular responses lead to luminal lesions. The relative contribution of these lesions to the failure of AV grafts is illustrated in Table 9.4. It is generally agreed that over 80% of thrombosed or flow-impaired synthetic grafts result from luminal lesions, with a majority of these occurring at the venous anastomosis. When these lesions are removed during access repair and subsequently evaluated histologically, most pathologists will return a finding of proliferative intimal hyperplasia. The abundance of cells described as myofibroblasts in the lesion is also commonly noted by most pathology services. Immunocytochemical characterization of these myofibroblasts using antibodies directed against alpha smooth muscle cell actin often establishes the presence of numerous cells with varying degrees of reactivity with these antibodies. Based on multiple laboratory studies evaluating not only AV graft–derived lesions but also intimal lesions from angioplasty-

TABLE 9.4 Site of Stenosis in ePTFE AV Grafts

Arterial Anastomosis (%)	Midgraft (%)	Venous Anastomosis (%)	Distal Venous Graft (%)	None (%)
18	7	62	9	4
1	6	71	16	4
7	0	58	0	35

injured arteries, venous peripheral grafts, and coronary artery bypass grafts, smooth muscle cell proliferation and cell metabolism resulting in extracellular matrix production are considered major mechanisms underlying the development of all these lesions. Numerous other cells may participate in lesion development, and studies evaluating the role of inflammatory cells and angiogenesis (new blood vessel development) are ongoing.

The mechanisms that explain the development of intimal thickening in AV grafts specifically and injured blood vessels in general are understandably the focus of numerous laboratory-based studies (38). Therapies directed at restenosis following blood vessel injury are being assessed for their effect on AV graft stenosis. Numerous mechanisms are being addressed, including therapies directed against platelet activation, leukocyte binding and recruitment, coagulation proteins (including thrombin), cellular proliferation, matrix production, and angiogenesis. A pharmacological intervention remains a future goal and—based on the level of current efforts—will undoubtedly be achieved. To date, no definitive pharmacological interventions have proven effective and surgical and/or radiological interventions remain the only tools currently available to restore appropriate blood flow in compromised AV grafts.

AV Fistula Failure

The choice of autogenous fistulae as a primary access is comparatively small in the United States as compared with European surgical centers. For this reason extensive data evaluating the mechanisms of failure in AV fistulae is developed predominantly through European centers. The observation that an AV fistula fails to mature is based upon a lack of venous response to increased blood flow. The desired response is a gradual expansion of the inner diameter of the vein, often described as dilatation with concomitant thickening of the vessel wall. This adaptive response requires arterial segments with significant vascular tone to provide the enhanced flow rate necessary to deliver fistula flow >500 mL/min while maintaining distal tissue perfusion. Lack of distal perfusion is defined as vascular steal and accounts for a component of AV fistula failures. Venous segments must be of significant size and exhibit cellular integrity to respond to increased flow. Vein segments that are too tortuous or are compromised due to inherent pathology will not dilate. During the early phases of maturation, the venous segment is susceptible to thrombosis. This is due in part to the tendency to use fistulas too early, in the maturation process; however, it must also be considered that the intimal endothelium may be exhibiting a prothrombogenic condition due to the presence of extremely high flow. Unlike the case with AV grafts, the first few weeks following fistula construction are critical with respect to thrombosis. Once a fistula successfully matures, the occurrence of thrombosis is significantly lessened.

Infection

The infection rate associated with different access types is disparate, with synthetic AV grafts exhibiting a much higher incidence as compared with native fistulas. In addition to the rarity of infections in AV fistulae, the living nature of these vessels permits treatment with standard antibiotic regimens. On the other hand, infections of synthetic grafts are much more problematic and relatively resistant to antibiotic eradication. Although thrombosis remains the major cause of AV graft failure, infection has been estimated to account for approximately 20% of such failures (33,39). Often bacteremia in dialysis patients is the result of primary graft infection, but this cause is frequently overlooked due to the lack of a visible response at the graft site. Occasionally the occurrence of an abscess or pustule may be observed in association with the graft. The porous nature of ePTFE grafts provides an excellent environment for bacterial expansion, with the ability to cause metastatic infections at numerous other sites. The onset of septic pulmonary emboli, endocarditis, osteomyelitis, empyema, and meningitis due to primary graft infection must be evaluated.

The causative bacterium in AV graft infections is most often *Staphylococcus aureus*, followed in frequency by *Staphylococcus epidermidis* (40,41). Gram-negative bacterial infections may also occur. The route of entry for these bacteria is often difficult to identify. Patient-related factors such as poor hygiene and intravenous drug use are possible factors. Skin preparation and graft cannulation are also possible routes of entry. The time from primary graft inoculation with bacteria and the incidence of symptoms of bacteremia may be quite long, making a determination of cause impossible. Treatment of AV graft infections must be aggressive, with intravenous antibiotic therapy. Often segmental or total removal of the involved graft must be performed. Since infected grafts are predisposed to thrombosis and occasionally exhibit a catastrophic blowout at the anastomotic site, the removal of infected grafts and placement of a new access device at a remote site is not uncommon and often advisable.

Aneurysms and Pseudoaneurysms

Two terms are used to describe the pathological dilatation of access vessels. *Aneurysms* occasionally occur in fistulae due to vessel wall degeneration. The formation of true aneurysms in synthetic AV grafts is now relatively uncommon owing to the rigid walls of these grafts. AV grafts constructed using bovine heterografts may exhibit aneurysm formation requiring excision. The formation of *pseudoaneurysms* is not common, but when these occur, they are most often observed in association with needle puncture sites. Again, bovine heterografts are susceptible to pseudoaneurysm formation at sites of frequent puncture. Expanded PTFE grafts will infrequently develop pseudoaneurysms at puncture sites when dialysis personnel use the same site chronically. A distinction can be made between a pseudoaneurysm, defined as the presence of a pulsating noncoagulated blood-filled space external to a graft, and an external graft hematoma, which is undergoing tissue integration. A pseudoaneurysm will exhibit extravasation of angiographic medium into the extravascular tissue surrounding the graft. The graft itself maintains material integrity and the luminal diameter does not increase at the site of blood loss and coordinate hematoma formation. Of concern, a pseudoaneurysm may continue to progress with increased expansion of the lesion. Figure 9.1 illustrates an AV graft which, presumably due to multiple needle punctures, has formed a stable hematoma. In contrast to a pseudoaneurysm, where a continuum of noncoagulated blood occurs between the intravascular and extravascular compartments, this lesion exhibits a stable hematoma undergoing tissue incorporation. Over an extended period of time and without additional trauma to this area of the graft, this lesion is likely to resolve. Treatment of ePTFE pseudoaneurysms involves suture repair of small defects or interposition of a small segment of new graft when the involved area is more extensive.

While stenosis and infection account for the majority of access failures, Table 9.1 lists numerous other possible mechanisms leading to failure. The key to the maintenance of vascular access is a complete understanding of graft failure modalities and constant surveillance of graft function. Optimal surgical creation of an access site followed by a team approach to access maintenance will avoid many complications. The biological response to access creation is often not preventable, but accurate diagnosis of access deterioration will yield timely interven-

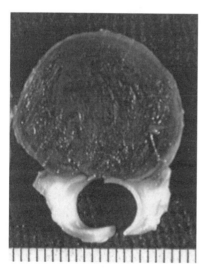

FIGURE 9.1   An AV graft that has formed a stable hematoma.

tion, resulting in prolonged assisted primary patency as well as prolonged secondary patency.

REFERENCES

1. Windus DW. Permanent vascular access: A nephrologist's view. Amer J Kid Dis. 21:457–471, 1993.
2. Bleyer AJ, Rocco MV Burkhart JM. The cost of hospitilizations due to hemodialysis access management. Nephrol News Issues 9:19–22, 1995.
3. Eggers PW. Internal Record HCFA 1992.
4. Wehrli H, Chenevard R, Zaruba K. Surgical experiences with the arteriovenous hemodialysis shunt (1970–1988). Helv Chir Acta 56:621–627, 1989.
5. Wellington JL. Expanded polytetrafluoroethylene prosthetic grafts for blood access in patients on dialysis. Can J Surg 21:420–422, 1978.
6. Wellington JL. Umbilical vein grafts for vascular access in patients on long-term dialysis. Can J Surg 24:608–609, 1981.
7. Taylor SM, Eaves GL, Weatherford DA, et al. Results and complications of arteriovenous access dialysis grafts in the lower extremity: A five year review. Am Surg 62:188–191, 1996.
8. Tordoir JH, Herman JM, Kwan TS, Diderich PM. Long-term follow-up of the polytetrafluoroethylene (PTFE) prosthesis as an arteriovenous fistula for haemodialysis. Eur J Vasc Surg 2(1):3–7, 1988.
9. Salmon PA. Vascular access for hemodialysis using bovine heterografts and polytetrafluoroethylene conduits. Can J Surg 24:59–63, 1981.
10. Munda R, First MR, Alexander JW, et al. Polytetrafluoroethylene graft survival in hemodialysis. JAMA 249:219–222, 1983.
11. Jaffers G, Angstadt JD, Bowman JS III. Early cannulation of plasma TFE and Gore-Tex grafts for hemodialysis: a prospective randomized study. Am J Nephrol 11: 369–373, 1991.
12. Jenkins AM, Buist TA, Glover SD. Medium-term follow-up of forty autogenous vein and forty polytetrafluoroethylene (Gore-Tex) grafts for vascular access. Surgery 88:667–672, 1980.
13. Jensen BV, Vestersgaard-Andersen TB, Nielsen PH. Arteriovenous shunts used in hemodialysis. A retrospective study of the results in 86 patients treated during a 5-year period Ugeskr Laeger 152:2169–2171, 1990.
14. Flores L, Dunn I, Frumkin E, et al. Dacron arterio-venous shunts for vascular access in hemodialysis. Trans Am Soc Artif Int Organs 19:33–37, 1973.
15. Baker LD Jr, Johnson JM, Goldfarb D. Expanded polytetrafluoroethylene (PTFE) subcutaneous arteriovenous conduit: An improved vascular access for chronic hemodialysis. Trans Am Soc Artif Int Organs 22:382–387, 1976.
16. Shack RB, Neblett WW, Richie RE, Dean RH. Expanded polytetrafluoroethylene as dialysis access grafts: Serial study of histology and fibrinolytic activity. Am Surg 43:817–825, 1977.
17. Ota K, Ara R, Takahashi K, et al. Clinical experience with circumferentially rein-

forced expanded polytetrafluoroenthylene (E-PTFE) graft as a vascular access for haemodialysis. Proc Eur Dialysis Transpl Assoc 14:222–228, 1977.

18. Elliott MP, Gazzaniga AB, Thomas JM, et al. Use of expanded polytetrafluoroethylene grafts for vascular access in hemodialysis: Laboratory and clinical evaluation. Am Surg 43:455–459, 1977.

19. Butler HG III, Baker LD Jr, Johnson JM. Vascular access for chronic hemodialysis: Polytetrafluoroethylene (PTFE) versus bovine heterograft. Am J Surg 134:791–793, 1977.

20. Wellington JL. Expanded polytetrafluoroethylene prosthetic grafts for blood access in patients on dialysis. Can J Surg 21:420–422, 1978.

21. Haimov M. Clinical experience with the expanded polytetrafluoroethylene vascular prosthesis. Angiology 29:1–6, 1978.

22. Burdick JF, Scott W, Cosimi AB. Experience with Dacron graft arteriovenous fistulas for dialysis access. Ann Surg 187:262–266, 1978.

23. Tellis VA, Kohlberg WI, Bhat DJ, et al. Expanded polytetrafluoroethylene graft fistula for chronic hemodialysis. Ann Surg 189:101–105, 1979.

24. Ackman CF, O'Regan S, Herba MJ, et al. Experience with polytetrafluoroethylene grafts in patients on long-term hemodialysis. Can J Surg 22:152–154, 1979.

25. Jenkins AM, Buist TA, Glover SD. Medium-term follow-up of forty autogenous vein and forty polytetrafluoroethylene (Gore-Tex) grafts for vascular access. Surgery 88:667–672, 1980.

26. Lilly L, Nighiem D, Mendez-Picon G, Lee HM. Comparison between bovine heterograft and expanded PTFE grafts for dialysis access. Am Surg 46:94–696, 1980.

27. Slater ND, Raftery AT. An evaluation of expanded polytetrafluoroethylene (PTFE) loop grafts in the thigh as vascular access for haemodialysis in patients with access problems. Ann R Coll Surg Engl 70:243–245, 1988.

28. Burger H, Kluchert BA, Kootstra G, et al. Survival of arteriovenous fistulas and shunts for haemodialysis. Eur J Surg 616(5):327–334, 1995.

29. Burkhart HM, Cikrit DF. Arteriovenous fistulae for hemodialysis. Semin Vasc Surg 10(3):162–165 1997.

30. Leapman SB, Boyle M, Pescovitz MD, et al. The arteriovenous fistula for hemodialysis access: Gold standard or archaic relic? Am Surg 62(8):652–656, 1997.

31. Hakaim AG, Nalbandian M, Scott T. Superior maturation and patency of primary brachiocephalic and transposed basilic vein arteriovenous fistulae in patients with diabetes. J Vasc Surg 27(1):154–157, 1998.

32. Schwab S. Hemodialysis vascular access. In Jacobson H, Stricker G, Klahr eds. The Principles and Practice of Nephrology. Philadelphia: Decker; 1990.

33. Hodges TC, Fillinger MF, Zwolak RM, et al. Longitudinal comparison of dialysis access methods: Risk factors for failure. J Vasc Surg 26(6):1009–1019, 1997.

34. Berardinelli L, Vegeto A. Lessons from 494 permanent accesses in 348 haemodialysis patients older than 65 years of age: 29 years of experience. Nephrol Dial Transplant 13(suppl 7):73–77, 1998.

35. Standage BA, Schuman ES, Ackerman D, et al. Does the use of erythropoietin in hemodialysis patients increase dialysis graft thrombosis rates? Am J Surg 165:650–654, 1993.

36. Sreedhara R, Himmelfarb J, Lazarus JM, Hakim RM. Anti-platelet therapy in graft thrombosis: Results of a prospective, randomized, double-blind study. Kidney Int 45:1477–1483, 1994.

37. Hakim R, Himmelfarb J. Hemodialysis access failure: A call to action. Kidney Int 54(4):1029–1040, 1998.

38. Hamon M, Lecluse E, Monassier JP, et al. Pharmacological approaches to the prevention of restenosis after coronary angioplasty. Drugs Aging 13(4):291–301, 1998.

39. Taylor SM, Eaves GL, Weatherford DA, et al. Results and complications of arteriovenous access dialysis grafts in the lower extremity: A five year review. Am Surg 62(3):188–191, 1996.

40. Albers FJ. Causes of hemodialysis access failure. Adv Renal Repl Ther 1(2):107–118, 1994.

41. Boelaert JR, Van Landuyt HW, De Baere YA, et al. Epidemiology and prevention of Staphylococcus aureus infections during hemodialysis. Nephrologie 15(2):157–161, 1994.

10

Short- and Long-Term Hemodialysis Catheters

Andrew T. Gentile
The University of Arizona Health Sciences Center, Tucson, Arizona

Scott S. Berman
The University of Arizona, Carondelet St. Mary's Hospital, The
Southern Arizona Vascular Institute, Tucson, Arizona

Catheters placed within the central venous system provide both short- and long-term access solutions for patients who require hemodialysis. The central venous approach for dialysis access has been available since the original description of femoral cannulation was provided by Shaldon et al. (1) in 1961. Their technique required placement of both arterial and venous cannulae to accomplish effective dialysis. It was not until Uldall (2) introduced a dual-lumen catheter for subclavian vein cannulation in 1980 that the modern era of percutaneous venous access for dialysis began. Further evolution in both catheter design and placement techniques has resulted in the more frequent and broader application of central venous catheters to maintain patients on hemodialysis.

CATHETER DESIGN

Materials

There are a number of catheter manufacturers in the marketplace, which is under-standably competitive, given that there are nearly 300,000 patients maintained on dialysis in the United States. Temporary catheters are usually constructed of polyurethane, which maintains a rigid structure at room temperature for ease of insertion but becomes flexible when exposed to body temperature, thereby reduc-ing the chance for vessel perforation (3). Polyurethane also offers the advantages of having relatively low thrombogenicity and structural stability when exposed to infusates. Long-term catheters, in contrast, are usually constructed of silicone elastomer (Silastic) (4). This polymer is softer, more flexible, and less thrombo-genic than the other available polymers, making it well suited for prolonged placement. However, these structural differences make insertion of Silastic cathe-ters more difficult, requiring the use of a peel-away sheath to manipulate the catheter into position (5).

Duration of Use

The distinction between a temporary and a long-term catheter is based upon its intended duration of use. Temporary catheters have no inherent barrier to infec-tion as part of their design. As such, these catheters are intended for use up to 2 weeks before either exchange or replacement is necessary. This factor justifies the use of a stiffer, usually smaller-diameter catheter that permits easy bedside placement. The addition of a silver-impregnated collagen cuff to the catheter shaft near the skin exit site may prolong the useful life of a temporary catheter up to 6 weeks by virtue of its protection against infection (6). Long-term cathe-ters are designed to be tunneled under the skin and typically include an external polyester felt cuff within the catheter shaft. As a result of incorporation of the cuff within the subcutaneous tissue, a barrier to infection is created, permitting these catheters to be used indefinitely. Long-term catheters are usually larger in diameter than temporary catheters. Because of this larger size combined with the need to tunnel the catheter and use a peel-away sheath introducer for placement, these catheters are usually inserted with the use of flouroscopic imaging. The exceptions to this design are the recently introduced completely implantable he-modialysis valves, which are discussed in a separate section below.

Lumen Configuration

Both temporary and long-term dialysis catheters are constructed with a dual-lumen configuration. In general, the lumens are designated as arterial and venous, based upon their function during the dialysis procedure. Blood withdrawal is usually accomplished through the proximal lumen designated as arterial, whereas venous return occurs through the more distal lumen. Three types of basic catheter design comprise the dual-lumen format: side by side, coaxial, and, more recently, individual lumen dual catheters.

The side-by-side configuration is used in most of the long-term catheters available. Subtle differences exist between the most popular catheters on the market. The PermCath (Quinton Instrument Co., Bothall, WA) has both of its lumens arranged side-by-side within an oval-shaped catheter (Figure 10.1). This offers the advantage of resistance to kinking when the catheter is placed in positions requiring acute angulation. That makes this catheter appealing for placement in the jugular system and allows the catheter to exit on the chest wall in an indiscriminate location. The disadvantage of this design is the requirement for a large peelaway sheath introducer (18F) with an oval lumen that is available only from Quinton. Standard and readily available round introducer sheaths will not work with this catheter; however, Quinton markets separately packaged introducer sheaths that the authors highly recommend be stocked and available if this cathe-

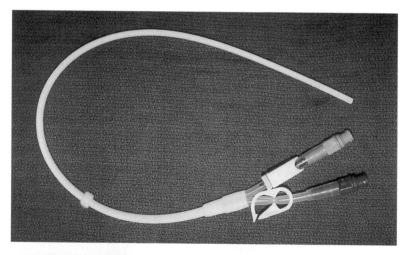

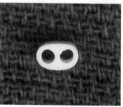

FIGURE 10.1 Quinton Permcath with side-by-side lumens, oval catheters, no kinking.

ter is chosen for use. Despite its large size, percutaneous placement is possible, and this is the authors' preferred route of placement of this catheter system.

The Hickman hemodialysis catheter (Bard Access Systems) incorporates the side-by-side dual-lumen design within a round Silastic catheter. Placement is simplified by the need for only a 14F introducer system. In addition, this catheter also incorporates a silver-impregnated VitaCuff to enhance protection against infection while the felt cuff becomes incorporated in the subcutaneous tissue. This somewhat complicates placement, since the collagen cuff is designed to be located just under the skin exit site, leaving little room for fine tuning of the catheter tip location once the catheter is inserted into the superior vena cava. Additionally, the rounded catheter is more susceptible to kinking when subjected to acute angulation or external compression. The Vas-Cath Soft-Cell PC catheter (Bard Access Systems, Salt Lake City, UT) incorporates the round dual-lumen side-by-side arrangement in a polyurethane catheter with a precurved shape to resist kinking. The stiffer catheter permits easy placement through a 13F sheath. The prefabricated curve is designed to be tunneled under the skin and contains a felt cuff for tissue incorporation. Careful selection of catheter length is necessary prior to placement, since adjustments for proper tip positioning are limited because the curved section of the catheter is fixed in relation to the cuff and the tip.

A new type of tunneled silastic catheter configuration has recently become available for long-term hemodialysis. The Schon, Tesio, and Ash Split Cath are all dual-lumen catheters comprising two separate Silastic tubes that are inserted through a single sheath (Figure 10.2) (7,8). The Schon catheter is joined at one point for a short distance with a triangular junction but has no fabric cuffs attached to the tubing. By contrast, the Tesio catheter consists of two individual pieces of tubing free of any connections; however, each tubing has a fabric cuff designed

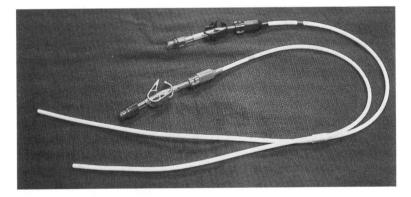

FIGURE 10.2 Schon, catheters illustrating separate lumens.

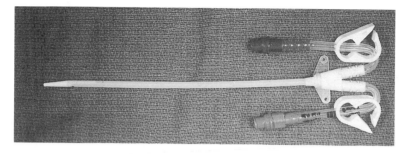

FIGURE 10.3   Quinton Mahurkar catheter side by side.

to be attached to the tubing by the operator and intended to function as a barrier to infection through tissue ingrowth. Finally, the Ash split cath combines the concept of dual free-floating lumens and an implantable cuff together with the ease of insertion of a round-body, flexible Silastic catheter. There are few studies on the performance of these new catheters. Our own anecdotal experience indicates that higher flow rates are more consistently achieved but that these catheters have been somewhat more tedious to insert and remove.

Temporary dual-lumen dialysis catheters are available in both side-by-side and coaxial configurations. The Quinton Mahurkar catheters are constructed with polyurethane in the side-by-side arrangement (Figure 10.3). They feature models available with molded curved extensions that provide consistent flow while keeping the access ports from interfering with patient comfort when placed in the jugular position. The rotating suture wing permits rotation and reversal of the catheter without the need for resuturing. The Flexicon II PC is similar in design, with molded curved extensions in a polyurethane catheter and freely rotating

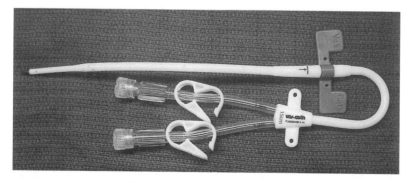

FIGURE 10.4   Vascath Flexicon coaxial catheter.

TABLE 10.1 Selected Dialysis Catheters

	Manufacturer	Lumen configuration	Material	Available lengths	Features
Temporary catheters					
Duo-Flow	Medcomp	Coaxial	Polyurethane	12, 15, 20 cm	Variable length extensions
Neostar	Horizon Medical Products	Coaxial	Polyurethane	4, 5, 6, 7, 8"	
Flexxicon II, II PC	Vas-Cath Inc.	Coaxial	Polyurethane	12.5, 15, 20, 24 cm	PC are precurved
Mahurkar dual lumen	Quinton Instrument Co.	Side by side	Polyurethane	10F(12, 15, 19.5 cm) 11.5F(13.5, 16, 19.5, 24 cm)	Available with VitaCuff, and precurved
Long-term catheters					
Soft-Cell PC	Vas-Cath Inc.	Side by side	Polyurethane	12, 19, 23 cm	Small 13F introducer
PermCath	Quinton Instrument Co	Side by side (oval catheter)	Silastic	28, 36, 40, 45 cm	Oval catheter resists kinking
Neostar	Horizon Medical Products	Side by side	Silastic	13, 19, 23 cm	Triple lumen available
Ash Split Cath Schon Twin Cath Tesio Twin Cath	Medcomp	Dual lumen Free-floating	Silastic	Ash: 11, 13" Schon: 14, 16, 1, 8, 20, 22 cm Tesio: 40 cm	Ash: Round body, easy insertion Schon: Single wire and sheath, no cuff on catheter Tesio: Dual wires and sheaths
Hickman hemodialysis/plasma-phoresis	Bard Access Systems	Side by side	Silastic	28, 36, 40, 45 cm	Comes with VitaCuff attached

suture wing. In contrast to the Mahurkar, the lumens of the Flexicon are configured in a coaxial format (Figure 10.4). Coaxial design may reduce flow disturbances caused by catheter angulation, since flow occurs in both lumens throughout the cross-sectional area of the catheter as opposed to being limited to one side or the other, as in the side-by-side arrangement (9).

Both temporary and long-term catheters have the lumen openings far enough away from one another to limit the amount of recirculation. All of the temporary and long-term catheters described are available as complete insertion trays or individual catheters in an assortment of catheter lengths. Table 10.1 displays a comparison of a number of the available catheters and their salient features. Although economic factors often determine decisions regarding the choice of vendor, costs are often quite comparable and negotiable with manufacturers. The best approach is a multidisciplinary assessment by both the physicians placing the catheters and the dialysis units using them on a regular basis. Once performance and satisfaction are assessed, cost decisions often have less of an impact on catheter selection.

CATHETER SELECTION

Acute Access

Central venous catheterization can provide vascular access for dialysis in a number of clinical settings. Our general approach to determining hemodialysis access routes is summarized in the algorithm which appears in Chapter 3 (see Figure 3.1). Once catheter access is deemed necessary, Table 10.2 provides a summary of indications for placement of both temporary and long-term catheters, which may guide device selection. For patients who develop acute renal failure and need urgent or emergent dialysis, temporary catheters play a central role in fulfilling this requirement. Box 10.1 displays the DOQI guidelines regarding the use of noncuffed catheters. Many of these patients will resolve their immediate need for renal replacement therapy and not need long-term access. Patients with chronic renal insufficiency who present with an acute deterioration are also candidates for temporary catheter placement. Careful consideration should be given to whether or not long-term access will be necessary for this category of patient, as this may impact upon the catheter selection. Temporary catheter placement is ideal for patients who will subsequently undergo construction of a prosthetic arteriovenous fistula. Most prosthetic fistulae can be accessed within 2 weeks thereby eliminating the need for exchange or replacement of the temporary catheter. If an autogenous fistula is planned for long-term access, the temporary catheter can be changed to a long-term catheter, which will provide an access route for ongoing dialysis while the native fistula matures. The extended period of access provided by the addition of a Vita Cuff to a temporary catheter may also exclude the need to place a long-term catheter. Temporary catheters are com-

Box 10.1   Acute Hemodialysis Vascular Access—Noncuffed Catheters

1. Hemodialysis access of less than 3 weeks' duration should be obtained using a noncuffed or cuffed double-lumen percutaneously inserted catheter.
2. These catheters are suitable for immediate use and should not be inserted before needed.
3. Noncuffed catheters can be inserted at the bedside in the femoral, internal jugular, or subclavian position.
4. The subclavian insertion site should not be used in a patient who may need permanent vascular access.
5. Prior to catheter use, chest x-ray is mandatory after subclavian and internal jugular insertion to confirm the catheter tip position at the caval atrial junction or the superior vena cava and to exclude complications prior to starting hemodialysis.
6. Where available, ultrasound should be used to direct insertion of these catheters into the internal jugular position to minimize insertion-related complications.
7. Femoral catheters should be at least 19 cm long to minimize recirculation. Noncuffed femoral catheters should not be left in place longer than 5 days and should be left in place only in bed-bound patients.
8. Nonfunctional noncuffed catheters can be exchanged over a guidewire or treated with urokinase as long as the exit site and tunnel are not infected.
9. Exit site, tunnel tract, or systemic infections should prompt the removal of noncuffed catheters.

Source: Modified from Ref. 10, Guideline 6.

TABLE 10.2   Catheter Selection Based on Indication for Placement

Indication	Expected duration of access	Catheter type
Acute renal failure	Less than 6 weeks	Temporary with Vitacuff
Acute/chronic renal failure	Indefinite	Long-term
Acute/chronic renal failure (not a candidate for autogenous graft)	Indefinite	Temporary with Vitacuff
Chronic renal failure (thrombosed chronic access)	Less than 2 weeks	Temporary
Plasmapheresis	More than 6 weeks	Long-term
Plasmapheresis	Less than 6 weeks	Temporary with Vitacuff

Box 10.2 Type and Location of Tunneled Cuffed Catheter Placement

1. Tunneled cuffed venous catheters are the method of choice for temporary access of longer than 3 weeks' duration (but are acceptable for access of shorter duration as well). In addition, some patients who have exhausted all other access options require permanent access via tunneled cuffed catheters. For patients who have a primary AV fistula maturing but need immediate hemodialysis, tunneled cuffed catheters are the access of choice.
2. The preferred insertion site for tunneled cuffed venous dialysis catheters is the right internal jugular vein. Other options include the right external jugular vein, the left internal and external jugular veins, subclavian veins, femoral veins, or translumbar access to the inferior vena cava. Subclavian access should be used only when jugular options are not available. Tunneled cuffed catheters should not be placed on the same side as a maturing AV access if possible.
3. Fluoroscopy is mandatory for insertion of all cuffed dialysis catheters. The catheter tip must be adjusted to the level of the caval atrial junction or beyond to ensure optimal blood flow.
4. Real-time ultrasound–guided insertion is recommended to reduce insertion-related complications.
5. There is currently no proven advantage of one cuffed catheter design over another. Catheter choice should be based on local experience, goals for use, and cost.

Source: Modified from Ref. 10, Guideline 5.

monly used as an interim mode of access for patients with complications of arteriovenous fistulae, such as thrombosis. In those patients in need of dialysis prior to treatment for a complication, temporary catheters provide expedient access for dialysis so that surgical or nonsurgical intervention to the fistula can proceed in a medically stable patient. Temporary catheters also provide a route to dialyze renal transplant patients who may present with acute renal failure as a complication of an episode of rejection or toxicity to immunosuppressant agents. Finally, temporary dialysis catheters are often used as venous access for patients in need of plasmapheresis (11). Catheter selection concerns are similar to those in the dialysis population (Table 10.2).

Chronic Access

Long-term dialysis catheters are commonly used in patients who need immediate access for hemodialysis but are concurrently undergoing construction of a native arteriovenous fistula for chronic venous access. Native fistulae require a period of time, usually 6 to 12 weeks, for adequate arterialization and hypertrophy of the venous outflow to permit safe and effective cannulation for dialysis. Long-term catheters function as an effective access bridge to maintain the patient on dialysis during this maturation period. Since roughly 30 to 50% of native fistulae fail to mature to the point of usable access, functional long-term catheters allow for more tolerance on the part of physicians and patients in waiting for autogenous fistulae to declare their ultimate outcome. Long-term catheters may also be the route of choice for maintaining hemodialysis access for patients who are frightened of repeated needle sticks, who have exhausted usable sites for peripheral access, or who have poor overall cardiopulmonary function with an expected short life expectancy on dialysis (12). Box 10.2 displays the DOQI guidelines surrounding the use of tunneled cuffed catheters.

CATHETER PLACEMENT

Specific details regarding anatomic sites and techniques for central venous catheter placement are discussed in Chapter 14. In considering placement of catheters for dialysis access, certain specific recommendations should be kept in mind. First and foremost, no patient who will likely need long-term access for hemodialysis and is a candidate for a permanent arteriovenous fistula should have a catheter placed by a subclavian approach. This point cannot be overstated. The incidence of subclavian stenosis related to previous dialysis catheter placement can be as high as 50% (13). Damage to and subsequent stenosis of the subclavian system can compromise the use of the ipsilateral extremity for chronic venous access. Though successful treatment of subclavian stenosis using percutaneous transluminal angioplasty with and without intravascular stent placement is well described in the literature, recurrence and failure of this intervention is significant. Since the subclavian vein is usually accessed as it passes through the thoracic outlet comprising the first rib and clavicle, this tight anatomical space is often the site of stenotic lesions. Despite technical successes with balloon dilation and stenting, recurrent stenosis and thrombosis limit the utility of this procedure and highlight the concern over indiscriminate use of this access site for catheter placement. Subclavian access does, however, have acceptable indications. When access in a particular extremity has been exhausted yet the ispsilateral subclavian vein remains patent, use of this vein for temporary or long-term catheterization would be appropriate. Moreover, if an extremity has been deemed unacceptable for chronic access due to arterial insufficiency, the subclavian approach would be suitable for establishing temporary or long-term venous access.

The usefulness of placing temporary and long-term catheters for hemodialysis rests on their ability to provide expedient and effective vascular access. Paramount to this end is selecting appropriate catheter lengths and accurate placement of catheter tips in the vena cava. Dialysis catheter selection definitely does not abide by the "one size fits all" dictum. Catheter length, which will be pivotal in determining catheter tip location, is a critical factor in achieving uninterrupted, consistent dialysis. It is similarly important to have a full selection of catheter sizes available before proceeding with central venous cannulation.

Temporary Catheters

For temporary catheters, which are more rigid due to their polyurethane construction, tip positioning within the superior vena cava (SVC) from the jugular approach or inferior vena cava from the femoral approach usually provides acceptable blood flow rates. The catheter must be sized with the patient's body habitus in mind. Tall, thin, asthentic builds often require a longer temporary catheter (15 cm) in even the right internal jugular position, which is usually the shortest pathway to the SVC. Likewise, accessing the SVC from the left jugular approach requires a longer catheter (19 to 20 cm). Femoral catheters at least 20 cm in length are necessary to access the inferior vena cava from the groin. Large panniculi of adipose tissue will also mandate the use of larger-than-expected catheters at all locations.

Long-Term Catheters

For long-term catheter placement, the most consistent function occurs when the tip is positioned at the junction of the right atrium and SVC. Catheter lengths up to 45 cm are necessary to achieve successful tip positioning while still allowing the catheter exit site to be placed in an unnoticeable area on the chest wall that can be concealed by clothing (Figure 10.5). This may seem like a minor point in regard to consistent catheter function; however, it can become a major consideration in patient satisfaction when deciding upon catheter selection. The PermCath and Hickman catheters are available in sufficient lengths to meet these criteria. One must be careful to accurately measure out length and expected tip location prior to catheter tunneling and placement, as—unlike other long-term central venous catheters—dialysis catheters cannot be trimmed to modify size. In general, a 40- or 45-cm catheter length is required when a left internal jugular approach is selected, while a 35- or 40-cm catheter length is adequate for the right internal jugular approach. Nuances related to placement of each type of long-term catheter occur, and specific attention should be paid to the product information provided with each type of catheter prior to insertion. For example, placement of a Schon catheter requires the use of a special guidewire with markings on it to determine the appropriate length of catheter for an individual patient. The catheters are packaged separately from the guidewire, which is contained in the insertion tray. Fluoroscopy is used to place the "j" portion of the guidewire in the proximal right atrium. The appropriate catheter length is thus determined by the exposed markings on the guidewire at the exit site of vessel cannulation. This technical detail helps to promote accurate and functional tip placement through fairly precise selection of the proper catheter length.

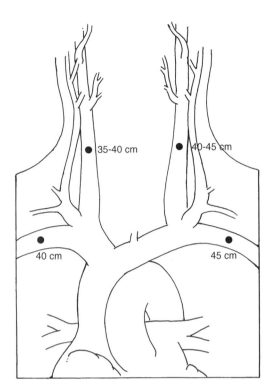

FIGURE 10.5   Illustration of catheter lengths based on position and exit site.

PEDIATRIC HEMODIALYSIS CATHETERS

When central venous access is necessary in the pediatric population for hemodialysis or plasmapheresis, the most common method utilized is the tunneled, cuffed silastic catheter (14,15). In the past, most central venous access in children was performed using cutdowns. However, with the availability of the peel-away sheath and smaller-size catheters as well as the ready accessibility of fluoroscopic imaging, most access procedures are now done percutaneously using the same approaches outlined for adults in Chapter 14. Once central venous access has been determined by the pediatric patient's care team to be the chosen route for dialysis, a tunneled, cuffed catheter can be placed using either the internal jugular, subclavian, or femoral vein percutaneous approaches. If a cutdown is necessary, alternative sites in children include the facial, external jugular, and cephalic veins. Pediatric dialysis catheters are available in a range of lengths (12, 18, and 24 cm) and diameters (6 through 11.5F). Care must be taken to make sure that the cuff is at least 2 cm from the exit site and that the catheter is tunneled and secured with the child's activity in mind.

IMPLANTED HEMODIALYSIS VALVES

Two new devices for hemodialysis access are being utilized in place of tunneled, cuffed external catheters. Both incorporate Silastic catheters and completely implanted titanium valves. The LifeSite system (Vasca Inc., Tewksbury, MA) is currently approved for use in the United States as a bridge for access while a fistula is maturing or other permanent access is planned (16). The LifeSite system comprises individual valves with individual catheters, each implanted through individual subcutaneous pockets into either the jugular or subclavian veins. The LifeSite system takes advantage of standard 14-gauge hemodialysis needles. In the only published experience with the LifeSite system, mean blood flow rates of 384.7 mL/min were achieved. Unlike the LifeSite system, the Dialock system (Biolink Corp, Norwell, MA) has both its valves and attached Silastic catheters incorporated into a single titanium housing (17). In addition to the single housing, the Dialock's major difference from the LifeSite system is the need to use a proprietary needle system to access the valves. As in the LifeSite system, blood flow with the Dialock system averages 300 mL/min. As of this writing, the Dialock system was not yet approved for use in the United States.

CONCLUSION

Central venous catheters have become an important adjunct in maintaining patients on hemodialysis. Temporary catheters are usually manufactured of stiffer polyurethane. By virtue of this design, temporary catheters are usually placed at the bedside in either the internal jugular or femoral position. Moreover, their inherent design characteristics limit their safe and recommended use for only short periods of time (<2 weeks) unless modified with a VitaCuff. By contrast, long-term catheters are fabricated of softer Silastic, which requires adjunctive use of peel-away sheath introducers for insertion, usually in an operating room or angiography suite with fluoroscopic imaging readily available. Long-term catheters incorporate into their design a portion of catheter that is tunneled subcutaneously, and most brands have fabric cuffs attached to the tubing near the designated exit site, which functions as a physical barrier to infection through tissue ingrowth. Together with their larger size and Silastic composition, these characteristics make long-term catheters an effective mode for maintaining vascular access for hemodialysis in appropriately selected patients. Though subtle differences in design and placement techniques exist between the available brands, no catheter to date has demonstrated overwhelming superiority in performance as compared with other brands. Completely implanted subcutaneous valves may offer a new alternative for hemodialysis access, not only as a bridge for patients with maturing fistulase but also as a solution for catheter-dependent patients.

REFERENCES

1. Shaldon S, Chiandussi L, Higgs B. Hemodialysis by percutaneous catheterization of femoral artery and vein with regional heparinization. Lancet 2:857–859, 1961.
2. Uldall PR, Woods F, Merchant N, et al. A double-lumen subclavian cannula for temporary hemodialysis access. Trans Am Soc Artif Organs 26:93–98, 1980.
3. Gravenstein N, Blackshear RH. In vitro evaluation of relative perforating potential of central venous catheters: Comparison of materials, selected models, number of lumens, and angles of incidence to simulated membranes. J Clin Monit 7:1–6, 1991.
4. Welch GW, McKeel DW, Silvestein P, et al. The role of catheter composition in the development of thrombophlebitis. Surg Gynecol Obstet 138:421–424, 1974.
5. Cohen AM, Wood WC. Simplified technique for placement of long-term central venous silicone catheters. Surg Gynecol Obstet 154:721–724, 1982.
6. Maki DG, Cobb L, Garmen JK, et al. An attachable silver-impregnated cuff for prevention of infection with central venous catheters: A prospective randomized multicenter trial. Am J Med 85:307–314, 1988.
7. Canaud B, Beraud JJ, Joyeux H, Mion C. Internal jugular vein cannulation using 2 silastic catheters: A new simple and safe long-term vascular access foe extracoporeal treatment. Nephron 43:133–138, 1986.
8. Millner MR, Kerns SR, Hawkins IF Jr, et al. Tesio twin dialysis catheter system: A new catheter for hemodialysis. Am J Roentgenol 164:1519–1520, 1995.
9. de Los Angeles A, Lerner A, Goldstein SJ, et al. Comparison of coaxial and side-by-side double lumen subclavian catheters with single lumen catheter. Am J Kidney Dis 3:221–224, 1986.
10. NKF-DOQI. Clinical Practice Guidelines for Vascular Access. New York: National Kidney Foundation, 1997.
11. Grishaber JE, Cunningham MC, Rohret PA, Strauss RG. Analysis of venous access for therapeutic plasma exchange in patients with neurological disease. J Clin Apheresis 7:119–123, 1992.
12. Gibson SP, Mosquera D. Five years experience with the Quinton PermCath for vascular access. Nephrol Dial Transplant 6:269–274, 1991.
13. Cimochowski GE, Worley E, Rutherford WE, et al. Superiority of the internal jugular over the subclavian access for temporary dialysis. Nephron 54:154–161, 1990.
14. Gibson TC, Dyer DP, Postlethwaite RJ, Gough DCS. Vascular access for acute hemodialysis. Arch Dis Child 62:141–145, 1987.
15. Donckerwolcke RA, Bunchman TE. Hemodialysis in infants and small children. Pediatr Nephrol 8:103–106, 1994.
16. Beathard GA, Posen GA. Initial clinical results with the LifeSite hemodialysis access system. Kidney Int 58:2221–2227, 2000.
17. Canaud B, My H, Morena M, et al. Dialock: A new vascular access device for extracorporeal renal replacement therapy. Preliminary clinical results. Nephrol Dial Transplant 14:692–698, 1999.

11

Accessing AV Accesses and Catheters

Rudy Mounia
IMPRA Inc., Tempe, Arizona

W. Bradford Carter
University of Maryland, Baltimore, Maryland

Blood access systems for hemodialysis and their associated devices have reached a high level of sophistication. Today's polymer engineered catheters and grafts offer many options for long-term access to supplement the natural arteriovenous (AV) fistula. The failure of these systems, however, represents the single leading cause of hospitalization for end-stage renal disease (ESRD) patients. The annual costs to Medicare for these procedures was conservatively estimated to be over $500 million (1). It is imperative that we continue to improve these systems, the techniques and means to competently install them, and the instructions and procedures provided for their optimal therapeutic use.

It is likely that most inconsistencies exist within "the instructions and procedures provided" in the scope of blood access care for ESRD patients. Much of what we give as instructions is based on incomplete references, anecdotal reports, our resignation to the reality that these systems do fail, and past successes with similar cases. For example, our approach to contemporary large-bore dialysis catheters is largely built upon experience gained with central venous monitoring and infusion catheters (2). Our solutions, however, frequently ignore the dissimilarities between the two; infusion catheters are single-lumen, single-

TABLE 11.1   Infection Control Measures

Staff and patient education should include instruction on infection control
measures for all hemodialysis access sites.

Source: Modified from Ref. 3, Guideline 13.

aperture, low-flow, continuously perfused, small-bore inpatient devices cared
for almost completely by professional medical staff. Surely a multilumen, multi-
apertured, high-flow, intermittently used, large-volume, large-bore devices subject to the rigors of outpatient wear require a different and specialized approach.
Similarly, interventions devised for use on the classic Brescia-Cimino fistula
guide nearly every procedure and directive towards an AV access. Just how similar is an AV fistula to its more frequently used replacement, the synthetic graft?
Knowing the similarities and differences of the available access systems and their
devices allows one to provide the most appropriate instructions and procedural
recommendations.

When the ESRD patient presents for a hemodialysis treatment, the assessment of his or her blood access system should be more than a cursory check for
patency. Every visit offers an opportunity to discern tactics for the present and
make plans for the future (Table 11.1).

CATHETERS

Assessment

With catheters, the integrity and appearance of the dressing may be the first indication of the need to counsel the patient on his or her role to keep the catheter
viable. A poorly applied and cared for dressing may be the first breakdown in
the barrier to infection for temporary catheters and may result in thrombosis or
vessel trauma, as described in subsequent sections. Exit-site infection, insertion
tract pain, and tenderness are best assessed predialysis after the dressing has been
removed. Any sign of catheter infection such as pericatheter drainage, erythema,
or pain should be brought to the attention of the patient's physician before com-
mencing the treatment. Interested readers are directed to Chapter 16 for a detailed
discussion on the diagnosis and management of catheter infections. Catheter patency is assessed just prior to treatment initiation and is described below (Table
11.2).

Initiating Dialysis

Soaking of the injection caps/Luer connectors with an effective bactericidal agent
prior to opening the catheter's female Luer connectors has become standard pro-

TABLE 11.2 Catheter Care and Accessing the Patient's Circulation

Catheter care and accessing the patient's circulation should be clean procedures.

1. Hemodialysis catheter dressing changes and catheter manipulations that access the patient's bloodstream should be performed only by trained dialysis staff.
2. The catheter exit site should be examine at each hemodialysis treatment for signs of infection.
3. Catheter exit site dressings should be changed at each hemodialysis treatment.
4. Use of dry gauze dressings and povidone-iodine ointment at the catheter exit site is recommended whenever possible.
5. Manipulating a catheter and accessing the patient's bloodstream should be performed in a manner that minimizes contamination.
6. During catheter connect and disconnect procedures, nurses and patients should wear surgical masks or face shields. Nurses should wear gloves during all connect and disconnect procedures.

Source: Modified from Ref. 3, Guideline 15.

cedure (Table 11.3). The operator should make certain that the bactericidal agent is left in place long enough to be effective. (Consult the agents' instructions for use for the appropriate amount of time.) Most dialysis units do not use a sterile technique to initiate dialysis with catheters. Sterile supplies (gauze sponges, syringes, needles, etc.) are delivered onto a clean or sterile field and typically han-

TABLE 11.3 Considerations for Accessing the Bloodstream Using Catheters

- The catheter hubcaps or bloodline connectors should be soaked for 3 to 5 min in povidone-iodine and then allowed to dry prior to separation.
- Catheter lumens should be kept sterile.
- To prevent contamination, the lumen and tip should never remain open to the air. A cap or syringe should be placed on or within the catheter lumen while maintaining a clean field under the catheter connectors.
- Patients should wear a surgical masks for all catheter procedures that remove the catheter caps and access the patient's bloodstream.
- Dialysis staff should wear gloves and surgical masks or face shields for all procedures that remove catheter caps and access the patient's bloodstream.
- A surgical mask for the patient and masks or face shields for the dialysis staff should be worn for all catheter dressing changes.

Source: Modified from Ref. 3, Table III-8.

dled with clean gloves. While this practice may have been driven by economics, it has not been directly correlated to a significant increase in catheter infections (4). In checking the patency of the lumen(s), use a syringe slightly larger than the stated priming volume of that lumen. If the lumen does not aspirate easily, be sure not to pull back on the catheter as you pull back on the plunger of the syringe. In this case, upon release of the plunger and syringe, the catheter surges forward. In a cuffed catheter configuration, this would place considerable stress on the cuff's ingrowth. The physical barrier to infection may be compromised. In a temporary catheter configuration, the risk of vessel perforation increases as well as the risk of damaging the retention sutures. It is important to know the construction of the catheter to determine any flow problem and specifically to know the number of holes in each lumen. When a catheter is easily irrigated but aspirates with difficulty, the thrombus is usually external to the lumen. Poor or no aspiration and irrigation are usually indicative of an intraluminal thrombus. If a thrombolytic agent is to be used, its primary effect will be on intraluminal clots, not external ones.

Air embolism is always a concern in handling internal jugular, femoral, and subclavian vein catheters. Use of the Trendelenburg position during manipulation of jugular and subclavian catheters is the simplest means available to the dialysis staff to minimize patient morbidity and mortality associated with an air embolism. Yet many dialysis units do not routinely use it to initiate (or discontinue) dialysis. We should not allow ourselves to be casual about this risk. Air embolism is the most serious complication associated with opening dialysis catheters. The Trendelenburg position offers reliable and inexpensive protection from serious morbidity and mortality, and its use should be mandatory in all treatment settings.

Engaging hemodialysis catheters is usually quick and painless. The number of problems that may arise are few compared with their internal AV counterparts; they include cracked or broken parts, clotted lumen(s), broken sutures, cuff erosion, infection, and air embolism. Except for clotted lumens, these complications can be minimized during the initiation of treatment. Physicians who place these catheters must be mindful of the "wearing position" of these devices as they relate to complications. If an outpatient's jugular catheter extension lines are secured at the base of the ear or the hairline, no one should expect the dressing to serve its intended functions and catheter thrombosis or infection should be expected. Precurved temporary jugular catheters allow for a functional dressing while diverting the extensions away from the patient's face and hair. Attention to detail in catheter selection and tunneling will be rewarded by prolonged and infection-free patency.

The caps used on catheters should be constructed of a material different than the catheters Luer extensions. Like materials tend to bind together and are much more difficult to remove. Recognizing this factor alone will prevent some of the creative repairs to Luer connectors and extension lines necessitated by the use of clamps to get "better" leverage and remove bound up caps.

Terminating Treatment

After reinfusion, the dialysis catheter requires special care. All lumens must be flushed vigorously with saline to ensure removal of blood components. The heparin-lock solution is instilled under pressure. The concentration of the solution is of little importance if the volume of the solution does not reach the entirety of the catheter's hole pattern. Over 90% of the stated volume of a catheter's lumen is without holes. If the lumen has more than one hole, a volume of solution greater than the stated volume must be used because solution will escape from the more proximal holes during infusion. This point cannot be overstated and needs to be taken into account in using concentrated heparin (10,000 U/mL) and urokinase dwells. Coaxial catheters with side holes will leak the dwell solution into the systemic circulation before the terminal holes are reached. This can result in a coagulopathic state and significant bleeding complications. Caution should be exercised in placing dwell solutions into catheters at the end of a procedure to avoid systemic anticoagulation. Since maintaining catheter patency is a function of displacing blood from the catheter and not a function of anticoagulating blood in the catheter, an argument can be made for simple saline flush at the end of the treatment and avoidance of other dwell formulas (5,6).

How the catheter is prepared for the patient to leave is another important issue. Dressings are used consistently on temporary central venous catheters and occasionally on permanent central venous catheters. They perform several important functions. They are used to create and maintain a healing environment for the exit site, provide protection from external sources, enhance patient comfort and wearability, secure the catheter, and help maintain the patency of the lumens. The healing environment is assured when the dressing allows aeration of the exit site. Protection from external sources allows the integrity of the catheter to remain intact. The catheter is a very important part of the patient's being but should not dominate it. The dressing must allow for as "natural" an existence as possible with regard to freedom of movement and the patient's wardrobe. Sutures and cuffs play the largest role in maintaining the position of hemodialysis catheters. A substantial dressing though, still serves as an important first line of defense.

One of the overlooked benefits of a dressing is its contribution to catheter patency. Before a catheter lumen clots, blood must enter the lumen. The dressing can play a major role in preventing blood from entering the lumen. The dialysis staff understand how opening the clamp on a catheter's extension line aspirates blood into the lumen. This same aspiration occurs when the catheter is bent or bowed through patient movement and allowed to relax below the level of the extension line clamps. A catheter's extension lines and any exposed length of cannula is easily moved when the patient moves—turning a page of a magazine, reaching forward, reaching up, hugging a child, getting dressed. Once the blood has displaced the catheter's priming or locking solution and no further aspiration occurs, there is very little chance of residual solution preventing a clot formation in this static flow environment. Permanent catheters tunneled onto the anterior chest wall, which are not usually provided a dressing but exhibit frequent clotting episodes, may benefit from a dressing trial. The dressing needs to prevent the cannula from being negatively affected by movement. This can be accomplished by curling the exposed cannula and securing it comfortably on the chest wall. The extension line clamps should be engaged as close to the catheters hub or exit site as possible. The extension lines can be turned down 180 degrees to lower their profile as well as secure them.

Finally, patients should be given specific instructions on how to handle any catheter-related issues away from the dialysis suite. Loose or displaced dressings should be replaced by trained staff. Breakage or laceration of an external catheter extension can be quickly managed by pinching the catheter into a fold and securing it with a rubber band until professional medical assistance is available. This simple maneuver not only avoids the potential life-threatening occurrence of an air embolism but can also treat or prevent significant hemorrhage from the catheter lumen. The single best piece of information to give patients is a reliable method to contact the dialysis staff in the event of any problems or questions.

ARTERIOVENOUS FISTULAE AND GRAFTS

AV Fistula Assessment

The creation of an AV fistula is a simple surgical procedure that can have a major effect on the operated extremity and patient. One of the first things to look for is the presence of any signs suggestive of a consequence of previous or concurrent ipsilateral internal jugular or subclavian vein catheter placement. The appearance of collateral venous circulation around the axilla and/or anterior chest areas is a certain indicator of central venous obstruction. Within the fistula itself, the pulsation (thrill) felt throughout will be more intense than usual. Normally, the thrill diminishes as flow enters the deep and collateral circulation.

The main trunk (primary vein) of a normally functioning AV fistula should offer several centimeters of relative straightness. If it is not easily seen, a mild restrictive tourniquet placed high on the proximal portion of the fistula can be used. Tributaries of the main trunk (runoffs) are easily evaluated for their suitability for venous cannulation. The hemodialysis staff should be encouraged to use the main trunk for ''arterial'' (outflow) sticks only whenever possible. Reducing trauma to the main trunk has the greater potential to extend the life of the fistula. Cannulation outside the main trunk would minimize recirculation as long as the draining vein empties into the deep circulation or to a more proximal area of the fistula.

An autogenous AV fistula is ready to be cannulated (mature) for the first time when it exhibits the following:

1. Uniform dilation—a result of increased blood flow
2. Wall thickening—a result of increased pressure
3. Crowning—a result of outflow tract resistance and the preceding factors

These conditions are too frequently left to develop passively. Satisfactory development of the fistula is often driven by the hope of superb vessel selection and good luck. Clinical experience and other authors have shown that the programmed use of a mild restrictive tourniquet can accelerate the maturation of an AV fistula (7). If a patient develops "arterialized" veins running distal to the anastomosis, venous hypertension may result. Ligation of those veins will prevent and/or correct venous hypertension. If these veins are present without attendant venous hypertension, they can be used for arterial sticks with the proviso that they meet the maturity criteria noted above.

Synthetic AV Grafts

Expanded polytetrafluorethylene (ePTFE) grafts have become the most frequently used chronic blood access devices for patients with ESRD (8). There are several different types available, which have been described in detail in Chapters 5 and 9, yet we have managed to lump them all together for our handling expediency. It is safe to propose we would use these grafts more effectively if we understood their characteristics better. This understanding need take place quickly, as new iterations of urethane composites, carbon coextruded, reinforced, wrapped, and multilayered grafts begin to compete for our patients.

An assessment of ePTFE grafts begins with knowing some general characteristics of the material. Most ePTFE grafts are noncompliant in the radial direction and nonelastic in the longitudinal. When the material is cannulated, an opening is left in the material. The material is incredibly inert. It is not biodegradable. It is naturally antithrombogenic and hydrophobic. When the grafts are expanded (pulled apart), fibrils (longitudinally oriented threads of material) and nodes (thicker transverse or radially oriented pieces of material linking the fibrils) are created. Open spaces within this wall structure result. The average distance between nodes is measured and reported as the internodal distance (IND). The porosity of ePTFE grafts is referred to as its IND. This differs considerably from the expression of porosity in polyester grafts; the amount of water that will pass through the wall of the graft measured in mL/min/cm^2 at 120 mmHg. This porous ePTFE surface serves as the first blood interface on all grafts. The transition of this interface and the true level of healing the graft subsequently undergoes directly affects how it should be engaged. Healing responses have been documented to affect the success or failure of ePTFE grafts. There are five types of healing responses that would affect ePTFE grafts. Some grafts undergo all five while others incur less (9,10). This is where knowledge of graft construction is invaluable in making an assessment. This is also where most of the similarities between ePTFE grafts end.

The level of healing, from a surgical procedure or a needle stick, is one of the first things evaluated when assessing an ePTFE graft. The risk of infection due to the constant trauma of needle sticks and the immunocompromised state of the patient is always great. Pseudoaneurysms result from graft design and needle-hole management techniques. When an ePTFE placement site is dramatically swollen postoperatively, the causes include tissue weeping, lymph node damage, bleeding associated with tunneling trauma, and physiological changes. More often than not, however, the cause is seroma leakage through the graft. This leakage is usually a result of breaking the hydrophobic barrier of the graft by changing its surface tension or displacing fibrils via pressure. It is often preventable. The presence of seroma can prevent a graft from being cannulated safely because of risk of the infection and hemorrhage involved. Seroma has been successfully resolved using elevation, fibrin glue, graft ligation and resection, and plasmapheresis.

The dialysis graft should be seen "crowning" on the implanted extremity. Its course is more straight than curved. It lies on a fairly consistent plane across its usable surface area. A crowning graft is more easily cannulated than others. When these conditions do not exist, the tunneling technique used during placement is the primary cause.

To determine the patency of an ePTFE graft, check the anastomosed *vein* by palpation and/or auscultation. Feeling the graft alone is not a reliable indicator due to the noncompliant property of ePTFE and the wide variety of graft wall thicknesses/layers. An organized thrombus in a partially occluded graft can conduct a transmitted pulse if the anastomosed artery is patent. Determining the direction of flow is best achieved by compressing the graft near its midpoint to impede flow. Palpate the graft proximal and distal to the area being compressed. The side with the strongest pulse is the arterial limb. An anatomical reference or drawing provided by the surgeon is always appreciated by the dialysis staff (Table 11.4).

Initiating Dialysis

Initiating treatment with an AV access begins with proper positioning. Whether the access is in the arm or leg, proper positioning offers benefits to the dialysis staff. Creating a firm anatomical base for cannulation is the first benefit. The

TABLE **11.4** Skin Preparation Technique for Permanent AV Accesses

A clean technique for needle cannulation should be used for all cannulation procedures.

Source: Modified from Ref. 3, Guideline 14.

access is less likely to retreat into the surrounding tissue. Immobilization of the access is another benefit. Limiting the fistula's or graft's ability to move or ''roll'' makes the cannulation attempt much easier. The better positions to use closely mimic those used during the surgery to implant the access. A medially placed upper arm graft is surgically installed with the patients arm extended from the body at close to a 90 degree angle. In cannulating to initiate dialysis, many patients' arms are extended less than 45 degrees. As much as one-third of the usable surface of the access is obscured by the lateral chest wall. By functionally shortening the graft, we accelerate and concentrate the trauma to the visible two-thirds. Our potential to acquire midgraft stenosis, hematoma, and pseudoaneurysm is increased. Another benefit of proper positioning is providing for the comfort of the dialysis staff. Cannulation is an invasive and stressful procedure for both the patient and the staff. It is the staff person, however, that has control of the ''weapon''—the dialysis needle. None of us would like to undergo a procedure where the person performing it was in any way uncomfortable. The same applies for the sticker. There are a variety of positions to use whereby both the patient and the staff are comfortable. We should strive to find them.

The final benefit of proper positioning is the identification of the usable surface area of the access. Before any AV access is cannulated, early or late, a stick-site rotation plan should be established. The natural AV fistula has the ability to fully repair itself from trauma. This has led some authors to suggest that rotating or varying stick sites is not necessary. As mentioned earlier, when an ePTFE graft is stuck, a hole remains. It is occupied by thrombus, fibrous tissue, and cellular debris. It does not repair itself. All graft manufacturers strongly recommend rotating stick sites. For consistency on the unit level, all types of AV access should be used on a rotating-site basis. Stick-site rotation plans allow 100% of the usable surface area on an access to be used in a logical and methodical fashion. There is a different type of plan for each access configuration, yet the design principle is the same. All AV accesses have no-stick zones and/or a midpoint. No-stick zones are areas within a dialysis needle's length of an obstruction, anastomosis, or anatomical flexure. The apex or loop portion of AV grafts is considered a no-stick zone. For straight and curved systems, divide the area between the no-stick zones in half. Designate one-half for venous sticks and one-half for arterial sticks. (With a natural AV fistula and sizable peripheral vessels for venous sticks, the arterial portion can be longer.) For loop-configured accesses, use the straight portion of the venous limb for venous and the other side for arterial sticks. If a loop graft has an external support at its apex, use the areas 1/4 to 1/2 in. away from the external support on each side as your beginning markers. The first venous stick is placed at the midpoint of a straight or curved system or at the edge of the no-stick zone on the venous limb near the loop. The first arterial stick is placed within 1/2 in. of the venous needle in straight and curved systems and at the edge of the no-stick zone on the arterial limb near the loop. The next treatments stick sites will be 1/4 to 1/2 in. distal from the previous sites on both limbs of the access. This progression should continue until an area is reached within a needle's length of an anastomotic or anatomical no-stick zone. If, during the site rotation plan, a stick is blown, the next attempt should be made at the next healthy site on that limb. If the most distal stick site is blown, the next attempt should be made at the limb's starting point. The key to this or any site-rotation plan is starting it correctly and having all staff members comply.

Cannulation

After a careful assessment of the access, successful and safe cannulation of permanent AV fistulae and grafts requires skin preparation to try to limit bacterial contamination of the site (Table 11.5). There are many experience-based theories on what is good cannulation technique. Most of these theories unfortunately are based on short term goals; "two sticks, good flow; short bleed, good show." Left out of these theories too, are the damage models of the accesses, especially for ePTFE grafts. Histopathological examinations of explanted grafts create a very vivid picture of how our interventions fare with these materials. The "per-

TABLE 11.5 Skin Preparation Technique for Permanent AV Accesses

- Locate and palpate the needle cannulation sites prior to preparation.
- Wash access site using an antibacterial soap or scrub (e.g., 2% chlorhexidine) and water.
- Cleanse the skin by applying 70% alcohol and/or 10% providone-iodine using a circular rubbing motion.
- Alcohol has a short bacteriostatic action time and should be applied in a rubbing motion for 1 min immediately prior to needle cannulation.
- Povidone iodine must be applied for 2 to 3 min for its full bacteriostatic action to take effect and must be allowed to dry prior to needle cannulation.
- Clean gloves should be worn by the dialysis staff for cannulation. Gloves should be changed if contaminated at any time during the cannulation procedure.
- New, clean gloves should be worn by the dialysis staff for each patient.

Source: Modified from Ref. 3, Table III-6.

fect technique'' needle mark in ePTFE is a crescent-shaped hole with a small flap. This mark is oriented in the transverse direction on the graft. The flap does not cover the hole completely. The noncompliant, nonelastic material is displaced. This mark is achieved through proper bevel orientation and angle of cannulation. When sticking a graft, the needle bevel should be up to the graft, not the sticker. This technique allows the tip of the bevel to enter the graft first. The graft material is then cut evenly on both sides of the tip, providing the crescent shape. When the bevel is up to the sticker and the graft is penetrated away from its apex, the side of the needle cuts through the graft, leaving a small longitudinal slit or ''smile.'' This hole is usually larger than its transverse counterpart. Sticking with the bevel down can also leave a crescent-shaped hole and flap, but the risk of coring (leaving a circular hole with no flap) is much greater. Obviously, of the three holes, this one would be the more difficult with which to achieve hemostasis.

Knowing the characteristics of the access is important when selecting the best angle of cannulation. The mature natural AV fistula is single walled, very peripheral and fairly well anchored in its anatomical bed by the surrounding tissue and deep run-offs. A shallow angle of 20 degrees is adequate. Single wall prosthetic grafts that are porous are well established in their anatomical bed because of connective tissue incorporation. This anchoring allows these grafts to be safely cannulated at a 20-degree angle as well. Low porosity wrapped or layered grafts delaminate more when stuck at lower angles. Because they are not anchored as well as single wall systems, higher approach angles are useful to cleanly penetrate these devices. Other factors that influence the angle of cannulation are internal diameter of the access, depth of placement, wall thickness of the access, length of the dialysis needle and the presence of any pseudoaneurysms. The use of a mild restrictive tourniquet high on the outflow tract can be very useful in cannulating an access because the resultant tenseness it creates make the access easier to penetrate. Never place a tourniquet on the synthetic graft. Localized flow disturbances may predispose the graft to thrombus attachment and potential occlusion.

The cannulation motion should be smooth with a constant forward pressure exerted. All accesses yield to the needle before giving way to penetration. If the forward pressure is relaxed, it is very possible that the needle may create a new hole as the graft springs back to its precannulation shape. Poking and probing of the graft must be discouraged. At the earliest objective indication of entering the bloodstream, the needle should be leveled off (lowered near parallel to the access). The needle is then inserted fully to its hub. *Do not flip the needle during cannulation*! The blind manipulation of a cutting instrument can never be condoned. Staff assumes that the graft is perfectly round and unobstructed. In reality, this is rarely the case in a mature access. So the threat of lateral and posterior wall laceration and the risk of embolizing luminally attached materials is significant.

If the arterial needle aspirates poorly, first check to see if the access is being sucked onto the bevel. If it is, break the attachment by infusing a small amount of saline or blood. Pull the needle back slightly or carefully rotate it. If it is not, pull the needle back slowly until the blood flows freely. The direction of needle placement has one constant: the venous needle is always placed antegrade. There have been no reports of increased pseudoaneurysm formation with retrograde cannulation of ePTFE grafts.

Early Cannulation

The issue of when to cannulate an ePTFE graft is a topic of considerable interest. While there have been no ePTFE grafts sent to the Food and Drug Administration claiming early cannulation characteristics, all manufacturers are quick to point out features that might make theirs the best choice. The true critical feature is weighing patient need versus the risks of early use. Perigraft hemorrhage, infection, premature loss of site, thrombosis, pseudoaneurysm, graft laceration, and hematoma formation are all complications associated with early use of ePTFE (11,12).

Again, knowledge of graft construction and healing will allow proper planning to avoid these complications. Of the complications listed, graft laceration and hematoma formation are directly attributable to cannulation. Graft laceration results from poor orientation of the needle bevel and the lack of subcutaneous tissue ingrowth or attachment to the graft wall. Without anatomical anchoring, the graft can be moved within its tunnel. There is greater resistance due compression before the point at which the graft yields to needle penetration. Hematoma formation during cannulation can result from prolonged attempts where the needle does not fill the hole in the graft quickly or when multiple holes are made. For this reason, the "dry stick" needle technique is most appropriate. Wet or "wet stick" techniques utilize saline-primed needles, often with syringes attached and tubing clamps engaged. Placement within the access is determined subjectively, by feel or observing a "pop." Aspiration is then attempted before final needle positioning. If needle placement is not correct, the risk of hematoma is great. The dry technique uses no priming solution, tubing clamp, or syringe. When the needle enters the graft a "flashback" or blood return is immediately seen in the needle tubing. This objective confirmation of needle placement allows swift and accurate placement. Final positioning of the needle is guided by a pulsating column of blood (in the tubing) visible to the operator. Other complications of early cannulation occur after the treatment is over. The management of needle holes plays a crucial role in the early (and late) survival of ePTFE grafts. Several authors have commented on the dangers of applying too much pressure to needle holes. What then is proper or adequate? Adequate compression is defined as *A pressure applied perpendicular to the needle hole at the vessel entry site that controls bleeding both internally and externally, while maintaining pulses of near equal intensity proximal and distal to the area being compressed.*

There are several key tenets to this definition. The perpendicular approach is necessary to prevent the eversion of the edges of the needle hole into the graft. The distance between the vessel entry site and the skin exit site can be as great as 2 cm with a 1-in. (2.54 cm) needle. Therefore, control of the source of bleeding is more important than control of the blood exit tract. All graft manufacturers recommend digital pressure be used to achieve needle-hole hemostasis. The ability to vary the pressure, compensate for patient comfort and movement are perceived advantages. The use of spring-and-strap type clamps have become very popular. The rigors of patient scheduling have made their use more of an economic factor—"a spare set of hands," than a clinical advantage. Still, the application of clamps must comply to the same adequate compression definition above. Moist wound dressings or collagen hemostats should not be used with early cannulation grafts. Their primary action is to seal the needle insertion tract by reacting to blood in it. Because there is no anatomical attachment to the graft via tissue ingrowth or attachment, there will be little chance of these devices sealing the hole in the graft as well. Again, graft construction has much to do with when the use of these devices is safe. The extent of cellular integration and the time interval necessary for it to occur should be known by all critical staff.

Terminating Treatment

Terminating treatment with an AV access begins with proper needle removal. Compression is applied to the insertion site after the needle has been extracted. If compression is applied over the bevel of the needle and the vessel entry site during needle removal, a posterior wall laceration may result. If compression is applied over the skin exit site during needle removal, an anterior wall laceration may result. Excessive bleeding can result, sometimes requiring surgical intervention. Again, adequate compression is defined as a pressure applied perpendicular to the needle hole at the vessel entry site that controls bleeding both internally and externally while maintaining pulses of near equal intensity proximal and distal to the area being compressed. Once hemostasis is achieved, the needle holes should be covered in a way that does not compromise the patency of the graft or comfort of the patient.

REFERENCES

1. Windus DW. Permanent vascular access: A nephrologist's view. Am J Kidney Dis 21:5, 1993.
2. Levin A, Mason AJ, Jindal KK, et al. Prevention of hemodialysis subclavian catheter infections by topical povidone-iodine. Kidney Int 40:934–938, 1991.

3. NKF-DOQI. Clinical Practice Guidelines for Vascular Access. New York, National Kidney Foundation, 1997:44–48.
4. Centers for Disease Control and Prevention. Draft guidelines for prevention of intravascular device related infections: Parts 1 and 2. Fed Reg 60:49978–50006, 1995.
5. Buturovic J, Ponikvar R, Kandus A, et al. Filling hemodialysis catheters in the interdialytic period: heparin versus citrate versus polygeline: A prospective randomized study. Artif Organs 11:945–947, 1008.
6. Stephens LC, Haire WD, Tarantolo S, et al. Transfus Sci 18:187–193, 1997.
7. McEwen DR. Arteriovenous fistula. Vascular access for long-term hemodialysis. AORN J 59:225–232, 1994.
8. Hurlbert SN, Mattos MA, Henretta JP, et al. Long-term patency rates, complications and cost-effectiveness of polytetrafluoroethylene (PTFE) grafts for hemodialysis access: A prospective study that compares Impra versus Gore-Tex grafts. Cardiovasc Surg 6:652–656, 1998.
9. Williams SK, Berman SS, Kleinert LB. Differential healing and neovascularization of ePTFE implants in subcutaneous versus adipose tissue. J Biomed Mat Res 35: 473–481, 1997.
10. Salzmann DL, Kleinert LB, Berman SS, Williams SK. Inflammation and neovascularization associated with clinically used vascular prosthetic materials. Cardiovasc Pathol 8:63–71, 1999.
11. Coyne DW, Lowell JA, Windus DW, et al. Comparison of survival of an expanded polytetrafluoroethylene graft designed for early cannulation to standard wall polytetrafluoroethylene grafts. J Am Coll Surg 183:401–405, 1996.
12. Hakaim AG, Scott TE. Durability of early prosthetic dialysis graft cannulation: Results of a prospective, nonrandomized clinical trial. J Vasc Surg 25:1002–1005, 1997.

12

Complications of Hemodialysis Access Fistulae and Grafts

Mark R. Sarfati
The University of Utah,
  Salt Lake City, Utah

Scott S. Berman
The University of Arizona, Carondelet St. Mary's Hospital, and The
  Southern Arizona Vascular Institute, Tucson, Arizona

Complications associated with surgically created arteriovenous (AV) access fistulae and grafts represent a significant source of morbidity and mortality in patients maintained on hemodialysis. A recent review of the Medicare End Stage Renal Disease (ESRD) Program database illustrates the magnitude of this problem (1). This database represents approximately 200,000 patients comprising 90% of ESRD patients in the United States. In 1986, access-related complications resulted in 29,741 hospital admissions, accounting for more than 17% of all hospitalizations in this population. From 1984 to 1986, the total number of access-related hospital days increased from 189,000 to over 208,000. During a 2-year period, 19% of patients on hemodialysis experienced an access-related complication requiring hospitalization, with a mean hospital stay of 7 days.

Moreover, the financial burden imposed by these complications is significant. In 1991, Medicare financed renal replacement therapy for over 215,000 patients at an annual cost in excess of $6 billion. Patients and third-party payers contributed an additional $2.4 billion (2). Morbidity managed both in the outpa-

TABLE 12.1 When to Intervene—Dialysis AV Grafts for Venous Stenosis, Infection, Graft Degeneration, and Pseudoaneurysm Formation

Appropriate intervention in AV grafts should be initiated upon identification of any of the following:
A. Hemodynamically significant stenosis (see Guideline 10, "Monitoring Dialysis AV Grafts for Stenosis").
B. Infection—an infected graft should be treated surgically.
C. Graft degeneration and pseudoaneurysm formation—grafts should be surgically revised when:
   1. Severe degenerative changes of the graft or overlaying skin are present.
   2. Skin above the graft is compromised.
   3. There is a risk of graft rupture due to the presence of a large (or multiple) pseudoaneurysm(s). (See Guideline 27, "Treatment of Pseudoaneurysm of Dialysis AV Grafts.")

Source: Modified from Ref. 3, Guideline 17.

tient and inpatient settings accounts for approximately 60% of these expenditures, with a significant proportion related to complications of dialysis access. By conservative estimates, over $150 million is spent annually treating dialysis access–related complications (1).

Access-related complications can be broadly classified as thrombotic, infectious, and hemodynamic. Few of these complications are completely avoidable over the course of a patient's dialysis lifetime; however, correct management of the complications can limit the degree of morbidity incurred. The epidemiology, pathophysiology, diagnosis, management, and prevention of these problems are

TABLE 12.2 When to Intervene—Primary AV Fistulae

Appropriate intervention in primary AV fistulae should be initiated upon identification of any of the following:
A. Inadequate flow to support the prescribed dialysis blood flow.
B. Hemodynamically significant venous stenosis.
C. Aneurysm formation—a primary AV fistula should be revised when an aneurysm develops if:
   1. The skin overlying the fistula is compromised.
   2. There is a risk of fistula rupture.
   3. Available puncture sites are limited.

Source: Modified from Ref. 3, Guideline 18.

addressed in this chapter. Native AV fistulae will be distinguished from prosthetic AV grafts throughout the discussion (Tables 12.1 and 12.2) (3).

THROMBOTIC COMPLICATIONS

Chapters 5 and 7 have addressed the management strategies for access thrombosis in detail; consequently, this section emphasizes prevention. Loss of hemodialysis access due to thrombotic occlusion is the most common complication encountered and could conceivably be considered as an inevitable event in any patient who has an AV access graft. Patency rates for autogenous fistulae and prosthetic grafts differ significantly. Although autogenous fistulae are at greater risk for early postoperative occlusion due to inadequate venous outflow and technical errors made during their construction, their long-term patency rates are superior to those of prosthetic grafts (Figure 12.1) (4). Zibari et al. (5) demonstrated a mean patency rate of 2.85 years for native fistulae versus 1.75 years for PTFE grafts. In the same study, access thrombosis was observed in only 11% of autogenous fistulae versus 64% of synthetic grafts.

Etiology

Thrombosis of prosthetic AV grafts may occur at any time during the life of the access. Early thrombosis, occurring within 1 month of surgery, is usually caused

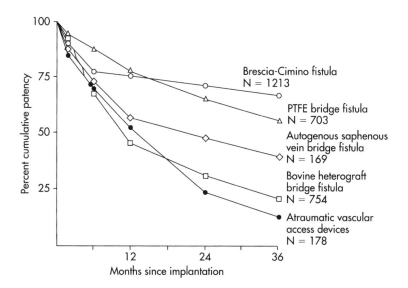

FIGURE 12.1   Actuarial survival of available access options (Cimino vs. bovine vs. ePTFE).

by either technical errors during creation of the access or inadequacy of the selected inflow artery or outflow vein unappreciated at the time of access construction. In our own experience, this occurs in less than 5% of prosthetic AV grafts. Early thrombotic failure of autogenous AV fistulae is more common than that seen with prosthetic grafts and occurs in 15 to 30% of cases, largely a consequence of poor venous outflow. Late thrombosis of both AV fistulas and grafts, defined as occurring more than 1 month postoperatively, is most commonly caused by venous outflow obstruction due to intimal hyperplasia (4). This time course, however, is subject to individual variation. Fibrotic stenosis within the access site secondary to repeated needle puncture may also lead to late thrombosis of either autogenous fistulae or prosthetic grafts.

Most episodes of early access thrombosis relate to errors committed during the planning and execution of the operative procedure. An awareness of potential technical errors combined with adherence to established vascular surgical principles and thoughtful preoperative planning should minimize the incidence of early graft thrombosis. Technical imperfections can cause stenosis or obstruction of the arterial or venous anastomosis resulting in early access thrombosis. The use of surgical loupe magnification may aid in accurate anastomotic construction. Catching the back wall of the vessel or raising an intimal flap must be avoided. Use of a single continuous or running suture can result in a purse-string effect, which narrows the anastomosis if too much tension is applied when the suture is secured. This pitfall may be avoided by the use of two sutures tied at two points or, in using a single suture, securing the knot after flow is established with the anastomosis under full distention. The anastomosis is gently dilated under arterial or venous pressure prior to tying the suture. Excessively large or numerous bites taken at either the heel of the arterial anastomosis or the toe of the venous anastomosis may lead to narrowing and subsequent thrombosis of a prosthetic graft (Figure 12.2). Following placement of these critical sutures, the anastomotic diameter may be assessed by gently probing with a coronary dilator.

Creation of a twist or kink of the conduit during subcutaneous tunneling of a prosthetic AV graft will result in early thrombosis. Expanded PTFE grafts are externally marked with a line that provides a means of orienting the graft to avoid twisting. Another technique used during AV graft construction that avoids twisting the graft is to perform the arterial anastomosis prior to tunneling the graft. With this method, the graft is pulled through the tunnel fully distended under arterial pressure, which protects the graft from twisting. Kinking in forearm loop AV grafts commonly occurs at the apex of the loop. This can be avoided by creating an adequately sized subcutaneous pocket at the apex of the loop, which allows the graft to assume a gradual curve. Graft redundancy will predispose to kinking and may be eliminated by applying gentle traction on the graft while it is trimmed to an appropriate length. Early thrombosis of autogenous fistulae may be caused by kinks or twists in the mobilized segment of vein used

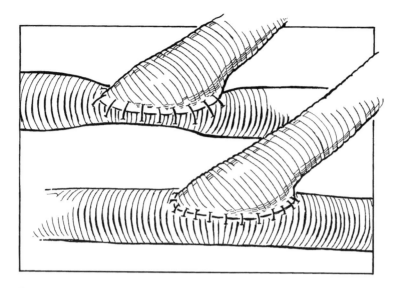

FIGURE 12.2   Excessively large bites at the toe of the venous anastomosis can result in severe narrowing of the outflow of an AV graft.

for the fistula. Care must be taken in configuring the fistula to avoid these defects. Marking the vein, gently distending it with heparinized saline, and/or passing a coronary dilator through it will confirm a smooth kink-and twist-free position prior to performing the anastomosis. The authors' preference for radiocephalic fistulae at the wrist is to perform a side-to-side anastomosis, which prevents any twisting of the vein segment. Once flow is established, the distal vein is ligated and divided, creating an end-to-side anastomosis. Careful visual inspection of the fistula and interrogation with Doppler will reveal any significant flow defects caused by position or adventitial bands requiring immediate attention to avoid early failure.

Poor venous outflow related to cephalic, basilic, axillary, or subclavian thrombosis, stenosis, or atresia is a common cause of early access failure for both native AV fistulae and prosthetic AV grafts. Accordingly, selection of an unobstructed venous outflow tract is essential in constructing dialysis access. The cephalic and basilic veins often have segmental stenoses or occlusions related to previous episodes of injury due to venipuncture, thrombosis, or thrombophlebitis. Preoperative physical examination of the cephalic and basilic veins should be performed using a tourniquet. This permits identification of segmental venous obstructions and is an essential part of planning the operation. Use of preoperative duplex venous mapping or venography in selected patients can aid in the identification of an unobstructed venous outflow tract (6). Once a patent venous outflow vessel has been identified, its course may be marked with an indelible felt-tipped pen, facilitating identification during surgery.

Of particular note is the recent demonstration of the high incidence of subclavian vein stenosis following central venous catheterization (7). If unrecognized, subclavian vein obstruction will result in early access thrombosis due to compromised outflow. Subclavian vein obstruction may often be clinically inapparent; however, when patients with a history of subclavian cannulation are evaluated with duplex ultrasonography or venography, the prevalence of this complication approaches 50% (8–10). Patients with a history of subclavian vein catheterization, documented subclavian vein thrombosis, arm edema, or superficial venous engorgement should be evaluated with a preoperative duplex examination or venography to identify subclavian vein obstruction prior to access construction. Since the incidence of central venous thrombosis is significantly less following internal jugular vein catheterization, this is the preferred site for central venous access in any patient who may require chronic renal replacement therapy (11,12). A policy of avoiding subclavian vein catheterization in this population can help limit this cause of access failure. Occult subclavian vein stenosis may manifest itself after angioaccess construction and present as ipsilateral arm edema or elevated venous pressures during dialysis. Correction of the subclavian obstruction may be accomplished using a combination of thrombolytic agents, balloon angioplasty, and endoluminal stent placement, although the long-term outcome of such interventions is unknown at this time (13–15).

Inadequate venous outflow may be recognized and corrected in the operating room. Before performing the venous anastomosis, the outflow vessel should be carefully probed with coronary dilators. An adequate vein should easily accept a 4-mm dilator. After the anastomosis is completed, the graft and venous outflow tract should be palpated and interrogated with Doppler. Doppler examination of a functional AV graft exhibits pulsatile flow and continuous flow through diastole together with a palpable thrill over the arterial anastomosis. Absence of these expected findings demands further investigation to delineate the underlying pathology. On-table fistulography provides a method to document any disturbances in the forearm and upper arm but offers only limited views of the central venous circulation with standard imaging equipment. A patent fistula with abnormal hemodynamics (i.e., absent thrill, poor Doppler flow) and no problems documented on intraoperative imaging should be immediately evaluated for outflow obstruction in the central venous circulation, so that prompt attention can be directed at the pathology. Otherwise access failure will be assured (Figure 12.3).

Generally, uninterrupted venous patency from the wrist to the antecubital fossa is requisite for a successful native radiocephalic AV fistula. Venous patency can be checked preoperatively by ballotting the vein from the wrist to the elbow with a tourniquet in place above the antecubital fossa. Local patency of the venous

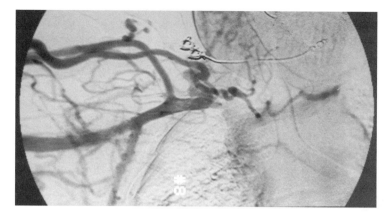

FIGURE 12.3   Subclavian vein stenosis proximal to a newly created forearm loop AV graft. This stenosis was subsequently balloon-dilated using the graft for percutaneous access.

outflow can be checked by passage of a small-diameter Fogarty balloon catheter or coronary dilator up the vein at the time of fistula construction. Poor hemodynamic performance in a newly constructed fistula demands further evaluation with fistulography and immediate revision to salvage the access site. As in the case of poorly functioning AV grafts, a full evaluation of the venous outflow including the central venous system is necessary to complete the workup of a poorly functioning native fistula.

Intimal hyperplasia resulting in venous outflow obstruction is the most common cause of late access thrombosis (16). This process most often occurs at the venous anastomosis but may also be seen more proximally along the venous outflow tract. Intimal hyperplasia is thought to represent an exaggerated and ultimately detrimental response to injury (17,18). The factors initiating and perpetuating this exaggerated response are unclear at this time. Current theories implicate a complex interaction between vascular endothelial cells, smooth muscle cells, leukocytes, and platelets. Furthermore, various growth factors, cytokines, and coagulation factors have been implicated as mediators of this process (19). To date, no effective therapy exists to combat intimal hyperplasia; however, numerous approaches to this problem are being explored. Treatments under consideration range from systemic drugs to local mechanical interventions.

Repeated needle puncture resulting in fibrotic stricture is another common cause of late AV access failure. Overzealous attempts to establish hemostasis after removing the dialysis needles by prolonged compression of the graft can result in stasis of flow and thrombosis. Premature use of an ePTFE graft prior

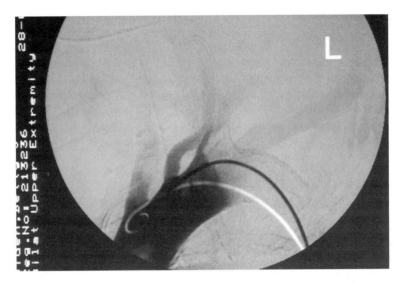

FIGURE 12.4   Occult left subclavian artery occlusion in a patient with normal, symmetrical arterial examination and subsequent failure of an upper arm AV graft.

to adequate healing and tissue incorporation may lead to bleeding from the needle holes, resulting in a perigraft hematoma. This can extrinsically compress and occlude the graft.

One way to avoid this complication is to wait 10 to 14 days before using a new ePTFE graft. However, if early cannulation is necessary, it may safely be accomplished by using small-guage needles and taking care not to puncture the back wall of the new graft. The Diastat graft, with its additional external layer of ePTFE, was designed for early use. Unfortunately, the enthusiasm with which its arrival was hailed has been subdued by emerging unfavorable complications with this prosthesis, particularly infection (20). Other potentially avoidable causes of graft thrombosis include hypotension, dehydration, low cardiac output, and inadvertent compression during general anesthesia. Insufficient arterial inflow is a less common cause of access failure and should largely be excluded by a careful physical examination prior to access construction. However, a well-collateralized proximal artery is an important factor to consider and should be assessed by arteriography in cases of difficult access when obstructive lesions are not found elsewhere (Figure 12.4).

Diagnosis and Management

Access occlusion is diagnosed by physical examination. Absence of a pulse, audible bruit, or palpable thrill indicates graft thrombosis. Absence of flow by Doppler examination further confirms the diagnosis. A careful history may elicit the cause of thrombosis. Recent prolonged episodes of bleeding from fistula access sites suggests venous outflow obstruction as an etiology of access thrombosis. Thrombosis within a month of placement of a prosthetic AV graft suggests either technical errors at the time of construction or selection of an inadequate venous outflow site. Surgical revision is mandatory to definitively address these problems; however, thrombolysis and fistulography with attention to the venous outflow prior to the surgical revision may help to direct the appropriate therapy. It may be more difficult to identify the etiology of early failure of an autologous fistula. Early failure of an initially functioning native AV fistula should be treated with thrombolysis, fistulography, and surgical revision if an anatomic lesion is identified. The more common scenario encountered comprises the native fistula that remains patent but fails to develop an arterialized segment suitable for access. In this circumstance, fistulography should be performed to assess the fistula for a correctable lesion (Figure 12.5). More often than not, the workup of native fistulae that fail to develop fails to reveal a correctable anatomic lesion. However, the superiority in long-term performance of native fistulae compared with prosthetic AV grafts explains our own aggressive approach to maintaining autologous access if at all possible, and, therefore, our determined use of fistulography in evaluating fistulae that fail to mature.

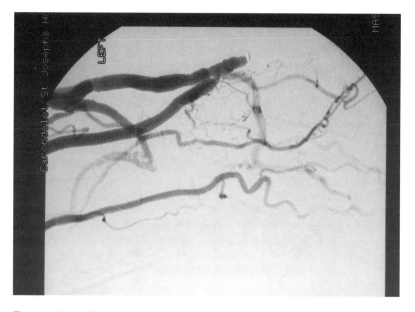

FIGURE 12.5   Fistulogram of poorly functioning 2-month-old snuffbox fistula showing anastomotic narrowing amenable to surgical correction and fistula salvage.

Management of AV graft and AV fistula thrombosis beyond 1 month after construction can be individualized and is discussed in detail in Chapters 7 and 8. Briefly, combinations of percutaneous and open surgical thrombectomy/thrombolysis, patch and balloon angioplasty, and revision have found varied success in disparate reports (21–23). When all the available literature is reviewed, whether percutaneous or surgical approaches are adopted, the end result is that patency of a thrombosed AV fistula or graft is restored for an average of 6 months before further interventions are required. Individual results will vary with the experience and the expertise of the specialty physicians available to care for the patient.

Our own approach centers on percutaneous techniques as the first line of treatment for all initial access thromboses. The findings are then reviewed by the interventional radiologists and surgeons so that future thrombotic events can be handled on an individual basis. Recurrent thrombosis within 30 to 60 days mandates assessment for surgical revision after patency is restored and dialysis is completed, if medically necessary. Otherwise surgical revision is performed without interval dialysis. Patients with a history of recurrent thrombosis without a clear etiology should be evaluated for hypercoagulability by assaying for protein C and S, antithrombin III, resistance to activated protein C, factor V Leiden level, and antiphospholipid antibodies (24,25).

Evidence is mounting that correction of venous outflow stenoses prior to access thrombosis is more cost-effective. Identifying patients at risk remains somewhat elusive. Sands (26) has championed an aggressive surveillance program that combines hemodynamic assessment with duplex sonography. A detailed discussion of graft surveillance techniques appears in Chapter 6. Correction of outflow obstruction prior to graft thrombosis may result in improved secondary patency. Early signs of venous outflow obstruction include elevated pressure in the venous dialysis line, increased relative graft resistance, and increased recirculation rate (27,28). If these measurements indicate outflow compromise, fistulography followed by revision is indicated.

ACCESS SITE INFECTION

Etiology

Infection is the most common reason for hospitalization and the second most common cause of death in hemodialysis patients. Infection accounts for 12% of mortality in this group, exceeded only by cardiovascular causes (29). Hemodialysis access sites are a common source of infection in this population. A recent multicenter prospective study demonstrated that up to 50% of documented bacteremias in hemodialysis patients originate in access grafts (30). Commonly encountered infectious complications include postoperative wound infection, cellulitis, puncture-site infection, perigraft abscess, graft erosion, or pseudoaneurysm. Patients may present with erythema, edema, warmth, tenderness, or fluctuance over the graft. Fever, leukocytosis, bacteremia, and frank sepsis may be seen. Alternatively, graft infections may be clinically indolent, presenting with fever and staphylococcal bacteremia but few local physical findings. Ultrasonographic demonstration of perigraft fluid or a positive radionuclide-tagged white blood cell scan may aid in the diagnosis of occult graft infection.

The vast majority of graft infections are caused by gram-positive cocci, with *Staphylococcus aureus* accounting for approximately 70% and *Staphylococcus epidermidis* responsible for only 10% in one series (31). It has been demonstrated that a significant percentage of dialysis patients are colonized with *S. aureus*; phage typing of pathogenic organisms indicates that the majority of staphylococcal infections in this population are caused by endogenous flora (32). Eradication of staphylococcal colonization through the use of prophylactic antibiotics may decrease the rate of access related infectious complications in dialysis patients (33). Graft infections caused by gram-negative rods, although uncommon, are difficult to treat and have been associated with anastomotic disruption and exsanguination (34).

Multiple factors inherent to ESRD patients contribute to the development of access-site infections. Chronic renal failure has various detrimental effects on immune function, including impaired lymphocyte-mediated cellular immunity, neutrophil chemotaxis, phagocytosis, and bacterial killing (35–38). These derangements in immune function predispose ESRD patients to access infection. However, despite its prevalence in ESRD, diabetes mellitus has not been shown to be an independent risk factor in the development of access infection (31).

Graft infection may occur during surgical implantation and may be associated with postoperative wound infection. This complication is seen in 3% of primary AV graft operations and in 0.4% of autogenous AV fistulae (31). Perioperative antibiotics have been shown to reduce the incidence of postoperative graft and wound infection following angioaccess surgery (39). Postoperative bleeding with perigraft hematoma formation is associated with a sevenfold increase in the incidence of graft infection (31). Since patients with chronic renal failure are often coagulopathic, adequate hemostasis must be assured prior to termination of the operative procedure to minimize the chance of hematoma formation and subsequent infection. We avoid the use of heparin in primary AV access procedures so as to minimize this risk.

Erosion of a prosthetic graft through the skin may either result from or be the cause of graft infection. Superficial tunneling of a prosthetic graft may lead to erosion, with subsequent infection of the exposed graft. Care must be exercised in placement of the graft in the subcutaneous space to avoid graft erosion. This may sometimes be difficult due to the fragile nature of the dermis and minimal subcutaneous tissue in some ESRD patients. In this subgroup, meticulous skin care must be emphasized, including the avoidance of adhesive dressings to reduce the chance of developing erosions, which can escalate to breakdown over the access site. In constructing a loop graft, the counterincision at the apex of the loop should not directly overlie the graft, as this may predispose to wound breakdown and graft exposure. To avoid incision breakdown directly over the apex of a loop graft, we position the counterincision several centimeters distal to the apex of the loop. Repeated access puncture provides numerous opportunities to introduce skin-borne bacteria. Adherence to strict aseptic technique during graft puncture is necessary. Premature puncture of ePTFE grafts prior to adequate healing and tissue incorporation may result in a perigraft hematoma and subsequent infection. It is ideal to wait 7 to 14 days after implantation before using ePTFE grafts. As with other foreign bodies, grafts can become infected secondary to transient bacteremias occurring during dental or other invasive procedures. Appropriate antibiotic prophylaxis should be administered prior to any procedure where transient bacteremia is anticipated.

Finally, the choice of conduit has a profound impact on the incidence of infectious complications. Infection is commonly seen in patients with synthetic grafts but is an uncommon complication of autogenous fistulae. The reported incidence of infection in ePTFE grafts is 5% per year. Consequently, the risk of a second infection dramatically rises to 12% per year. In contrast, infection occurring at the site of an autogenous fistulae is exceedingly uncommon, with a reported incidence 0.02% per year (31).

Presentation and Management

Access-site infection can vary in severity and presentation. Note should be made of an inflammatory response seen in roughly one-third of newly placed ePTFE AV grafts. This response manifests itself as intense erythema over the course of loop AV grafts in the forearm and is often associated with significant pain, fever, and edema. This response is usually self-limited and clears within 2 weeks, but it often provokes concern over early graft infection and is treated with a course of empiric antibiotics against gram-positive organisms. We have not appreciated a relationship between this inflammatory response and subsequent emergence of infectious complications. True access-site infection may range in presentation from localized erythema over the course of the access or the surgical incision to frank graft erosion to perigraft or incisional abcesses. Equally varied in presentation are systemic signs of infection such as fever, leukocytosis, pain, and—in patients with diabetes—poor glycemic control.

The management of access-site infections varies according to the type of conduit, extent of infection, and causative organism. Table 12.3 summarizes the DOQI guideline for prosthetic AU graft infection treatment. If possible, the inciting organism should be identified and appropriate antibiotics initiated. As the vast majority of access infections are caused by gram-positive cocci, we often

TABLE 12.3 Treatment of Infection of Dialysis AV Grafts

1. Local infection of a dialysis AV grafts should be treated with appropriate antibiotics based on culture results and by incision/resection of the infected portion of the graft.
2. Extensive infection of a dialysis AV graft should be treated with antibiotics and total resection of the graft.
3. Infection of a newly placed graft (i.e., within 1 month) should be treated with antibiotics and by removing the graft regardless of the extent of the infection.
4. Initial antibiotic treatment should cover both gram-negative and gram-positive organisms and *Enterococcus*.

Source: Modified from Ref. 3, Guideline 24.

treat patients empirically with intravenous vancomycin, since a single dose will remain therapeutic for 7 days in the ESRD patient. If a gram-negative organism is identified, we initiate aminoglycoside therapy.

Infection, which occurs infrequently in native AV fistulae, most often presents as an infected perigraft hematoma or abscess (Table 12.4). Many infected autogenous fistulae can be salvaged. Incision and drainage of the perigraft collection is followed with routine local wound care. Specimens for Gram's stain and culture are obtained at the time of surgical drainage. Intravenous vancomycin is begun empirically and is adjusted as indicated by Gram's stain and culture results. Perianastomotic involvement with or without pseudoaneurysm formation usually requires dismantling the anastomoses. In appropriately selected patients, the fistula can be reconstructed with an autogenous vein graft tunneled through an non-infected field. The presence of marked systemic sepsis or extensive graft involvement would preclude attempts at salvage.

Although more difficult to manage than infected autogenous fistulae, prosthetic graft salvage can be accomplished in a significant proportion of appropriately selected patients (31). One of the overwhelming advantages of ePTFE grafts compared with bovine grafts is the ability to salvage a ePTFE access should a portion become infected (40,41). By contrast, infected bovine AV grafts usually

TABLE 12.4 Treatment of Infection of Primary AV Fistulae

1. Infections of primary AV fistulae are rare and should be treated as subacute bacterial endocarditis with 6 weeks of antibiotic therapy.
2. Fistula take-down is required in cases of septic emboli.

Source: Modified from Ref. 3, Guideline 25.

require removal of the entire prosthesis, including the arterial and venous anastomoses, to completely eradicate the infection. Attempts at graft salvage are contraindicated in patients with significant sepsis, persistent bacteremia, and extensive graft involvement, particularly if the arterial anastomosis is involved. Since graft infections with gram-negative rods are notoriously difficult to eradicate and because of their association with anastomotic disruption, their presence is considered a further contraindication to graft preservation (34).

Attempts at salvage often require a combination of local abscess drainage and segmental excision of infected graft material. A number of scenarios come to mind. Localized small abscesses overlying a segment of well-incorporated ePTFE graft can often be treated with incision and drainage. If adequate healthy subcutaneous tissue exists in proximity to the infection, culture-specific antibiotics and local wound care may result in secondary healing without the need for any graft removal. More extensive infection in a segment of AV graft remote from the anastomoses can be treated with excision of the infected segment and reconstruction with a new graft segment interposed through noninfected fields. Whether reconstruction is performed concurrently with excision of the infected segment depends somewhat on the degree of infection. Our preference is to proceed with reconstruction if the graft is patent and the infection is manifest only as exposed graft without gross purulence. If the graft is thrombosed and the infected segment surrounded by purulent material, graft excision and reconstruction are performed as staged procedures with reconstruction conducted once the wounds have completely healed. This usually requires interval placement of a temporary jugular venous catheter for dialysis until permanent access continuity can be restored.

Anastomotic involvement with or without pseudoaneurysm formation requires segmental graft resection and closure of the anastomosis. If only the venous anastomosis is involved, it is possible to limited resection to this area and reestablish access continuity with a jump graft to a new venous outflow site once the infected wounds are healed. If the arterial anastomosis is involved in the infection, it is often difficult to salvage the access site and complete removal of all unincorporated graft material will be necessary. Graft resection and primary closure can be applied to the venous anastomosis; however, vein patch angioplasty is usually necessary when the arterial anastomosis is involved so as to avoid distal ischemic complications. One basic principle that must be adhered to is the complete removal of all unincorporated graft material. Occasionally, an access graft will be infected except for the arterial and venous anastomoses. In this circumstance, complete graft removal is performed save for a cuff of graft at both the venous and arterial anastomoses.

Wound closure covers this area with both subcutaneous and dermal tissues, thereby avoiding the need to dissect out the arterial and venous anastomoses, which can be difficult and may be associated with significant bleeding and the potential for nerve injury. In managing infected forearm AV grafts, we have broadly applied the use of a sterile pneumatic tourniquet for vascular control (42). Use of the pneumatic tourniquet permits avascular dissection and control while accomplishing eradication of infected material without the need for excessive dissection through scarred, noninfected planes to establish proximal and distal vascular control. Moreover, we apply the principles for managing vascular graft infection developed at our own institution with the use of intraoperative vascular wall cultures to guide the duration of postoperative antibiotic therapy (43,44). Rarely, coverage of exposed conduit may require the use of local soft tissue flaps.

HEMODYNAMIC COMPLICATIONS

Construction of an AV access, whether configured as an autogenous fistula or a prosthetic graft, "short circuits" the circulation in the extremity where the access is placed. This occurs by the shunting of blood from a muscular high-pressure artery into a low-pressure vein, effectively eliminating the high-resistance arterioles and capillary beds from the circulation of the inflow artery. Therefore the end result of a successful access is high flow, which manifests itself as a palpable thrill in the fistula. The thrill is the tactile representation of the turbulence through the access due to the high level of blood flow into a low-resistance runoff bed.

A functioning fistula must provide blood flow rates on the order of 400 to 600 mL/min in order for effective dialysis to be accomplished. Three untoward complications may develop as a consequence of a functioning access site with or without pathological implications that may require intervention. The three complications are steal, venous hypertension, and congestive heart failure. Fortunately, the incidence of each complication is relatively low; however, their management poses significant challenges to access surgeons, as described in the following sections (Table 12.5).

Steal

Arterial insufficiency or "steal syndrome" is an uncommon but potentially devastating complication of angioaccess surgery. The syndrome derives its name from the reversal of flow seen in the inflow artery of an AV fistula or graft, distal to the anastomosis. This flow reversal may result in the actual stealing of nutrient blood flow from the tissue beds distal to the arterial anastomosis. Asymptomatic or physiological steal is a common finding and can be appreciated by noninvasive testing in up to 90% of AV access sites (45). Symptomatic arterial insufficiency, however, is seen in less than 5% of patients following Brescia-Cimino or forearm loop PTFE fistulae. The incidence is higher, at 8 to 10%, in more proximally based autogenous or prosthetic fistulae (5). This syndrome may be more common

TABLE 12.5 Managing Potential Ischemia in a Limb Bearing an AV Access

All patients, particularly those in high-risk groups, should be monitored for the development of limb ischemia following AV access construction.

1. Patients in high-risk groups (diabetic, elderly, those with multiple access attempts in an extremity) should be monitored closely for the first 24 h postoperatively. Monitoring should include the following:
   a. Subjective assessment of complaints, including sensations of coldness, numbness, tingling, and impairment of motor function (not limited by postoperative pain).
   b. Objective assessment of skin temperature, gross sensation, and movement and distal arterial pulses in comparison to the contralateral side.
   c. Teaching patients to immediately report any coldness, loss of motion, or significant reduction in sensation.
2. Patients with an established fistula should be assessed monthly. The following are recommended as part of this assessment:
   a. Obtaining an interval history of increased distal coldness or distal pain during dialysis, decreased sensation, weakness or other reduction in function, or skin changes.
   b. Confirming any abnormalities by physical examination.

Patients with new findings suggestive of ischemia should be referred to a vascular access surgeon emergently. Reduced skin temperature as an isolated finding requires follow-up observation but no emergent intervention.

Source: Modified from Ref. 3, Guideline 16.

in patients with severe atherosclerosis and diabetes (46). Previously occult arterial occlusive disease of the extremity inflow arteries may become manifest following fistula construction and should be carefully looked for preoperatively (47).

Steal syndrome, or ischemia related to a patent dialysis access site, declares itself with severe pain in the distal extremity. In the most severe cases, the pain is unrelenting and very similar in character to ischemic rest pain of the foot (Figure 12.6). In milder cases, the patient may exhibit pain and/or paresthesias only during dialysis treatments. The mechanism of dialysis-induced ischemia is unknown but likely related to changes in volume, electrolytes, and systemic blood pressure commonly seen during a dialysis session. Since blood flow through the access does not change appreciably during a dialysis treatment compared with the pretreatment level, it is unlikely that flow disturbances alone result in treatment-related symptoms. Ischemic symptoms in dialysis patients are often confused with or dismissed as neuropathy, which is another common phenomenon in ESRD patients (48,49). Careful evaluation of patients exhibiting pain and par-

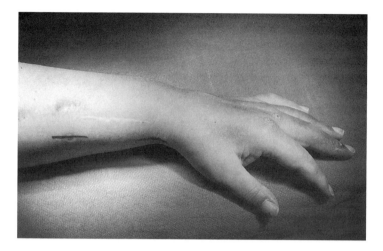

FIGURE 12.6 Severe ischemia secondary to steal from a Cimino fistula with hyperemia and early gangrene.

esthesias in the extremity distal to the site of an AV access fistula or graft, however, may uncover an ischemia component that may be treatable (50).

Access-related ischemia may appear acutely after fistula construction, subacutely within the first few weeks after fistula placement, or chronically several years after fistula placement (51). In our own experience with 21 cases, patients were more likely to present with pain and paresthesias in the acute and subacute setting. Those patients experiencing chronic ischemia often had evidence of tissue loss with either ischemic ulcerations or digital gangrene. There are two challenges the clinician must overcome related to access induced ischemia. The first challenge comprises a careful preoperative evaluation and attention to detail in access construction to minimize the incidence of clinically significant ischemia. The second and more formidable challenge is successfully treating clinically significant access-related ischemia.

The preoperative assessment of a patient undergoing an AV access placement has been discussed in detail in Chapter 2. A brief summary of the issues related to minimizing extremity ischemia is given in this section. A careful examination of all peripheral pulses is the first component in reducing the likelihood of ischemia developing after AV access placement. For the upper extremity, specific note should be made of the presence and character of the axillary, brachial, radial, and ulnar pulses. A simple hand-held Doppler examination should be performed to characterize the presence and quality of palmar arch and digital arterial flow. Performance of an Allen's test is particularly important if a Cimino-type autogenous AV fistula is planned. A positive Allen's test suggests inadequate collateral flow to the hand, thereby eliminating a radiocephalic fistula at the wrist as an access option (52). A similar evaluation of the lower extremities is required when a thigh AV graft is planned. A simple segmental Doppler examination with digital pressures will suffice in identifying patients with significant lower extremity occlusive disease in the absence of easily palpable pedal pulses.

A normal preoperative arterial examination in the chosen extremity, however, does not preclude the development of access-induced ischemia. In our own series, 3 of 10 patients who developed acute ischemia had occlusive disease documented arteriographically, despite normal preoperative examinations (Figure 12.7) (51). This finding highlights the complexity of "steal" physiology, which results in ischemia despite the absence of occlusive disease in the majority of patients. The etiology remains unclear, but the strength and adequacy of collateral arterial flow around the arterial anastomosis of the access seems suspect. Unfortunately, at this time there are no provocative tests available to predict ischemia prior to access construction in a patient without preoperative signs of arterial insufficiency. By contrast, chronic ischemia in the access extremity is more likely related to the presence of arterial occlusive disease. All 11 of the patients with chronic access-induced ischemia in our series had occlusive disease in the affected extremity (51). Given the time course of symptom development in these patients, it is likely that the "steal" physiology acts in concert with underlying

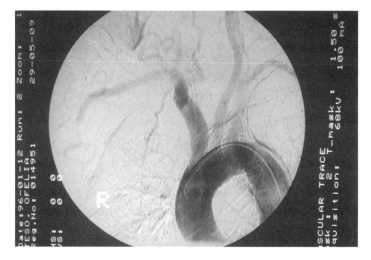

Figure 12.7 Occult axillary artery stenosis above a patent forearm loop AV graft discovered when the patient exhibited severe steal.

arterial occlusive disease, leading to the tissue loss that is appreciated in these patients (Figure 12.8).

The second and more overwhelming challenge facing surgeons who must deal with access-related ischemia revolves around the reversal of the ischemia as well as the maintenance of a functional access site. A number of treatment options for symptomatic steal exist, including simple ligation or takedown of the

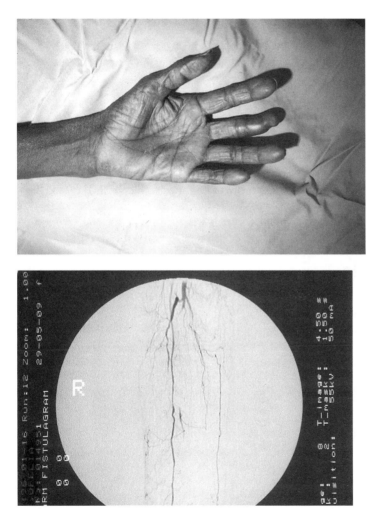

FIGURE 12.8   Chronic ischemia in a patient with a patent AV fistula and atherosclerotic occlusive disease of the infrabrachial arteries.

fistula, flow reduction through the fistula by either banding or interposing a flow restrictor, or revascularization of the extremity distal to the AV access (51,53–60). Ligation or dismantling of the fistula or access is the simplest form of treatment and invariably eliminates the ischemia (53). Unfortunately, this leaves the patient and surgeon with the perplexing problem of reestablishing access at another site, which carries the consequent risk of recurrent ischemic symptoms. Ligation may assume another form for patients with steal related to a patent Cimino fistula. Here the radial artery just distal to the fistula at the wrist is ligated, thereby eliminating the pathway for steal through the palmar arch. This specific technique is applicable in patients with pure steal unrelated to occlusive disease and is classically described for radiocephalic fistulae at the wrist whereby hand perfusion is preserved through the ulnar artery feeding the palmar arch and symptoms are related to the overwhelming flow reversal through the fistula in the radial artery distal to the AV anastomosis (61).

Unlike fistula ligation or takedown, an alternative technique for treating steal syndrome—which centers upon the principle of reducing flow through the AV fistula or access graft by increasing the resistance in the fistula or graft—seeks to preserve the access site. By either lengthening the segment of prosthetic graft or, more commonly, narrowing a portion of the access by either banding or interposition of a tapered segment of prosthesis (Figure 12.9), total flow through the fistula can be reduced (54–57). Despite the initial success with a tapered graft reported by Rosenthal et al. (54), consistent protection from ischemic complications has not been demonstrated as experience with the clinical use of tapered grafts has grown (62). Failure of flow reduction alone, through

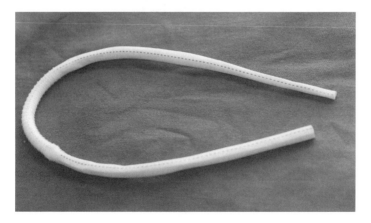

FIGURE 12.9 Tapered 4-mm arterial limb to 7-mm venous limb ePTFE graft designed to limit steal by providing a smaller, high-resistance arterial segment.

the use of tapered grafts, to consistently correct or avoid steal complications highlights the complexity of this problem and suggests that multiple physiological factors need to be addressed to effectively treat significant ischemia.

A comparable inference can be made from a review of the experience with banding techniques (Figure 12.10). Few objective data are available to calibrate the amount of banding necessary to reliably eliminate the distal ischemia while maintaining flow through the fistula. As a result of the subjective nature of this treatment, access thrombosis is a common complication. Jain et al. (56) recently published their limited experience of three patients, using intraoperative angiodynography to gauge the amount of banding required to eliminate flow reversal in the distal artery, in which ischemia was relieved and access function preserved. Our own experience with the banding technique more closely correlates with that reported in the literature. Successful treatment of ischemia and maintenance of the access site was achieved in only 15 of 29 patients treated with banding (51). Moreover, access thrombosis was the prevalent outcome achieved once flow was reduced enough to relieve the ischemia (63).

The last technique described to deal with significant steal was originally presented by Schanzer et al. (58,59). We have recently reviewed our own experience with this technique and have called it the distal revascularization–interval ligation (DRIL) procedure (51). It involves revascularization from the artery

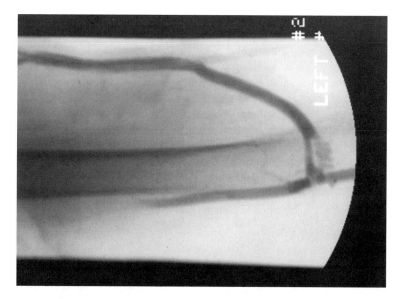

FIGURE 12.10 Banding of an AV access accomplished with application of clips to narrow the flow channel in the arterial limb.

above the fistula to an artery below the fistula accompanied by interval ligation of the artery between the origin of the AV access and the distal anastomosis of the bypass (Figure 12.11). In 1992, Schanzer's group reported their experience to date with 14 patients, of which 13 achieved limb salvage and preservation of a functional access with a 1-year patency of 84% (59). An additional series of six patients was recently added to the published experience with this procedure by Katz and Kohl and furnished further support for the reliability in treating ischemia and preserving the AV access site that the DRL procedure makes possible (60).

We recently published our own series of 21 patients treated with the DRL technique and demonstrated consistency in resolving limb ischemia without sacrificing a functioning AV access. With the support of the reports of Schanzer et al. (58,59) and Katz and Khol (60) as well as our own published experience (51), we believe that the DRL procedure is the method of choice for treating access-induced ischemia. None of the alternative methods described for managing steal have achieved the consistent results realized with the DRIL procedure in salvaging both a viable extremity and a functional AV access site, and we commend the DRIL procedure to all access surgeons as the first choice for dealing with the complex problem of steal syndrome induced by a functioning AV access.

Venous Hypertension

Venous hypertension is an uncommon complication of dialysis angioaccess. Two clinical syndromes may be recognized. The first occurs in the setting of a side-to-side fistula and affects the extremity distal to the fistula (64). High-pressure arterial blood flows into the low-resistance venous bed results in venous hypertension, which is manifest as progressive extremity swelling, hyperpigmentation, induration, cyanosis, and—if allowed to progress—skin ulceration. The hand is most commonly affected. The clinical appearance is similar to that seen in chronic lower extremity venous insufficiency. Resolution is typically seen following ligation of the vein distal to the anastamosis, converting the side-to-side anastomosis to a functional side-of-artery to end-of-vein configuration.

The second syndrome of venous hypertension is related to venous outflow obstruction. This more common form of venous hypertension may present acutely when an arteriovenous anastomosis is constructed distal to an unrecognized proximal venous stenosis or occlusion. More often, however, venous hypertension develops chronically in the extremity with a patent AV fistula and proximal venous obstruction. The most common site of venous obstruction is at the axillary–subclavian vein level. Stenoses and occlusions at this site have been correlated with prior placement of temporary dialysis catheters through a subclavian vein approach. Increased venous flow under arterial pressure in the face of venous outflow obstruction results in marked venous hypertension. Massive upper ex-

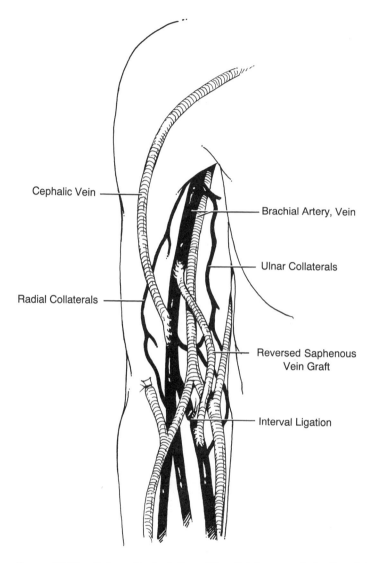

FIGURE 12.11 Schematic depiction of the distal revascularization–interval ligation (DRIL) procedure for access steal. Courtesy of the Journal of Vascular Surgery.

tremity edema in the immediate postoperative period after placement of AV access is suggestive of proximal venous obstruction and should trigger further evaluation. If the subclavian vein occlusion is located proximal to the internal mammary vein, ipsilateral breast edema may be seen (65).

Treatment of venous hypertension secondary to a patent and functioning AV access is contingent upon the severity of the symptoms. Mild symptoms may respond to elevation of the extremity which usually requires the limb to be kept almost continuously above the level of the heart. Occasionally, venous collaterals around the shoulder develop sufficiently to permit the resolution of symptoms without intervention (Figure 12.12). Severe symptoms, such as pain and ulceration, require further evaluation and treatment.

The first step in managing severe venous hypertension includes accurate anatomical delineation of the site and severity of the venous obstruction. Although duplex scanning can visualize the axillary and portions of the subclavian veins, the best method to image the complete peripheral and central venous system is through venography. This can often be accomplished through the venous limb of the fistula. Occasionally, a severe, acute stenosis or occlusion of the subclavian vein is not well collateralized and thereby provides poor visualization of the central venous system. In this circumstance it becomes necessary to image central venous system through a transfemoral approach. A number of anatomical findings maybe encountered to account for the venous hypertension and that individually have therapeutic implications.

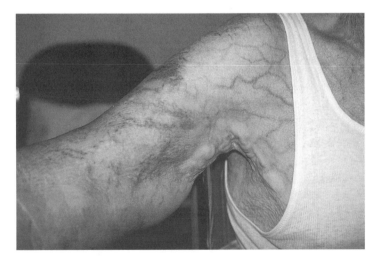

FIGURE 12.12   Chronic venous hypertension secondary to an AV graft. Note massive subcutaneous venous collaterals in the shoulder.

The venous hypertension may be secondary to a high-grade stenosis in the subclavian or brachiocephalic venous system (Table 12.6). These lesions are often treated by percutaneous balloon angioplasty (PTA) at the time of fistulography, as described in detail in Chapter 8. Acute lesions usually have few collaterals around the shoulder. By contrast, chronic lesions may produce findings suggestive of postphlebitic recanalization of the central vein with marked venous collaterals around the shoulder. As with angioplasty in other locations, focal lesions tend to respond well to balloon treatment. Second-and third-time recurrent lesions following successful primary or secondary PTA are often treated with adjunctive stenting. Repeat angioplasty of stent lesions is also possible to maintain long-term patency. In general, central venous stenotic lesions are considered to be nonsurgical because of the significant morbidity associated with their reconstruction. As such, aggressive use of PTA and stents may salvage an extremity and functioning access when venous obstruction is encountered. Procedural success rates approach 80% with 6-month patency rates reaching 50 to 60% in this difficult population.

In contrast to a subclavian or brachiocephalic stenosis, correction of a subclavian occlusion maybe somewhat more difficult. If other clinical signs of chronicity are absent, a trial of thrombolytic therapy may be required to determine whether the occlusion is acute or chronic. Acute occlusions that are successfully opened with thrombolysis and reveal a precipitating stenosis are managed as described in the preceding paragraph. Chronic subclavian vein occlusions are more difficult to treat successfully. One surgical option that has met with moderate success is the jugular vein turndown procedure, similar to the technique described for the treatment of chronic venous insufficiency of the upper extremity caused by thoracic outlet syndrome. With this technique, the internal jugular (IJ) vein is mobilized from the base of the neck to the base of the skull and divided proximally. The IJ is then swung down laterally to be anastomosed to the axillary-subclavian vein to effectively bypass the proximal subclavian vein occlusion. An alternative technique employs a prosthetic graft extension off the venous limb of an upper arm AV graft, which courses across the shoulder joint and over the clavicle; it is anastomosed to the IJ vein at the base of the neck (Figure 12.13).

These bypass techniques are usually reserved for patients with functioning

TABLE **12.6** Treatment of Central Vein Stenosis

1. Percutaneous intervention with transluminal angioplasty is the preferred treatment for central vein stenosis.
2. Stent placement combined with angioplasty is indicated in elastic central vein stenoses or if a stenosis recurs within a 3-month period.

Source: Modified from Ref. 3, Guideline 20.

AV fistulae and few options for future access sites. Both techniques rely on a patent ipsilateral IJ vein. This should be verified by venography to be in continuity with the superior vena cava. Although duplex scanning can determine the status of the cervical portion of the IJ, the mediastinal section cannot be adequately imaged with this modality and requires confirmatory venography prior to surgical intervention. Moreover, patency of the contralateral IJ vein is desirable to avoid massive head edema in the event of failure or thrombosis of the IJ used for the bypass procedure. It is not uncommon for dialysis patients to have undergone multiple central venous access procedures during their dialysis lifetimes and similarly not uncommon for them to have multiple silent central venous occlusions, which only become apparent during the evaluation and treatment of venous hypertension. Both of these bypass techniques offer methods of salvage for these complex patients, though limited experience with these techniques appears in the literature for review or comparison.

When complete subclavian or brachiocephalic occlusion is encountered in a patient whose contralateral extremity is free of any contraindications for use as an AV access site, the most reliable method to eliminate venous hypertension in the involved extremity is simple access ligation. We generally place the new access graft and confirm is functionality prior to proceeding with access ligation in patients whose inciting fistula remains patent. This usually requires staging the procedures a few weeks apart. Fistula ligation can be accomplished under local anesthesia. When severe venous engorgement is present, limb exsanguination and tourniquet placement can simplify the ligation procedure by decompressing the giant venous collaterals. Paramount in the postoperative care is the use of elastic wrappings to facilitate resolution of the chronic edema, often in a few weeks.

Congestive Heart Failure

Congestive heart failure in the dialysis patient is most frequently due to volume overload caused by inadequate dialysis, myocardial ischemia, anemia, or poorly controlled hypertension. Uncommonly, the hemodynamic effects of a surgically created arteriovenous fistula will precipitate congestive heart failure. The hemodynamic consequences of dialysis angioaccess include an increase in resting cardiac output and heart rate and a fall in systemic vascular resistance, with no significant change in mean arterial or central venous pressure (66). The observed increase in cardiac output is due to an increase in venous return to the heart, which is proportional to the diameter of the feeding artery and the size of the arteriovenous anastomosis. In patients with compromised cardiac function, increased venous return results in ventricular volume overload and high-output cardiac failure. The incidence of this complication is likely related to the fistula flow rates and the degree of underlying cardiac dysfunction. Congestive heart failure is unusual in fistulae with flow rates less than 20 to 50% of cardiac output (67). In one reported series, all patients developing congestive heart failure had fistula flow rates greater than 600 mL/min. The often mentioned Nicaladoni-Branham sign, a fall in heart rate with temporary fistula occlusion, is rarely observed (67). Correction requires either fistula ligation or flow reduction, as described in the section on steal syndrome, above (68).

OTHER COMPLICATIONS

Pseudoaneurysm

Pseudoaneurysm formation secondary to graft infection or trauma occurs in 2 to 10% of patients and is more commonly seen in prosthetic grafts (5). Pseudoaneurysm formation at the arterial anastomosis is often due to local infection, with partial disruption of the suture line. This complication may lead to anastomotic disruption or graft rupture, with resultant exsanguination. Anastomotic pseudoaneurysms are treated by dismantling the anastomosis. In selected patients, the fistula may be salvaged with a jump graft. Pseudoaneurysms may also form along the length of the graft due to laceration during needle puncture. Pseudoaneurysms along the length of the graft are treated with either local suture repair or local excision and reconstruction with interposition or jump grafting. Critical in the treatment of any pseudoaneurysm is the assessment of graft incorporation. Any sign of poor graft incorporation should signal the possibility of graft infection and suggest the need for adequate debridement, intraoperative cultures, and the application of reconstructive techniques described in the earlier section on access infection (Table 12.7).

Access Aneurysm

True aneurysms (Table 12.8) are more likely to occur in native AVFs, although their overall incidence is poorly defined, since there are no clear criteria distinguishing the usual diffuse enlargement seen in a native AVF from an actual aneurysm. Aneurysms in native AVFs become troublesome when they are focal in

TABLE **12.7** Treatment of Pseudoaneurysms of Dialysis AV Grafts

1. Needle insertion into the area of pseudoaneurysm should be avoided.
2. Pseudoaneurysm of a dialysis AV graft should be treated by resection and insertion of an interposition graft if the pseudoaneurysm (a) is characterized by rapid expansion in size, (b) exceeds twice the diameter of the graft, (c) threatens viability of the overlying skin, or (d) is infected.

Source: Modified from Ref. 3, Guideline 27.

TABLE 12.8 Aneurysm of Primary AV Fistulae

1.	Aneurysms of primary AV fistulae require surgical intervention only when the aneurysm involves the arterial anastomosis.
2.	Venipuncture should avoid the aneurysm.

Source: Modified from Ref. 3, Guideline 28.

that the wall of the aneurysmal segment is thin and weak and poses problems for hemostasis after cannulation. More commonly, diffuse aneurysmal enlargement of an AVF limits available stick sites for dialysis treatments. Management of AVF aneurysms depends upon their size and extent. Focal aneurysms can be managed with either interposition replacement with vein or a prosthesis or, if the wall is fairly thick, resection and imbrication to a size that matches the remainder of the access. Diffuse aneurysmal degeneration of an AVF will require either bypass with a prosthetic graft or placement of a new access at a new site.

REFERENCES

1. Feldman HI, Held PJ, Hutchinson JT, et al. Hemodialysis vascular access morbidity in the United States. Kidney Int 43:1091–1096, 1993.
2. The United States Renal Data System's 1994 Annual Data Report. Am J Kidney Dis 24:S33–S47, 1994.
3. NKF-DOQI. Clinical Practice Guidelines for Vascular Access. New York: National Kidney Foundation; 1997.
4. Kherlakian GM, Roedersheimer LR, Arbaugh JJ, et al. Comparison of autogenous fistula versus expanded polytetrafluoroethylene graft fistulas for angioaccess in hemodialysis. Am J Surg 152:238–243, 1986.
5. Zibari GB, Rohr MS, Landreneau MD, et al. Complications from permanent hemodialysis vascular access. Surgery 104:681–686, 1988.
6. Comeaux ME, Bryant PS, Harkrider WW. Preoperative evaluation of the renal access patient with color Doppler imaging. J Vasc Tech 17:247–250, 1993.
7. Vanherweghem JL, Yassine T, Goldman M, et al. Subclavian vein thrombosis: A frequent complication of subclavian vein cannulation for hemodialysis. Clin Nephrol 26:235–238, 1986.
8. Spinowitz BS, Galler M, Golden RA, et al. Subclavian vein stenosis as a complication of subclavian catheterization for hemodialysis. Arch Intern Med 147:305–307, 1987.
9. Barrett N, Spencer S, McIvor J, Brown EA. Subclavian stenosis: A major complication of subclavian dialysis catheters. Nephrol Dial Transplant 3:423–425, 1988.
10. Surratt RS, Picus D, Hicks ME, et al. The importance of preoperative evaluation of the subclavian vein in dialysis access planning. Am J Roentgenol 156:623–625, 1991.

11. Cimochowski GE, Worley E, Rutherford WE, et al. Superiority of the internal jugular over the subclavian access for temporary dialysis. Nephron 54:154–161, 1990.

12. Schillinger F, Schillinger D, Montagnac R, Milcent T. Post catheterization vein stenosis in haemodialysis: Comparative angiographic study of 50 subclavian and 50 internal jugular accesses. Nephrol Dial Transplant 6:722–724, 1991.

13. Schwab SJ, Quarles LD, Middleton JP, et al. Hemodialysis-associated subclavian vein stenosis. Kidney Int 33:1156–1159, 1988.

14. Glanz S, Gordon DH, Lipkowitz GS, et al. Axillary and subclavian vein stenosis: Percutaneous angioplasty. Radiology 168:371–373, 1988.

15. Kovalik EC, Newman GE, Suhocki P, et al. Correction of central venous stenoses: Use of angioplasty and vascular Wallstents. Kidney Int 45:1177–1181, 1994.

16. Munda R, First MR, Alexander JW, et al. Polytetrafluoroethylene graft survival in hemodialysis. JAMA 249:219–222, 1983.

17. Rekhter M, Nicholls S, Ferguson M, Gordon D. Cell proliferation in human arteriovenous fistulas used for hemodialysis. Arterioscler Thromb 13:609–617, 1993.

18. Sottiurai V, Yao J, Batson R, Sue S, Jones R, Nakamura Y. Distal anastomotic intimal hyperplasia: Histopathologic character and biogenesis. Ann Vasc Surg 3: 26–33, 1989.

19. Clowes AW. Pathologic intimal hyperplasia as a response to vascular injury and reconstruction. In Rutherford RB, ed. Vascular Surgery, 4th ed, Philadelphia: Saunders; 1995:285–295.

20. Bartlett ST, Schweitzer EJ, Roberts JE, et al. Early experience with a new ePTFE vascular prosthesis for hemodialysis. Am J Surg 170:118–122, 1995.

21. Kanterman RY, Vesely TM, Pilgram TK, et al. Dialysis access grafts: Anatomic location of venous stenosis and results of angioplasty. Radiology 195:135–139, 1995.

22. Katz SG, Kohl RD. The percutaneous treatment of angioaccess graft complications. Am J Surg 170:238–242, 1995.

23. Beathard GA. Thrombolysis versus surgery for the treatment of thrombosed dialysis access grafts. J Am Soc Nephrol 6:1619–1624, 1995.

24. Prieto LN, Suki WN. Frequent hemodialysis graft thrombosis: Association with antiphospholipid antibodies. Am J Kidney Dis 23:587–590, 1994.

25. Svensson PJ, Dahlback B. Resistance to activated protein C as a basis for venous thrombosis. N Engl J Med 330:517–522, 1994.

26. Sands J, Young S, Miranda C. The effect of Doppler flow screening studies and elective revisions on dialysis access failure. ASAIO J 38:M524–M527, 1992.

27. Schwab SJ, Raymond JR, Saeed M, et al. Prevention of hemodialysis fistula thrombosis. Early detection of venous stenosis. Kidney Int 36:707–711, 1989.

28. Van Stone JC, Jones M, Van Stone J. Detection of hemodialysis access outlet stenosis by measuring outlet resistance. Am J Kidney Dis 23:562–568, 1994.

29. Port FK. Mortality and causes of death in patients with end-stage renal failure. Am J Kidney Dis 3:215–217, 1990.

30. Kessler M, Hoen B, Mayeux D, et al. Bacteremia in patients on chronic hemodialysis. Nephron 64:95–100, 1993.

31. Taylor B, Sigley RD, May KJ. Fate of infected and eroded hemodialysis grafts and autogenous fistulas. Am J Surg 165:632–636, 1993.

32. Ena J, Boelaert JR, Boyken LD, et al. Epidemiology of Staphylococcus aureus infections in patients on hemodialysis. Infect Control Hosp Epidemiol 15:78–81, 1994.

33. Yu VL, Goetz A, Wagener M, et al. Staphylococcus aureus nasal carriage and infection in patients on hemodialysis. N Engl J Med 315:91–96, 1986.

34. Ballard JL, Bunt TJ, Malone JM. Major complications of angioaccess surgery. Am J Surg 164:229–232, 1992.

35. Wilson WEC, Kirkpatrick CH, Talmage DW. Suppression of immunologic responsiveness in uremia. Ann Intern Med 62:1–14, 1965.

36. Peresecenschi G, Blum M, Aviram A, Spirer ZH. Impaired neutrophil response to acute bacterial infection in dialyzed patients. Arch Intern Med 141:1301–1302, 1981.

37. Salant DJ, Glover AM, Anderson R, et al. Depressed neutrophil function in patients with chronic renal failure and after renal transplantation. J Lab Clin Med 88:536–545, 1976.

38. Hanicki Z, Cichocki T, Komorowska Z, et al. Some aspects of cellular immunity in untreated and maintenance hemodialysis patients. Nephron 23:273–275, 1979.

39. Bennion RS, Hiatt JR, Williams RA, Wilson SE. A randomized, prospective study of perioperative antimicrobial prophylaxis for vascular access surgery. J Cardiovasc Surg 26:270–274, 1985.

40. Doyle DL, Fry PD. Polytetrafluoroethylene and bovine grafts for vascular access in patients on long-term hemodialysis. Can J Surg 25:379–382, 1982.

41. Hurt AV, Batello-Cruz M, Skipper BJ, et al. Bovine carotid artery heterografts versus polytetrafluoroethylene grafts. A prospective, randomized study. Am J Surg 146:844–847, 1983.

42. Berman SS, Lopez J. Use of a pneumatic tourniquet for vascular control in the management of vascular access for hemodialysis. In Henry ML, Ferguson RM, eds. Vascular Access for Hemodialysis V. Chicago: Gore; 1997:307–315.

43. Malone JM, Lalka SG, McIntyre KE, et al. The necessity for long-term antibiotic therapy with positive arterial wall cultures. J Vasc Surg 8:262–267, 1988.

44. Durham JR, Malone JM, Bernhard VM. The impact of multiple operations on the importance of arterial wall cultures. J Vasc Surg 5:160–169, 1987.

45. Kwun KB, Schanzer H, Finkler N, et al. Hemodynamic evaluation of angioaccess procedures for hemodialysis. Vasc Surg 13:170–177, 1979.

46. Connolly JE, Brownell DA, Levine EF, McCart M. Complications of renal dialysis access procedures. Arch Surg 119:1325–1328, 1984.

47. Calligaro KD, Ascer E, Veith FJ, et al. Unsuspected inflow disease in candidates for axillofemoral bypass operations: a prospective study. J Vasc Surg 11:832–837, 1990.

48. Bosanac PR, Bilder B, Grunberg RW, et al. Post–permanent access neuropathy. Trans Am Soc Artif Intern Organs 23:162–167, 1977.

49. Wytrzes L, Markley HG, Fisher M, Alfred HJ. Brachial neuropathy after brachial artery–antecubital vein shunts for chronic hemodialysis. Neurology 37:1398–1400, 1987.

50. Hye RJ, Wolf YG. Ischemic monomelic neuropathy: An underrecognized complication of hemodialysis access. Ann Vasc Surg 8:578–582, 1994.

51. Berman SS, Gentile AT, Glickman MH, et al. Distal revascularization–interval liga-

tion (DRIL) for limb salvage and maintenance of dialysis access in ischemic steal syndrome. J Vasc Surg 26:393–404, 1997.

52. Fuhrman TM, Reilly TE, Pippin WD. Comparison of digital blood pressure, plethysmography, and the modified Allen's test as a means of evaluating the collateral circulation to the hand. Anaesthesia 47:959–961, 1992.

53. Corry RJ, Patel NP, Natvarlal P, West JC. Surgical management of complications of vascular access for hemodialysis. Surg Gynecol Obstet 151:49–54, 1980.

54. Rosenthal JJ, Bell DD, Gaspar MR, Movius HJ, Lemire GG. Prevention of high flow problems of arterio-venous grafts. Development of a new tapered graft. Am J Surg 140:231–233, 1980.

55. West JC, Evans RD, Kelly SE, et al. Arterial insufficiency in hemodialysis access procedures: Reconstruction by an interposition polytetrafluoroethylene graft conduit. Am J Surg 153:300–301, 1987.

56. Jain KM, Simoni EJ, Munn JS. A new technique to correct vascular steal secondary to hemodialysis grafts. Surg Gynecol Obstet 175:183–184, 1993.

57. Ebert A, Saranchak HJ. Banding of a PTFE hemodialysis fistula in the treatment of steal syndrome. Clin Exp Dial Apheresis 5:251–257, 1981.

58. Schanzer H, Schwartz M, Harrington E, Haimov M. Treatment of ischemia due to "steal" by arteriovenous fistula with distal artery ligation and revascularization. J Vasc Surg 7:770–773, 1988.

59. Schanzer H, Skladany M, Haimov M. Treatment of angio-access induced ischemia by revascularization. J Vasc Surg 16:861–866, 1992.

60. Katz S, Kohl RD. The treatment of hand ischemia by arterial ligation and upper extremity bypass after angioaccess surgery. J Am Coll Surg 183:239–242, 1996.

61. Storey BG, George CRP, Stewart JH, et al. Embolic and ischemia complications after anastomosis of radial artery to cephalic vein. Surgery 66:325–327, 1969.

62. Shaffer D. A prospective randomized trial of 6 mm versus 4–7 mm PTFE grafts for hemodialysis access in diabetic patients. In Henry ML, Ferguson RM, eds. Vascular Access for Hemodialysis V. Chicago: Gore; 1997:91–94.

63. Humphries AL Jr, Nesbitt RR Jr, Rogers BC, et al. Use of Weck clips to adjust flow in an A-V PTFE bridge graft. In Henry ML, Ferguson RM, eds. Vascular Access for Hemodialysis IV. Chicago: Gore; 1995:219–224.

64. Haimov M, Baez A, Neff M, Slifkin R. Complications of arteriovenous fistulas for hemodialysis. Arch Surg 110:708–712, 1975.

65. Topf G, Jenkins P, Gutmann FD, Rieselbach RE, Saltzstein EC. Unilateral breast enlargement: A complication of an arteriovenous fistula and coincidental subclavian vein occlusion. JAMA 237:571–572, 1977.

66. Johnson G, Blythe WB. Hemodynamic effects of arteriovenous shunts used for hemodialysis. Ann Surg 171:715–723, 1970.

67. Anderson CB, Codd JR, Graff RA, et al. Cardiac failure and upper extremity arteriovenous fistulas. Arch Intern Med 136:292–297, 1976.

68. Anderson CB, Groce MA. Banding of arteriovenous dialysis fistulas to correct high-output cardiac failure. Surgery 78:552–554, 1975.

13

Biomaterials in Vascular Access: Selection, Function, and Host Response

Stuart K. Williams
The University of Arizona,Tucson, Arizona

Bruce E. Jarrell
The University of Maryland, Baltimore, Maryland

HISTORICAL PERSPECTIVE

The development of the first chronic arteriovenous (AV) fistula is attributed to Scribner and colleagues, who described the use of a polymer-based shunt (1). This shunt was established outside the body and provided access to the bloodstream. Initial work with this device was designed to evaluate the feasibility of establishing a long-term vascular access based on polymer implants (2,3). The use of an external shunt permitted vascular access but was problematic for several reasons, including, initially, the development of infection at the polymer–subcutaneous tissue interface, thrombosis within the graft, lack of control of bleeding at puncture sites, and the development of anastomotic complications related to polymer–tissue interactions (4,5). While these initial results were not optimal, they were encouraging enough to prompt a search for other materials suitable for access construction. Two basic material groups were subsequently evaluated: synthetic polymer-based materials and grafts made of natural materials. The selection, use, and clinical outcome of all these materials is based primarily on the lack of suitable vessels available for construction of an autogenous fistula, which has remained the "gold standard" for vascular access since its introduction by Brescia et al. 30 years ago (6).

The development of materials used to construct artificial AV fistulae follows the development of materials for all vascular replacements. Historically, new vascular graft designs and materials have been evaluated in either peripheral or aortic applications first, followed by evaluation of their potential as AV fistulae (7). Table 13.1 illustrates the different types of fistulae, including autogenous, heterologous, and prosthetic fistulae developed for the purpose of dialysis access. This table also provides information concerning the current status of the use of these different fistulae. The initial polymeric vascular grafts were constructed of nylon, but they exhibited poor healing characteristics and therefore the use of nylon was quickly abandoned (12,13). Subsequent materials tested for use as vascular grafts including AV fistulae have included silicone, (3,14–18) expanded polytetrafluoroethylene (ePTFE) (19–31), polyethylene terephthalate (PET)

TABLE 13.1   Fistulae Used for Dialysis Access

Material	Author/Manufactuerer	Specialized Characteristics
Autogenous vessel	May (8)	Most commonly saphenous vein
Silastic	Scribner	Original external AV shunt
Expanded PTFE	Atrium	External surface with high porosity
	Impra, Inc.	
	W. L. Gore	External wrap
Polyethylene terephthalate (PET)		
	Golaski Laboratories	Low-inflammatory PET
	Meadox Inc.	
	Vascutek	PET with fluorine passivation
Polyurethane	Ota et al. (9)	Experimental
Hybrid graft	Possis Inc.	Venturi flow restrictor incorporated in
Bovine carotid artery	Haimov (10)	Glutaraldehyde cross-linked
Umbilical vein	Dardik (11)	

(26,32,33), polyurethane (PU) (23), polyesters, and polycarbonates. Nonsynthetic materials have also been evaluated, including bovine carotid artery (23,34) and umbilical vein (35,36). All of these materials are considered "biomaterials" simply because they have been used as implants. It is important to note that the term *biomaterial* does not connote anything concerning whether a material is biocompatible. A truly biocompatible material would provide a replacement with healing and functional characteristics identical to the tissue being replaced (37). Thus very few if any materials currently used as implants can be considered biocompatible. The lack of compatibility remains a major focus of biomaterials research today.

Each of the base polymers defined above has been manufactured for AV grafts in a number of different configurations. The design and manufacture of these different polymer configurations is often driven by a concern for several graft-related functions, including kink resistance (38), suturability (39), and response to continuous needle puncture (40,41). With a few exceptions (42,43), little attention has been directed to developing AV grafts with more optimal healing characteristics. This lack of attention to healing has resulted in numerous graft configurations with excellent physical strength and good handling characteristics but relatively poor healing characteristics. The physical structure of several AV grafts, as analyzed by scanning electron microscopy, is illustrated in Figure 13.1. These scanning electron micrographs illustrate the unique differences in polymers all manufactured for use as AV fistulae. Many of these structural characteristics are discussed further on.

MATERIAL DEVELOPMENT

The clinical disadvantages of polymer-based AV grafts were observed with the earliest devices and include infection (44,45), thrombosis on the blood-contacting surface (46,47), poor healing of the external (abluminal) graft surface (48–50), and finally the development of occlusive intimal thickening (51–54). All of these complications have been the target of intense research activities, with progress made in all areas. However, significant complications remain as a direct result of the relative nonbiocompatibility of prosthetic grafts. All currently available prosthetic grafts are made of base polymers that were never originally developed for implantation in humans. These materials in general have been adapted from other uses and were chosen for their expected durability. The earliest grafts were external devices made of silicone tubing. Silicone remains a generally inert polymer with superior long-term survival in implants. Later developments included the use of polyethylene terephthalate (PET), most often described as Dacron, its trademarked name (7). This material has unique properties permitting extrusion as fine fibers with excellent durability and the ability to weave or knit these fibers into tubes of several different designs. Figure 13.1 illustrates the structure of

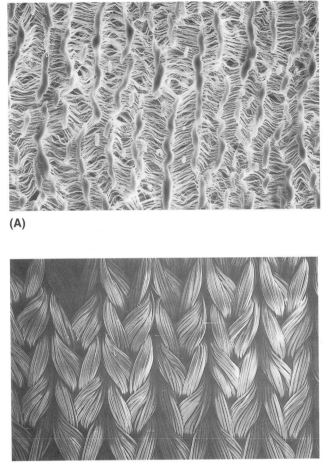

(A)

(B)

FIGURE 13.1 Scanning electron micrographs illustrating the luminal blood-contacting surface of vascular graft materials. These materials include (A) Atrium ePTFE, (B) Dacron knit, (C) Dacron weave, and (D) Meadox Hemashield Dacron.

knitted and woven Dacron (7) fabric. The major difference observed is the relatively high porosity of knitted fabrics, necessitating preclotting of this material before implantation. Without preclotting, a significant amount of transmural bleeding occurs until the pores of the graft are filled. Newer designs of knitted Dacron include the incorporation of a chemically cross-linked collagen matrix, precluding the need to preclot the grafts.

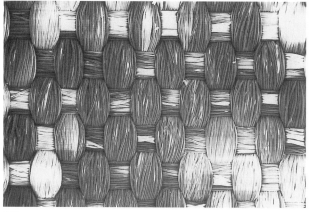

(C)

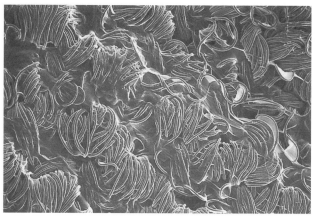

(D)

MATERIAL SELECTION

Synthetic Polymers

Silastic

Although *Silastic* is the name most commonly used to describe material manufactured from silicone, Silastic is actually a silicone-based material that is polymerized into an elastomeric material and is more appropriately known as silicone elastomer. Silicone elastomer is widely used in the manufacture of biomedical implants with multiple applications. Considering the current concerns with silicone-based implants, it is important to note that silicone can be used to manufacture implants using gels, elastomers, and oils. Of these three materials, the silicone elastomer is among the most inert of those used in medical implants. In vascular access, Silastic is the most commonly used material for indwelling catheters. Silastic material also has the distinction of being the first to be used as a chronic, albeit external, vascular access fistula. Scribner described the use of silastic as an AV shunt for end-stage renal disease (ESRD) patients and reported the first successful dialysis using a synthetic fistula (1). Complete internalization of this fistula within a subcutaneous pocket was impeded by the difficulty in cannulating these devices once implanted.

A complete description of the differences in the available forms of silicone is beyond the scope of this chapter but should be reviewed for those patients who have concerns related to the use of Silastic. In any case, silicone elastomer remains a highly stable synthetic polymer of great utility, especially in the manufacture of catheters. It is among the most biocompatible polymers available. This biocompatibility is due in part to the relative lack of inflammatory response associated with silicone elastomeric implants—a characteristic that would be desirable in other synthetic polymers used in the manufacture of implantable AV fistulae.

Composite AV fistulae made of both Silastic and ePTFE have been reported (17). The most significant advantage of these grafts is the ability of the silicone elastomer to self-seal needle puncture holes following cannula removal. The clinical use of these grafts has not been widely reported and they remain experimental.

Polyethylene

This polymer is synthesized from monomeric ethylene with varying degrees of branching. The degree of branching is an important consideration in the clinical use of polyethylene, since highly branched polyethylene results in a pliable material, while more linear, nonbranched polyethylene is relatively rigid. Highly branched polyethylene is also called low-density polyethylene and is a major component of central venous catheters. The more linear polyethylene is produced in two major forms and is commonly referred to as either high-density or ultra-high-density polyethylene (HDPE and UHDPE respectively). This high-density polyethylene is not highly inflammatory and is used as a permanent implant in both orthopedic and plastic surgery applications. The more pliable low-density polyethylene would have certain applications as an AV fistula; however, this material is highly inflammatory when used as a chronic implant. Use of low-density polyethylene remains in short-term catheter placements but not chronic placements because of complications resulting from inflammation (55).

Polyethylene Terephthalate

This polymer (often abbreviated PET or PETE) is more commonly known as Dacron, its trademarked name (7). PET is a widely used polymer—most commonly, for example, in the manufacture of disposable drink containers. The history of the development and use of synthetic materials for vascular grafts saw experimentation with both the textile Dacron and ePTFE grafts. Dacron grafts, created initially from Dacron fabric, have seen widespread use in large vessel reconstructions and, more recently, as components of stent grafts (56–58); however, the use of PET for small-diameter grafts and AV grafts has not been extensive (59–61).

Dacron AV grafts of various designs were actively evaluated clinically during the 1970s and '80s (26,32,33). Many of these studies were comparative evaluations using other synthetic and natural AV grafts. The Dacron velour graft was used in several trials and exhibited significant improvement in resistance to infection compared with natural heterografts (26,32,33). The reasons these grafts did not receive active clinical acceptance are probably severalfold. First, the initial Dacron grafts were manufactured using a highly porous knit or weave requiring a preclotting step. The time to preclot the graft was not long but placed it at a significant disadvantage to grafts that did not require this additional procedure (e.g., bovine heterografts and ePTFE). Other problems noted were the increased difficulty in placing dialysis needles through the graft interstices and unraveling the textile fibers if the graft had not been handled carefully. These difficulties were noted in studies where a direct comparison was made with natural vessel and remains a significant difference for all synthetic grafts.

One feature of Dacron grafts that provides superiority over other nontextile synthetic grafts is that the material can be easily sutured. Modifications in the design of Dacron have continued since its initial use. These include inclusion of an external velour (33); prepackaged preclotting with either collagen or gelatin gels (62,63); and surface modification using a technique known as radiofrequency glow discharge (64,65). This latter technique has been used to incorporate highly negative fluoroethylene or fluorene groups onto the internal surface of the grafts, theoretically providing a more thromboresistant surface via a charge repulsion process. Clinical trials of fluorine-passivated surfaces have not indicated that this modification provides any specific improvement in graft function (64).

Expanded Polytetrafluoroethylene

Of all the synthetic grafts used in vascular surgery, expanded polytetrafluoroethylene has seen the most widespread clinical use and acceptance. Like all other synthetics used as vascular conduits, this material was originally designed for other commercial uses but was borrowed for clinical testing by an astute surgeon (19). The emergence of ePTFE as a synthetic conduit is based on several factors, including the stability of this polymer during long-term implantation; its relatively low cost as compared with natural vessel heterografts; its ease of handling, especially the lack of necessity to preclot the material before use; and finally its relative lack of inflammatory response following implantation. The term *relative* is used, since, as with all synthetic materials used as implants, some degree of inflammation is observed.

Expanded polytetrafluoroethylene (ePTFE) is a material manufactured and supplied as vascular grafts by several corporations including Impra, Atrium, and W.L. Gore. Unlike Dacron, which is extruded as a fiber and subsequently processed into a tube, ePTFE is extruded as solid tubes of PTFE and subsequently expanded at an elevated temperature to create the unique porous characteristics of ePTFE (66). Manufacturers of ePTFE have developed different methods for expanding PTFE. Figure 13.2 illustrates the luminal, abluminal, and cross-sectional morphology of Atrium, Gore, and Impra grafts. Two physical characteristics are most often mentioned in describing ePTFE. First, grafts are described according to their wall thickness as either of regular thickness or thin-walled. For AV access, grafts of regular thickness are generally used owing to the belief that these grafts will exhibit greater resistance to the formation of false aneurysms and tearing during puncture as part of the dialysis process.

The second general structural characteristic is the relative porosity of the grafts based upon direct measurement of polymer density on the luminal and abluminal surface. It is in this respect that the greatest difference in grafts supplied from different manufacturers is observed. The description of graft porosity is often provided as a statement of graft internodal distance. The measurement of this parameter is illustrated in Figure 13.3, with bars illustrating the internodal distance. Commercially available ePTFE grafts are generally referred to in the literature as grafts with 30-μm internodal distances. However, since the original introduction of ePTFE, the internodal distance on commercially supplied grafts has slowly been reduced to a distance of approximately 20 μm. In Figure 13.2, the internodal distances between grafts from different manufactures can be compared. Impra grafts exhibit a uniform internodal distance on both the luminal and abluminal surfaces. The Atrium AV graft is manufactured with a unique design incorporating a narrow luminal internodal distance of 20 μm with a transinterstitial graft transition to an outer surface with an internodal distance of approximately 60 μm. Grafts constructed with this transitional porosity are believed to exhibit better healing characteristics owing to the high porosity of ePTFE interacting with tissue for healing. The Gore ePTFE is constructed of an ePTFE with an approximately 20-μm internodal distance throughout the graft. However, during manufacture, the Gore graft receives an external wrap of an additional layer of ePTFE with an extremely small internodal distance. The manufacturer believes that this external wrap provides superior resistance to aneurysm formation as well as to damage from needle puncture during dialysis. Resistance to aneurysm formation, occurrence of seromas, and resistance to damage due to needle punc-ture appear to be quite similar in all the currently available ePTFE. Anecdotal evidence exists; but in the absence of a study that directly compares the function of these grafts, the general conclusion to be drawn is that all of these materials perform acceptably as AV fistulas. However, this is not to suggest that significant improvement in synthetic fistula design and manufacture cannot be achieved.

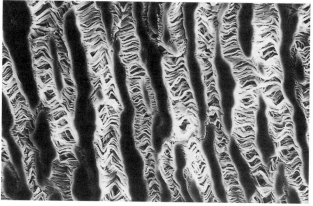

(A)

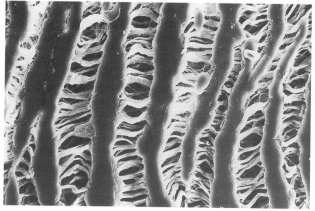

(B)

FIGURE 13.2 Scanning electron micrographs comparing the luminal and abluminal surface of commonly used ePTFE grafts: (A) Atrium lumenal surface, (B) Atrium abluminal surface, (C) Impra luminal surface, (D) Impra abluminal surface, (E) Gore luminal surface (F) Gore abluminal surface, (G) cross section through wall of Atrium ePTFE, and (H) cross section through wall of Impra ePTFE.

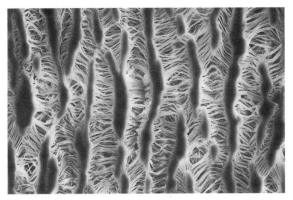

(C)

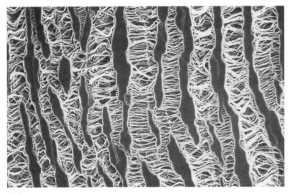

(D)

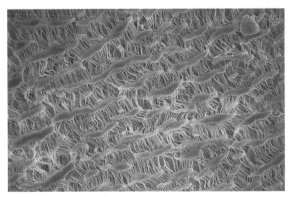

(E)

FIGURE 13.2   Continued

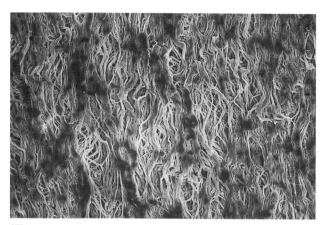

(F)

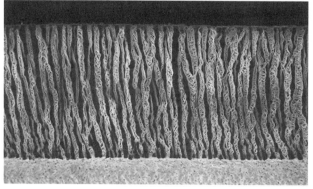

(G)

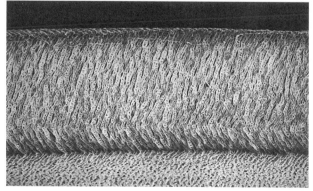

(H)

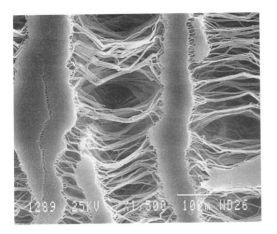

FIGURE 13.3 Measurement of internodal distance on ePTFE grafts is performed by measuring the distance between the centers of two opposing nodes in the extruded polymer.

NATURAL TISSUE AV GRAFTS

During the development of AV grafts, within the period initiated by Scribner (5) and the external synthetic shunt and ending with the utilization and acceptance of ePTFE grafts, several natural vessel AV grafts were evaluated. These grafts represented both natural autografts [i.e., autogenous saphenous vein (8,67–70)] and heterografts [i.e., umbilical vein (36,11) and bovine carotid artery (10,23,34,71)].

Autogenous Saphenous Vein

This vessel source is the same as that used in any vascular procedure employing saphenous vein interposition grafts. Veins are harvested from the thigh and used most commonly as fistulae between brachial vessels. The major disadvantage of this procedure is the use of autogenous vessel, which may be needed for subsequent coronary or peripheral vascular reconstructions. Moreover, greater effectiveness of autogenous vein over synthetic fistulae has not been observed (67,70).

In contrast, the saphenous vein may actually be an inferior conduit, as the incidence of puncture-related complications may be elevated in autogenous saphenous vein grafts (69). On the other hand, saphenous vein grafts exhibit minimal infection as compared with synthetic grafts (67). The use of the saphenous vein graft has been extremely limited, but—interestingly—extensive use of these grafts in Europe and Japan has been reported (68,70). Again, differences in patient selection between the United States and other countries must be considered in comparing graft use and performance.

HETEROGRAFTS

Bovine Carotid Artery

The bovine heterograft is manufactured using segments of carotid arteries harvested from cows. This artery is subsequently ''tanned'' by a process involving treatment with a cross-linking agent, which is most commonly glutaraldehyde. This tanning process is essentially identical to the preparation of natural tissue heart valves and leaves a biological material that is composed of predominantly extracellular matrix. Cells present in the artery are destroyed during the tanning process, leaving a cross-linked matrix with extensive cellular debris. These heterografts were used extensively for a period of time but are now used infrequently (30,31,34,72,73). Their infrequent use can be attributed to many factors, including their relatively high cost of manufacture, incidence of infection, the occurrence of aneurysms, and the occurrence of punctate intimal thickening, most commonly observed at the venous anastomotic site (72). The higher cost and perception that the incidence of complications is higher with the bovine heterograft have contributed significantly to its reduced use in clinical practice.

Umbilical Vein

The use of human umbilical vein as an alternate source of a biological conduit was first attempted in the late 1970s (11,35,36). The use of these grafts was based upon the belief that grafts of a biological nature would exhibit improved patency as compared with synthetic grafts. However, comparison of patency between heterografts and synthetic grafts indicates little difference (35,36). Concerns related to the use of umbilical vein grafts are similar to those involving the bovine carotid heterograft, namely cost and problems with infection. For both of these heterografts it is important to note that infections can be devastating, since bacteria produce proteolytic enzymes that can essentially destroy the structure of the graft. Incidents of early hemorrhage relating to infection in heterografts have been reported.

PREVALENCE OF DIFFERENT GRAFT TYPES

Current data to establish the relative frequency of the type of graft used for either first or subsequent vascular access procedures provide equivocal conclusions. The most extensive data exists in the form of the Medicare End-Stage Renal Disease program (75) as well as in recent reviews (74,75). These data suggests that at least 50% of all first-time AV fistulae are prosthetic, with the trend toward increased placement of prosthetic fistulae in first-time patients. The Medicare data also suggest that in 1990, approximately 83% of grafts placed in established chronic hemodialysis patients were prosthetic. Of these prosthetic grafts, ePTFE grafts were the predominant type. Data from countries other than the United States are less conclusive but again provide some suggestions. Outside the United States the use of autogenous arteriovenous fistulae predominate in first-time as well as chronic dialysis patients (74–77). However, comparison of patient selection criteria for dialysis between the United States and other countries provides several reasons for this difference in type of fistula. The primary difference is the age of patients selected for dialysis, where the patient population in the United States is dramatically older in mean age and thus presents a patient population that often does not have usable autogenous vessels for fistula construction (77). Thus the predominance of prosthetic fistula use in U.S. patients appears to result primarily from the types of patients selected for initial dialysis as well as the types of current dialysis methods available in the United States as compared with other countries. While autogenous arteriovenous fistulae remain the fistulae of choice, prosthetic fistulae and predominately ePTFE fistulae remain the most common alternative; in compromised patients, these prosthetic grafts often provide the only type of fistula material.

GRAFT CHARACTERISTICS CONSIDERED TO AFFECT HEALING AND PATENCY

Compliance

The failure of synthetic fistulae has been attributed to many mechanisms, including what is termed a compliance mismatch between graft and natural vessel (78,79). Synthetic grafts have very little compliance, defined as the ability of a material to expand and contract both radially and tangentially as compared with native blood vessels. Some investigators have hypothesized that compliance mismatch, especially at the anastomosis, leads to a chronic tissue response that is clinically observed as intimal thickening (78,79). This hypothesis remains essentially untested owing to the difficulty in manufacturing highly compliant synthetic grafts that both maintain their compliance once implanted and also exhibit biological stability. Considering that an anastomosis from a natural vein to an artery also exhibits intimal thickening, the compliance mismatch hypothesis has not received significant support. Undoubtedly compliance is one of several mechanisms that collectively affect vessel response to injury.

Stability

The stability of materials used in currently available and experimental AV grafts is a significant concern. With AV grafts, stability is of paramount importance, since grafts are physically penetrated when dialysis cannulas are placed. This penetration results in a cylindrical deformation in the graft wall, leaving a hole approximately 200 μm in diameter on cannula removal. An example of a puncture hole in a graft which has healed is shown in Figure 13.4. The hole is replaced initially by thrombus, followed by varying degrees of tissue ingrowth. Again, each graft material has varying degrees of tissue ingrowth. Several manufacturers have evaluated graft materials that have self-closing characteristics. Materials such as silicone or soft polyurethanes have a "memory" and will partially fill the cylindrical channel formed when the dialysis cannula is removed. This design parameter has theoretically significant value, since the incidence of bleeding would be markedly reduced.

Stability—defined as the ability of grafts to resist either chemical or physical degradation—has been a major concern in AV graft development and has

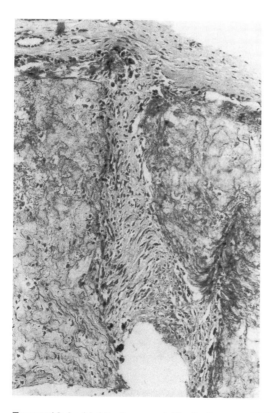

FIGURE 13.4   Light micrograph illustrating an ePTFE graft punctured by a dialysis needle and the healing response that occurs via ingrowth of surrounding tissue.

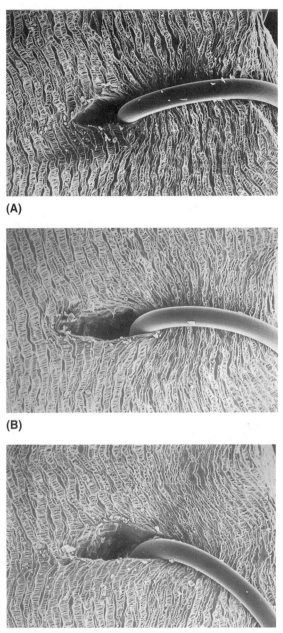

(A)

(B)

(C)

FIGURE 13.5 Examples of the physical damage to ePTFE AV graft material that occurs during suturing.(A) suture placed with maximal attention to minimize needle tension on graft material. (B) Suture placed forcing the needle directly through the graft without rotating the needle as it passes through the material.(C) Suture placed with tangential strain placed on the ePTFE by the needle.

resulted in a limited number of materials available for clinical use today. Materials such as polyurethane and biodegradable materials have not reached clinical use as AV grafts due to lingering concerns regarding the stability of these materials in long-term implants. Synthetic grafts of ePTFE remain the most widely used AV grafts.

Suturing and Graft Handling

The process of constructing an anastomosis from a synthetic graft to a vessel subjects both the graft and the vessel to significant physical manipulation. One aspect of this manipulation is placement of sutures through the interstices of the graft, with subsequent approximation of graft and vessel. Several aspects of suture placement should be considered with respect to the effects on graft structure and subsequent healing. Since most synthetic grafts used are ePTFE, this material is the focus of this discussion. The ePTFE material can be stretched in a three-dimensional coordinate; thus, the amount of tension placed on each suture will result in variable amounts of ePTFE distortion. Sutures placed with extensive tangential strain will open the ePTFE structure, resulting in prolonged bleeding. Secondarily, the formation of granulation tissue will be more extensive in this area. Figure 13.5A illustrates the placement of a suture with maximal attention to minimizing needle tension on the graft material. Figure 13.5B shows the suture being placed, forcing the needle directly through the graft without rotating the needle as it passes through the material. Finally, Figure 13.5C illustrates the damage that occurs when the suture is placed with tangential strain placed on the ePTFE by the needle. This disruption in the ePTFE surface structure results in increased surface area for platelet and fibrin deposition. Suture retention strength in commercially available ePTFE grafts is quite similar. However, comparative studies will be necessary to determine whether suture hole bleeding is different between materials.

Another aspect of polymer design that is affected by physical manipulation during anastomosis construction is the effect on ePTFE caused by handling with forceps and clamps. The ePTFE material is easily deformable, and this deformation, when applied with significant force, will remain following release of the clasping device. The healing characteristics of ePTFE are affected by all these physical manipulations (80). One cause for poor incorporation of grafts can be the overmanipulation of the material in this fashion, which should be avoided.

POLYMER-TISSUE INTERACTIONS

Following implantation of a synthetic AV fistula, a healing response is observed, which—with respect to cellular and extracellular components—is similar in many ways to normal wound healing. The most significant difference observed following synthetic fistula implantation is the prolongation of the inflammatory phase (81). In essence, synthetic polymers elicit a chronic inflammatory response that remains active for the duration of the life of the implant. As diagrammed in Figure 13.6, the normal response to injury involves a programmed sequence of cellular and extracellular responses leading to the formation of replacement tissue similar in structure to the tissue prior to damage. Figure 13.7 illustrates the current state of knowledge of how the presence of a synthetic fistula alters the healing response, leading to both heightening of inflammatory components and their subsequent prolongation. The cellular nature of this response is illustrated morphologically in Figure 13.8, which demonstrates the cellular response on the outer surface of an ePTFE graft. The most prominent feature is the presence of numerous macrophages, with the common appearance of foreign-body giant cells. This reaction is constant and is observed in implants that have been evaluated years after their primary implantation.

The presence of these foreign-body reactions is coordinate with the synthesis and secretion of numerous cytokines—such as interleukins, tumor necrosis factor, transforming growth factor beta, and interferon gamma—as well as numerous other growth factors and chemoattractants (81–84). The net result of these factors is chronic recruitment of additional inflammatory cells and often the development of a fibrous capsule around the implant. This capsule is seen as an attempt by the tissue to wall off the highly inflammatory material. Essentially the tissue response has evolved to encapsulate foreign bodies that cannot be effectively degraded by the action of cell-associated digestive enzymes and chemicals. In summary, the environment surrounding an implanted synthetic AV

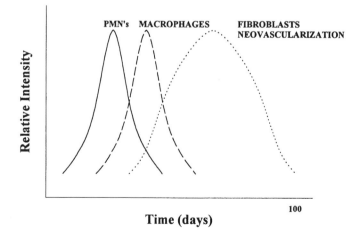

FIGURE 13.6 Cellular events that occur during normal wound healing.

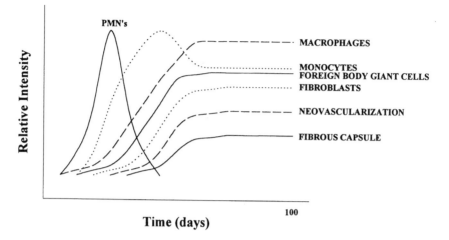

FIGURE 13.7 Cellular events associated with wound healing when a biomaterial is present.

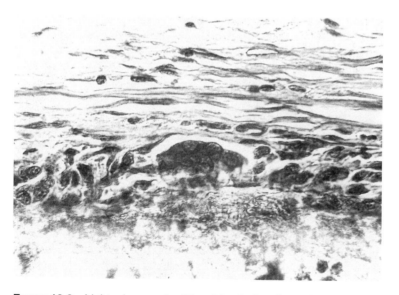

FIGURE 13.8 Light micrograph of the abluminal surface of an AV graft illustrating the presence of inflammatory cells, including a foreign body giant cell.

fistula is initially composed of inflammatory cells that persist, resulting in a chronically inflamed implant. This inflammation may be reduced by the encapsulation of the implant in an acellular extracellular matrix–rich capsule. The inflammatory tissue environment surrounding a synthetic fistula is also characterized by a lack of microvascular elements, indicating that this region is poorly perfused.

The implantation of AV fistulas results in protein and cellular responses on the luminal and abluminal surfaces as well as a tissue reaction at the anastomotic site. These distinct sites all exhibit different responses, since one surface, the lumen, is interacting with blood components while the abluminal surface is interacting with surrounding tissue. The graft-vessel interface at the anastomosis is a third unique site of healing as the blood vessel wall responds to both surgical injury and the presence of a foreign material.

Endothelialization

The formation of a natural endothelial cell lining on the luminal surface of prosthetic fistulae has been hypothesized as a means to improve the long-term function of these grafts (85). The accelerated formation of this cellular lining has been evaluated using both endothelial cell transplantation (86–88) as well as polymer modifications to improve spontaneous formation of luminal linings with endothelial cells (89–90). Endothelial cell transplantation has reached the point of clinical evaluation, with continued development of procedures to improve the rate and stability of the endothelial cell lining (87,91). In Figure 13.9, a scanning electron micrograph of the flow surface of an endothelial cell transplanted graft is illustrated, providing an example of the cellular lining that can be established with this technique. The modification of polymers to improve healing characteristics and promote spontaneous endothelialization is predominantly in the preclinical stage. Exceptions include the development of ePTFE grafts with high external porosity to accelerate healing (43). Significant efforts are ongoing to improve the healing of both the luminal and abluminal surfaces of synthetic grafts, with particular emphasis on the cellular response following synthetic AV fistula implantation.

Blood-Materials Interactions

The initial response following restoration of blood flow through AV fistulae is the interaction of blood components with the luminal flow surface (92–97). Synthetic AV grafts are uniformly nonbiological, and thus the initial interactions are characterized as an activation of blood cells and plasma proteins. The initial surface interactions have been characterized to involve the absorption of plasma proteins in a sequence directly related to the relative concentration of the protein in the blood (94,96,97). Serum albumin, the most abundant plasma protein, inter-

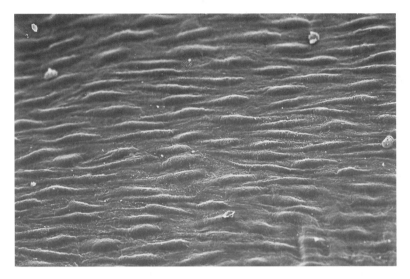

FIGURE 13.9   Scanning electron micrograph of the luminal surface of an AV (eP-TFE) graft that received transplanted endothelial cells at the time of graft implantation.

acts with the luminal surface first, and it is sequentially followed by immunoglobulins and fibrinogen. Other proteins—such as factor VIII, Hageman factor, and circulating fibronectin—are also absorbed by the luminal surface. The net result of this protein deposition is a complex surface of absorbed proteins. Individually, these proteins exhibit both nonthrombogenic characteristics, as exemplified by serum albumin, and prothrombogenic characteristics, as exemplified by factor VIII, Hageman factor, and fibronectin (93). The net thrombogenicity of the lumen surface of a vascular graft is dependent upon the protein surface exposed to blood. Several attempts have been made to reduce the thrombogenicity of grafts by either bonding serum albumin to the luminal surface or imparting a negative surface charge to the polymer surface to mimic the charge of albumin (98,99). Mixed results with these types of modifications have been reported (100).

Cell-Material Interactions

Following the deposition of proteins, circulating platelets as well as leukocytes contact the lumenal surface of vascular grafts. Figure 13.10 illustrates the association of platelets and leukocytes with grafts following their implantation. The interactions of platelets and leukocytes is modulated by specific interactions between plasma membrane proteins in platelets and leukocytes with the proteins

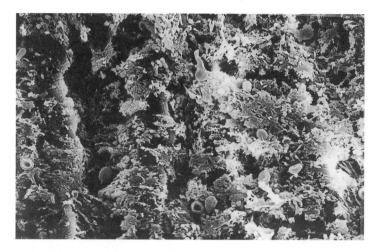

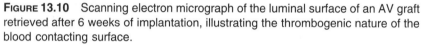

FIGURE 13.10   Scanning electron micrograph of the luminal surface of an AV graft retrieved after 6 weeks of implantation, illustrating the thrombogenic nature of the blood contacting surface.

associated with the graft surface (92,93). For example, von Willebrand factor, another plasma protein that associates with graft surfaces, exhibits affinity for platelet GPIb, a protein found on the surface of platelets. This interaction leads to the binding of platelets to the graft surface and is further accelerated by platelet-platelet interactions. Continued deposition of platelets leads to the formation of platelet aggregates that grow in size until the force of detachment created by the shear force in the fistula surpasses the force of attachment anchoring the platelet aggregate (101). Platelet microemboli are subsequently released, leading to a continuous cycling of platelet aggregation and embolization in a process believed to continue for the life of the implanted device.

Leukocyte deposition, and especially monocyte adherence, is not as well characterized but does occur even at the high flow rates observed in AV grafts. Leukocytes express integrin protein heterodimers on their plasma membranes with known binding affinity for immunoglobulins, fibronectin, and fibrinogen (102). The mechanisms regulating leukocyte-integrin interactions have been established in the microcirculation but are poorly understood in the high-flow-rate environment common in large blood vessels and especially as observed in AV fistulae.

The surgical implantation of any material results in a wound healing response, with components common to all wound healing. However, a significant difference in material-related wound healing is the prolongation of cellular processes seen during granulation tissue formation (81,82). Specifically, the recruitment of monocytes and the transformation of these cells into macrophages is prolonged (83,84). With many material implants, the subsequent formation of foreign-body giant cells from monocytes is extremely common (84). Proliferation of fibroblasts and the formation of extracellular matrix is another cellular process that is prolonged (82). The formation of a fibrous capsule around the external, abluminal surface of AV grafts is common; however, the extent of this fibrous capsule varies depending on the type of synthetic polymer.

Intimal Thickening

The earliest responses on the blood-contacting surfaces of synthetic AV fistulae are characterized as sequentially serum protein deposition, fibrin deposition, and finally platelet and leukocyte deposition. Subsequent cellular reactions on the blood-flow surface in the portion of the graft more than 1 cm from the anastomoses do not change significantly during the ensuing months to years. The blood-flow surface remains highly thrombogenic, with continual deposition of activated platelets and fibrin and with embolization of these aggregates in the form of microemboli. This process of deposition and embolization continues for the life of the implant; thus the luminal surface is never quiescent. The blood-flow surface of a fistula is often characterized as a pseudointima; however, this term is inherently incorrect, since the surface is essentially acellular and thus is not an intimal lining.

A most characteristic feature of the blood-flow surface distant from the anastomosis is the complete absence of an endothelial cell lining even in grafts that have been evaluated after more than 10 years of implantation. This lack of spontaneous endothelialization is a hallmark of the blood-flow surface (103). Interestingly, other nonhuman animal species exhibit the ability to form spontaneous endothelial cell linings on synthetic grafts. Certain animal species such as the baboon exhibit extremely rapid spontaneous endothelialization rates. Unfortunately, the human species lacks the ability to spontaneously endothelialize the lumenal blood-flow surface, and the mechanism of this failure to endothelialize is currently under active investigation.

Anastomotic healing of synthetic AV fistulae exhibits cellular and extracellular responses common to all vascular grafts, including the occurrence of a progressive intimal thickening at the distal (venous) anastomosis. The occurrence of intimal thickening is a significant cause of fistula failure. These anastomotic lesions were originally defined as intimal hyperplastic lesions, suggesting that their presence was the result of cellular proliferation, with smooth muscle cells being considered the major cell found in hyperplastic lesions. Indeed, immunocytochemical staining of tissue samples from anastomotic lesions from AV grafts exhibits the presence of the cytoskeletal protein known as alpha smooth muscle cell actin. Investigators are generally agreed that this marker confirms that cells in these lesions were derived from smooth muscle cells activated by the process of AV fistula implantation.

Our current concept of the mechanism of anastomotic lesion formation is undergoing significant reconsideration for a number of reasons. First, many cells of mesenchymal origin exhibit alpha smooth muscle cell actin staining, suggesting that cells in the intimal lesions are not definitively of smooth muscle cell origin (104). Second, evaluation of the proliferation rate of cells in AV fistula intimal lesions indicates that proliferation of cells is very rare. Moreover, many of the cells observed to be proliferating in intimal lesions are microvascular endothelium and not cells generally described as myofibroblasts (105). Finally, the cell density found in AV fistula intimal lesions is not quantitatively in the range of a hyperplastic response but must be described more accurately as an extracellular hypertrophic response. The intimal lesions are predominantly extracellular matrix when the distribution of components is quantified on the basis of a unit volume of lesions. The anastomotic response following the implantation of an AV fistula is currently most accurately described as an intimal thickening composed of a luminal lining of endothelial cells. These endothelial cells rarely penetrate onto the luminal surface of the fistulae more than 1 cm from the anastomosis. The intimal thickening under the endothelial cell lining is composed of numerous cell types, including microvascular endothelium, inflammatory cells, myofibroblasts, and a rich investment of extracellular matrix. Future studies will be imperative to understand the mechanisms of this, which result in the formation of intimal thickening.

COMPLICATIONS

Infection

Material-based infections are a significant complication of synthetic grafts, and they are compounded by the relative cellularity of these implants. Studies have reported infection rates for AV grafts at 1 year between 10 and 35% (106–111). Bacterial infection come from several sources, including abluminal sources during graft placement and luminal sources due to bacterial-polymer interaction. The most significant bacterial infections are due to *Staphylococcus epidermidis* and *aureus* (112). The mechanisms of bacterial-polymer interactions are under active evaluation (113–115). Interestingly, it appears that this interaction may not be passive but may involve utilization of specific receptor interaction between proteins on the surface of grafts and receptors found on the surface of bacteria. The most effective barrier to bacterial–vessel wall interaction remains the endothelial cell. In the absence of this cellular barrier, bacteria can invade the porous polymer, resulting in colonization and drug resistance.

Pretreatment of synthetic grafts with antibiotics has been suggested as a prophylaxis against infection (115). Such treatment varies from antibiotic binding techniques to simple preimplant immersion. Types of antibiotics for this treatment also vary and include surfactants (116), pennicillins, cephalosporins (117,118), and rifampin (119). To date, the effectiveness of antibiotic treatment is undetermined. Careful attention to sterile technique remains the method of choice when synthetic grafts are used.

Seroma

The porous nature of synthetic grafts results in the ability of both plasma and formed elements to penetrate the luminal surface of the graft and to varying degree penetrate its interstices, giving them access to the abluminal surface. Massive penetration of plasma and cells does not occur for several reasons. First, although the porosity of ePTFE is often quoted as approximately 30 μm, this represents the average distance between nodes on the surface of the graft. This value suggests that the grafts would impose little restriction on erythrocytes or plasma; however, the internodal distance is not the major determinant of graft porosity. As observed in Figures 13.1 and 13.2, the density of fibers between nodes is a more significant factor affecting edema formation. Chronic penetration of grafts with catheters leads to a breakdown in the structural integrity of grafts and can lead to several complications, including aneurysms, hematomas, and seromas (120).

REFERENCES

1. Quinton WE, Dillard D, Scribner BH. Cannulation of blood vessels for prolonged hemodialysis. Trans Am Soc Artif Intern Organs 6:104, 1960.
2. Graham WB. Historical aspects of hemodialysis. Transplant Proc 9(1):xlix–li, 1977.
3. McDonald HP Jr, Gerber N, Mishra D, et al. Subcutaneous Dacron and Teflon cloth adjuncts for Silastic arteriovenous shunts and peritoneal dialysis catheters. Trans Am Soc Artif Intern Organs 14:176–180, 1968.
4. Blackshear PJ, Dorman FD, Blackshear PL Jr, et al. The design and initial testing of an implantable infusion pump. Surg Gynecol Obstet 134(1):51–56, 1972.
5. Niederhuber JE. Totally implanted venous and arterial access system to replace external catheters in cancer treatment. Surgery 92(4):706–712, 1982.
6. Brescia MJ, Cimino JE, Appel K, Hurwich BJ. Chronic hemodialysis using venipuncture and a surgically created arteriovenous fistula. N Engl J Med 275(20): 1089–1092, 1966.
7. Bothe A Jr, Piccione W, Ambrosino JJ, et al. Implantable central venous access system. Am J Surg 147(4):565–569, 1984.

8. May J, Tiller D, Johnson J, et al. Saphaneous vein arteriovenous fistula in regular dialysis treatment. N Engl J Med 280(14):770, 1969.

9. Ota K, Nakagawa Y, Kitano Y, et al. Clinical application of modified polyurethanegraft to blood access. Artif Organs 15:449–453, 1991.

10. Haminov M, Jacobson JH. Experience with the modified bovine arterial heterograft in peripheral vascular reconstruction and vascular access for hemodialysis. Ann Surg 180(3):291–295, 1974.

11. Dardik H, Ibrahim IM, Dardik I. Arteriovenous fistula constructed with modified human umbilical cord vein graft. Arch Surg 111(1):60–62, 1976.

12. Smith SR. The principles underlying graft selection for arterial reconstruction. Br J Hosp Med 38(4):358–363, 1987.

13. Vorhees AB, Jaratzki A, Blackmore AW. The use of tubes constructed from Vinyon-"N" cloth bridging arterial grafts. Ann Surg 135:332–336, 1952.

14. Schanzer H, Martinelli GP, Bock G, Peirce EC. PTFE-silicone self-sealing dialysis prosthesis. ASAIO Trans 32(1):297–299, 1986a.

15. Schanzer H, Martinelli GP, Bock G, Peirce EC. A self-sealing dialysis prosthesis. Coaxial double PTFE-silicone graft. Ann Surg 204(5):574–579, 1986b.

16. Moss AH, McLaughlin MM, Lempert KD, Holley JL. Use of a silicone catheter with a Dacron cuff for dialysis short-term vascular access. Am J Kidney Dis 12(6): 492–498, 1988.

17. Schanzer H, Martinelli G, Chiang K, et al. Clinical trials of a new polytetrafluoroethylene-silicone graft. Am J Surg 158(2):117–120, 1989b.

18. Moss AH, Vasilakis C, Holley JL, et al. Use of a silicone dual-lumen catheter with a Dacron cuff as a long-term vascular access for hemodialysis patients. Am J Kidney Dis 16(3):211–215, 1990.

19. Baker LD Jr, Johnson JM, Goldfarb D. Expanded polytetrafluoroethylene (PTFE) subcutaneous arteriovenous conduit: An improved vascular access for chronic hemodialysis. Trans Am Soc Artif Intern Organs 22:382–387, 1976.

20. Shack RB, Neblett WW, Richie RE, Dean RH. Expanded polytetrafluoroethylene as dialysis access grafts: Serial study of histology and fibrinolytic activity. Am Surg 43(12):817–825, 1977.

21. Ota K, Ara R, Takahashi K, et al. Clinical experience with circumferentially reinforced expanded polytetrafluoroethylene (E-PTFE) graft as a vascular access for haemodialysis. Proc Eur Dial Transplant Assoc 14:222–228, 1977.

22. Elliott MP, Gazzaniga AB, Thomas JM, et al. Use of expanded polytetrafluoroethylene grafts for vascular access in hemodialysis: Laboratory and clinical evaluation. Am Surg 43(7):455–459, 1977.

23. Butler HG, Baker LD Jr, Johnson JM. Vascular access for chronic hemodialysis: Polytetrafluoroethylene (PTFE) versus bovine heterograft. Am J Surg 134(6):791–793, 1977.

24. Wellington JL. Expanded polytetrafluoroethylene prosthetic grafts for blood access in patients on dialysis. Can J Surg 21(5):420–422, 1978.

25. Haminov M. Clinical experience with the expanded polytetrafluoroethylene vascular prosthesis. Angiology 29(1):1–6, 1978.

26. Burdick JF, Scott W, Cosimi AB. Experience with dacron graft arteriovenous fistulas for dialysis access. Ann Surg 187(3):262–266, 1978.

27. Tellis VA, Kohlberg WI, Bhat DJ, et al. Expanded polytetrafluoroethylene graft fistula for chronic hemodialysis. Ann Surg 189(1):101–105, 1979.
28. Ackman CF, O'Regan S, Herba MJ, et al. Experience with polytetrafluoroethylene grafts in patients on long-term hemodialysis. Can J Surg 22(2):152–154, 1979.
29. Jenkins AM, Buist TA, Glover SD. Medium-term follow-up of forty autogenous vein and forty polytetrafluoroethylene (Gore-Tex) grafts for vascular access. Surgery 88(5):667–672, 1980.
30. Lilly L, Nighiem D, Mendez-Picon G, Lee HM. Comparison between bovine heterograft and expanded PTFE grafts for dialysis access. Am Surg 46(12):694–696, 1980.
31. Salmon PA. Vascular access for hemodialysis using bovine heterografts and polytetrafluoroethylene conduits. Can J Surg 24(1):59–63, 1981.
32. Flores L, Dunn I, Frumkin E, et al. Dacron arterio-venous shunts for vascular access in hemodialysis. Trans Am Soc Artif Intern Organs 19:33–37, 1973.
33. Lindenauer SM, Williams R. Dacron velour arteriovenous fistula for hemodialysis access. Ann Surg 193(1):43–48, 1981.
34. Kaplan MS, Mirahmadi KS, Winer RL, et al. Comparison of "PTFE" and bovine grafts for blood access in dialysis patients. Trans Am Soc Artif Intern Organs 22: 388–393, 1976.
35. Wellington JL. Umbilical grafts for vascular access in patients on long-term dialysis. Can J Surg 24(6):608–609, 1981.
36. Mindich BP, Silverman MJ, Elguezabal A, Levowitz BS. Umbilical cord vein fistula for vascular access in hemodialysis. Trans Am Soc Artif Intern Organs 21: 273–280, 1975.
37. Williams DF. Concensus and definitions in biomaterials. In DePutter C, deLange GL, DeGroot K, Lee AJC, eds. Implant Materials in Biofunction: Advances in Biomaterials. Amsterdam: Elsevier; 1988:11–71.
38. Drasler WJ, Wilson GJ, Stenoien MD, et al. A spun elastomeric graft for dialysis access. ASAIO J 39(2):114–119, 1993.
39. Pourdeyhimi B, Kern S. Ease of suturing surgical fabrics: A quantitative evaluation. Am J Surg 149(3):387–389, 1985.
40. Nemcek A Jr. Vascular graft puncture. J Vasc Intervent Radiol 7(3):377–378, 1996.
41. Olofsson P, Rabahie GN, Matsumoto K, et al. Histopathological characteristics of explanted human prosthetic arterial grafts: Implications for the prevention and management of graft infection. Eur J Vasc Endovasc Surg 9(2):143–151, 1995.
42. White RA. The effect of porosity and biomaterial on the healing and long-term mechanical properties of vascular prostheses. ASAIO Trans 34(2):95–100, 1988.
43. Martakos P, Karwoski T. Healing characteristics of hybrid and conventional polytetrafluoroethylene vascular grafts. ASAIO J 41(3):M735–M741, 1995.
44. Taylor SM, Weatherford DA, Langan EM, Lokey JS. Outcomes in the management of vascular prosthetic graft infections confined to the groin: a reappraisal. Ann Vasc Surg 10(2):117–122, 1996.
45. Strachan CJ. The prevention of orthopaedic implant and vascular graft infections. J Hosp Infect 30(suppl):54–63, 1995.
46. Taylor SM, Eaves GL, Weatherford DA, et al. Results and complications of arterio-

venous access dialysis grafts in the lower extremity: A five-year review. Am Surg 62(3):188–191, 1996.

47. Tordoir JH, Herman JM, Kwan TS, Diderich PM. Long-term follow-up of the poly-tetrafluoroethylene (PTFE) prosthesis as an arteriovenous fistula for haemodialysis. Eur J Vasc Surg 2(1):3–7, 1988.

48. Headley JL, Cole GW. The development of pseudo-Kaposi's sarcoma after place-ment of a vascular access graft. Br J Dermatol 102(3):327–331, 1980.

49. Keough EM, Callow AD, Connolly RJ, et al. Healing pattern of small caliber Da-cron grafts in the baboon: An animal model for the study of vascular prostheses. J Biomed Mater Res 18(3):281–292, 1984.

50. Guidoin R, Chakfe N, Maurel S, et al. Expanded polytetrafluoroethylene arterial prostheses in humans: Histopathological study of 298 surgically excised grafts. Bio-materials 14(9):678–693, 1993.

51. Rekhter M, Nicholls S, Ferguson M, Gordon D. Cell proliferation in human arterio-venous fistulas used for hemodialysis. Arterioscler Thromb 13(4):609–617, 1993.

52. Zamora JL, Gao ZR, Weilbaecher DG, et al. Hemodynamic and morphologic fea-tures of arteriovenous angioaccess loop grafts. Trans Am Soc Artif Intern Organs 31:119–123, 1985.

53. Puckett JW, Lindsay SF. Midgraft curettage as a routine adjunct to salvage opera-tions for thrombosed polytetrafluoroethylene hemodialysis access grafts. Am J Surg 156(2):139–143, 1988.

54. Taber TE, Maikranz PS, Haag BW, et al. Maintenance of adequate hemodialysis access. Prevention of neointimal hyperplasia. ASAIO J 41(4):842–846, 1995.

55. Tang L, Ugarova TP, Plow EF, Eaton JW. Molecular determinants of acute in-flammatory responses to biomaterials. J Clin Invest 97(5):1329–1334, 1996.

56. Sterpetti AV, Hunter WJ and Schultz RD. Congenital abdominal aortic aneurysms in the young. Case report and review of the literature. J Vasc Surg 7(6):763–769, 1988.

57. Kanda T, Kaneko K, Yamauchi Y, et al. Indium[111]-labeled platelets accumulation over abdominal aortic graft with chronic disseminated intravascular coagulation— A case history. Angiology 44(5):420–424, 1993.

58. May J, White GH, Yu W, Waugh RC, et al. Results of endoluminal grafting of abdominal aortic aneurysms are dependent on aneurysm morphology. Ann Vasc Surg 10(3):254–261, 1996.

59. Laborde JC, Parodi JC, Clem MF, et al. Intraluminal bypass of abdominal aortic aneurysm: Feasibility study. Radiology 184(1):185–190, 1992.

60. Parodi JC. Endovascular repair of aortic aneurysms, arteriovenous fistulas, and false aneurysms. World J Surg 20(6):655–663, 1996.

61. Mathisen SR, Wu HD, Sauvage LR, et al. The influence of denier and porosity on performance of a warp-knit Dacron arterial prosthesis. Ann Surg 203(4):382–389, 1986.

62. Kadoba K, Schoen FJ, Jonas RA. Experimental comparison of albumin-sealed and gelatin-sealed knitted Dacron conduits. Porosity control, handling, sealant resorp-tion, and healing. J Thorac Cardiovasc Surg 103(6):1059–1067, 1992.

63. Westaby S, Parry A, Giannopoulos N, Pillai R. Replacement of the thoracic aorta

with collagen-impregnated woven Dacron grafts. Early results. J Thorac Cardiovasc Surg 106(3):427–433, 1993.

64. Farmer DL, Goldstone J, Lim RC, Reilly LM. Failure of glow-discharge polymerization onto woven Dacron to improve performance of hemodialysis grafts. J Vasc Surg 18(4):570–576, 1993.

65. Kiaei D, Hoffman AS, Hanson SR. Ex vivo and in vitro platelet adhesion on RFGD deposited polymers. J Biomed Mater Res 26(3):357–372, 1992.

66. Heydorn WH, Geasling JW, Moores WY, et al. Changes in the manufacture of expanded microporous polytetrafluoroethylene: Effects on patency and histological behavior when used to replace the superior vena cava. Ann Thorac Surg 27(2): 173–177, 1979.

67. May J, Harris J, Patrick W. Polytetrafluoroethylene grafts for hemodialysis: Patency and complications compared with those of saphenous vein grafts. Aust NZ J Surg 49(6):639–642, 1979.

68. Lornoy W, Becaus I, Gillardin JP, et al. Autogenous saphenous vein AV fistulae for hemodialysis: Eight years experience with 30 patients. Proc Eur Dial Transplant Assoc 19:227–233, 1983.

69. Haimov M, Burrows L, Baez A, Neff M, Slifkin R. Alternatives for vascular access for hemodialysis: Experience with autogenous saphenous vein autografts and bovine heterografts. Surgery 75(3):447–452, 1974.

70. Valenta J, Bilek J, Opatrny K. Autogenous saphenous vein graft as a secondary vascular access for hemodialysis. Dial Transplant 14:567, 1985.

71. Garcia-Rinaldi R, Von Koch L. The axillary artery to axillary vein bovine graft for circulatory access. Am J Surg 135(2):265–268, 1978.

72. Burbridge GE, Biggers JA, Remmers AR Jr, et al. Late complications and results with bovine xenografts. Trans Am Soc Artif Intern Organs 22:377–381, 1976.

73. Mohaideen AH, Mendivil J, Avram MM, Mainzer RA. Arterio-venous access utilizing modified bovine arterial grafts for hemodialysis. Ann Surg 186(5):643–650, 1977.

74. Bleyer AJ, Rocco MV, Burkart JM. The costs of hospitalizations due to hemodialysis access management. Nephrol News Issues 9(1):19–22, 1995.

75. Feldman HI, Held PJ, Hutchnson JT, et al. Hemodialysis vascular access morbidity in the United States. Kidney Int 43(5):1091–1096, 1993.

76. Eggers PW. A quarter century of medicine expenditures for ESRD. Semin Nephrol 20(6):516–522, 2000.

77. Windus DW. Permanent vascular access: A nephrologists view. Am J Kidney Dis 21(5):457–471, 1993.

78. Okuhn SP, Connely DP, Calakos N, et al. Does compliance mismatch alone cause neointimal hyperplasia? J Vasc Surg 9(1):35–45, 1989.

79. Kinley CE, Marble AE. Compliance: A continuing problem with vascular grafts. J Cardiovasc Surg 21(2):163–170, 1980.

80. Holubec H, Hunter GC, Putnam CW, et al. Effect of surgical manipulation of polytetrafluoroethylene grafts on microstructural properties and healing characteristics. Am J Surg 164(5):512–516, 1992.

81. Anderson JM. Inflammatory response to implants. ASAIO Trans 34(2):101–107, 1988.

82. Schreuders PD, Salthouse TN, von Recum AF. Normal wound healing compared

to healing within porous Dacron implants. J Biomed Mater Res 22(2):121–135, 1988.

83. Anderson JM, Ziats NP, Azeez A, et al. Protein absorption and macrophage activation on polydimethylsiloxane and silicone rubber. J Biomater Sci Polymer Ed 7(2): 159–169, 1995.

84. Miller KM, Anderson JM. Human monocyte/macrophage activation and interleukin 1 generation by biomedical polymers. J Biomed Mater Res 22(8):713–731, 1988.

85. Williams SK, Jarrell BE, Rose DG, et al. Human microvessel endothelial cell isolation and vascular graft sodding in the operating room. Ann Vasc Surg 3(2):146–152, 1989.

86. Williams SK. Endothelial cell transplantation. Cell Transplant 4(4):401–410, 1995.

87. Park PK, Jarrell BE, Williams SK, et al. Thrombus-free, human endothelial surface in the midregion of a Dacron vascular graft in the splanchnic venous circuit—observations after nine months of implantation. J Vasc Surg 11(3):468–475, 1990.

88. Williams SK, Jarrell BE. Tissue-engineered vascular grafts. Nature Med 2(1):32–34, 1996.

89. Salzmann DL, Kleinert LB, Berman SS, Williams SK. The effects of porosity on endothelialization of ePTFE implanted in subcutaneous and adipose tissue. J Biomed Mater Res 34(4):463–476, 1997.

90. Clowes AW, Kirkman TR, Reidy MA. Mechanisms of arterial graft healing: Rapid transmural capillary ingrowth provides a source of intimal endothelium and smooth muscle cells in porous PTFE prostheses. Am J Pathol 123(2):220–230, 1986.

91. Berman SS, Jarrell BE, Raymond MA, et al. Early experience with ePTFE dialysis grafts sodded with liposuction-derived microvascular endothelial cells. In Henry ML, Ferguson RF, eds. Vascular Access for Hemodialysis IV. Chicago: Precept Press. Precept; 1995:292–302.

92. Baier R. The organization of blood components near interfaces. Ann NY Acad Sci 283:17–36, 1976.

93. Grinnel F. Blood material interactions: adsorption of fibronectin. Summary of the Devices and Technology Branch Contractors Meeting, December, 1982. Publication No 84-1651. Bethesda, MD: NIH/National Heart Lung and Blood Institute; 1984.

94. Lyman DJ, Knutson K, MeNeil B, et al. The effect of chemical structure and surface properties of synthetic polymers on the coagulation of blood. IV. The relation between polymer morphology and protein absorption. Trans Am Soc Artif Intern Organs 21:49–54, 1975.

95. Merrill EW. Properties of materials affecting the behavior of blood at their surfaces. Ann NY Acad Sci 283:6–16, 1977.

96. Pankowsky DA, Ziats NP, Topham NS, et al. Morphological characteristics of absorbed human plasma proteins on vascular graft biomaterials. J Vasc Surg 11(4): 599–606, 1990.

97. Weathersby PK, Horbett TA, Hoffman AS. A new method for analysis of the absorbed plasma protein layer on biomaterial surfaces. Trans Am Soc Artif Intern Organs 22:242–252, 1976.

98. Domurado D, Guidoin R, Marois M, et al. Albuminated Dacron protheses as improved blood vessel substitutes. J Bioeng 2(1–2):79–91, 1978.

99. Boerboom LE, Olinger GN, Karas BJ, et al. Heparinization of biological vascular graft reduces fibrin deposition. Int J Artif Organs 16(5):263–267, 1993.

100. Freischlag JA, Moore WS. Clinical experience with a collagen-impregnated knitted Dacron vascular graft. Ann Vasc Surg 4(5):449–454, 1990.

101. Slack SM, Cui Y, Turitto VT. The effects of flow on blood coagulation and thrombosis. Thromb Haemost 70(1):129–134, 1993.

102. Goodman SL, Cooper SL, Albrecht RM. Integrin receptors and platelet adhesion to synthetic surfaces. J Biomed Mater Res 27(5):683–695, 1993.

103. Berger K, Sauvage LR, Rao AM, Wood SJ. Healing of arterial prosthesis in man: Its incompleteness. Ann Surg 175(1):118–127, 1972.

104. Kocher O, Madri JA. Modulation of actin mRNAs in cultured vascular cells by matrix components and TGF-beta 1. In Vitro Cell Dev Biol 25(5):424–434, 1989.

105. Rekhter M, Nicholls S, Ferguson M, Gordon D. Cell proliferation in human arteriovenous fistulas used for hemodialysis. Arterioscler Thromb 13(4):609–617, 1993.

106. Jenkins AM, Buist TA, Glover SD. Medium-term follow-up of forty autogenous vein and forty polytetrafluoroethylene (Gore-Tex) grafts for vascular access. Surgery 88(5):667–672, 1980.

107. Palder SB, Kirkman RL, Whittemore AD, et al. Vascular access for hemodialysis. Patency rates and results of revision. Ann Surg 202(2):235–239, 1985.

108. Raju S. PTFE grafts for hemodialysis access. Techniques for insertion and management of complications. Ann Surg 206(5):666–673, 1987.

109. Munda R, First MR, Alexander JW, et al. Polytetrafluoroethylene graft survival in hemodialysis. JAMA 249(2):219–222, 1983.

110. Steed DL, McAuley CE, Rault R, Webster MW. Upper arm graft fistula for hemodialysis. J Vasc Surg 1(5):660–663, 1984.

111. Kherlakian GM, Roedersheimer LR, Arbaugh JJ, et al. Comparison of autogenous fistula versus expanded polytetrafluoroethylene graft fistula for angioaccess in hemodialysis. Am J Surg 152(2):238–243, 1986.

112. Ludwicka A, Jansen B, Wadstrom T, Pulverer G. Attachment of stahphylococci to various polymers. Zbl Bakt Hyg (Med Micro, Inf Dis, Virol, Parasitol) 256(4): 479–489, 1984.

113. Gristina AG, Rovere GD, Shoji H, Nicastro JF. An in vitro study of bacterial response to inert and reactive metals and to methyl-methacrylate. J Biomed Mater Res 10(2):273–281, 1976.

114. Gristina AG, Dobbins JJ, Giammara B, et al. Biomaterial-centered sepsis and the total artificial heart. Microbial adhesion vs tissue integration. JAMA 259(6):870–874, 1988.

115. Greco RS, Harvey RA. The role of antibiotic bonding in the prevention of vascular prosthetic infections. Ann Surg 195(2):168–171, 1982.

116. Rodriguez JL, Trooskin SZ, Greco RS, et al. Reduced bacterial adherence to surfactant-coated catheters. Curr Surg 43(5):423–425, 1986.

117. Powell TW, Burnham SJ, Johnson G Jr. A passive system using rifampin to create an infection-resistant vascular prosthesis. Surgery 94(5):765–769, 1983.

118. Sobinsky KR, Flanigan DP. Antibiotic bonding to polytetrafluoroethylene via gly-cosaminoglycan-keratin luminal coating. Surgery 100:629–634, 1986.

119. Moore WS, Chvapil M, Seiffert G, Keown K. Development of an infection-resistant vascular prosthesis. Arch Surg 116(11):1403–1407, 1981.

120. Delorme JM, Guidoin R, Canizales S, et al. Vascular access for hemodialysis: Pathologic features of surgically excised ePTFE grafts. Ann Vasc Surg 6(6):517–524, 1992.

III

Central Venous Access

14

Central Venous Catheters: Selection and Placement Techniques

Kenneth Fox
Children's Hospital of Austin/Cardiothoracic and Vascular Surgeons, Austin, Texas

Donald J. Roach
Radiology Limited, Tucson, Arizona

Scott S. Berman
The University of Arizona, Carondelet St. Mary's Hospital, and The Southern Arizona Vascular Institute, Tucson, Arizona

The placement of central venous access devices has become an everyday component of the management of a significant proportion of patients suffering from a variety of maladies in a number of diverse treatment environments. Central venous access is routinely used in the treatment of critically ill intensive care unit patients for both durable intravenous access as well as a route for measurement of central hemodynamics. In less critically ill hospitalized patients, central venous access is frequently applied to difficult intravenous access situations or where prolonged intravenous administration of medications such as antibiotics or nutrition is required. Finally, as more and more treatment is transitioned from inpatient to outpatient settings, central venous access devices are commonly seen in ambulatory patients receiving chemotherapy for malignancies and infections, prolonged intravenous nutrition, and as a means to perform renal replacement therapy.

The placement and maintenance of a functional central venous access device can become a formidable challenge in patients who need these appliances for prolonged periods of time. This chapter reviews the general points for catheter selection and focuses on catheter placement techniques for central venous catheters (CVC). Since most catheter insertions are done using percutaneous techniques, our own general procedure for most CVC insertion is described in detail under "Percutaneous Insertion," below. The specific considerations related to central venous catheters used for hemodialysis have already been discussed in Chapter 10 and interested readers are referred there for details regarding these special catheter types. Moreover, Chapter 17 comprises an explicit discussion of the prevention and treatment of catheter-related complications, which are not repeated here.

CATHETER SELECTION

Central venous catheters are used in a broad number of applications. The type of catheter placed is somewhat dependent upon the specific needs of each clinical scenario. For instance, catheters inserted in the intensive care unit and used for hemodynamic monitoring are usually required for only short periods of time and are rarely needed beyond a few days after placement. By contrast, catheters inserted for chemotherapy to treat solid tumors may be left in place for months or years. The details surrounding each catheter's clinical indication help determine appropriate catheter specifications required.

For simplicity, we have grouped the catheters into three general categories based upon duration of access required. Our discussion of catheter specifications centers on catheters designed for temporary use (less than 1 week), short-term use (one to 6 weeks) and long-term use (more than 6 weeks). Common clinical circumstances that may predicate catheter criteria are mentioned. Another factor that must be considered is the number of lumens required. This component is also guided by the clinical circumstances. In general, multilumen catheters have a higher infection rate than their single-lumen counterparts (1–3). This holds true whether one considers temporary or long-term CVCs and is related to the higher incidence of catheter access with multilumen devices. Multilumen catheters are available in a number of configurations, including the double-D, circular, and coaxial designs. Lumen configuration becomes a significant issue when high flows are required through the catheter, as in hemodialysis or plasmapheresis. A detailed discussion of lumen configuration appears in Chapter 10.

Temporary Catheters

Establishment of central venous access for periods of time measured in days is usually required for central hemodynamic monitoring in critically ill or injured patients or in patients undergoing major surgical procedures. By contrast, CVCs are not considered the first choice for vascular access for the resuscitation of trauma victims, whereas large-bore antecubital intravenous catheters are still the mainstay in these patients. Catheters used for temporary access range from simple single-lumen CVCs to complex combinations of introducer sheaths and multilumen catheters. These catheters are commonly made of stiff polyurethane for easy placement. Most catheters are supplied as self-contained insertion trays allowing for ease of placement at the patient's bedside. Temporary catheters are designed for percutaneous insertion using the Seldinger technique, as described in greater detail further on.

Temporary CVCs are typically placed via the internal jugular or subclavian route, depending on the clinical situation. Occasionally, in patients with severe coagulation abnormalities or in those who lack available jugular or subclavian access routes, femoral vein access is required. Most single and multilumen temporary CVCs have a fixed length and require careful attention to tip location during placement to avoid atrial or ventricular tip positioning. Instances of atrial perforation have occurred most frequently with polyurethane catheters, prompting the Food and Drug Administration to recommend not letting any catheter tip come to rest in the right atrium (4). Introducer sheaths, ranging in size from 9 to 11 F, not only function as large-bore CVCs for fluid resuscitation but can also provide a conduit for the introduction of pulmonary artery catheters into the central venous circulation.

Temporary catheters are intended for short periods of use, usually less than 7 days. Beyond this time frame, the risk of catheter infection increases. By design, the catheters lack any barrier to infection, as in permanent or degradable cuffs. Although protocols for catheter care vary, most institutions recommend removal or replacement of a temporary CVC at 7 days. In an effort to reduce the infection risk of CVCs, some manufacturers have incorporated antimicrobial components into the catheter construct. One example of this technology is the ArrowgardBlue antiseptic surface applied to a number of catheters available from Arrow International, Inc., Reading, PA (Figure 14.1). The coating consists of chlorhexidine-silver sulfadiazine molecularly bonded to the external surface of the catheter, which provides a prolonged antiseptic effect to the intravascular portion of the CVC. In both in vitro and in vivo experiments, a reduction in catheter-related bacteremias has been correlated with the use of this antiseptic surface (4,5).

Polyurethane, the base polymer utilized in most temporary CVCs, limits the duration of cannulation of these devices. By virtue of its rigidity, catheters

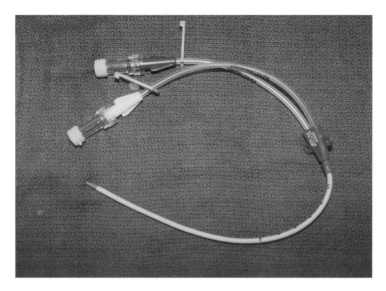

FIGURE 14.1   Arrow blue catheter.

made of polyurethane are predisposed to vessel perforation acutely during placement and to vessel erosion when left in place for prolonged periods of time.
Moreover, polyurethane is associated with a higher rate of fibrin sheath formation
and intimal reaction compared with silicone, the base polymer frequently employed in most long-term intravascular devices (6). Both of these responses limit
the functionality of the device through either catheter thrombosis or vessel thrombosis, respectively. A predilection for these adverse reactions limits the safety
and durability of polyurethane catheters beyond 1 to 2 weeks of use.

Short-Term Catheters

Few catheter designs address the need for intravascular access for the intermediate time period of 1 to 6 weeks. Clinical scenarios that might call for this include
infections requiring prolonged intravenous antibiotic administration, such as osteomyelitis, endocarditis, or intravascular device–related infections. Other indications for this interval of access comprise total parenteral nutrition in a patient
with ischemic colitis or short-bowel syndrome. Short-term access is largely
achieved with either a modified temporary catheter or a long-term catheter, as
described below. We are aware of only one device designed for a limited period
of prolonged access—the Hohn catheter (Bard Access Systems, Salt Lake City,
UT) (7).

The Hohn catheter shares a number of characteristics with both temporary and long-term catheters. It is available as either a 5F single-lumen or 7F dual-lumen device (Figure 14.2). Both sizes are provided as self-contained placement kits that allow for bedside insertion. The small size of the Hohn catheter and over-the-wire placement makes bedside insertion feasible and safe, a trait shared with temporary catheters. Both models come with a variable-length intravascular portion that necessitates trimming the catheter to an estimated length for tip placement in the superior vena cava (SVC). Prolonged use of the Hohn catheter is enhanced by its construction of soft Silastic, which minimizes intravascular intimal trauma and risk of catheter erosion. Unlike traditional long-term catheters, no portion of the Hohn catheter is designed for subcutaneous tunneling. However, each Hohn catheter is equipped with a Vitacuff (see Figure 14.2) to provide a barrier to infection for up to 6 weeks. The Vitacuff is a silver-impregnated collagen cuff attached to the catheter just under the skin by the exit site. During the 6-week degradation of the collagen cuff, continuous release of silver ions provides a barrier to infection along the shaft of the catheter (8).

One nuance of the Hohn catheter deserving of mention centers on insertion problems. The tip of the catheter is a blunt cylinder that sometimes makes penetration through the subcutaneous tissue and into the vessel lumen difficult. This is aggravated by the soft pliability of the Silastic catheter. We have overcome this problem by using 6F (single-lumen) and 8F (double-lumen) peel-away sheath introducers to traverse the subcutaneous tissue and enter the vessel lumen whenever resistance is encountered. Because no tunneling is required, catheter removal is simple and straightforward, requiring only removal of an anchoring stitch or two and gentle traction. Aside from the technical point with insertion mentioned above, the Hohn catheter provides an excellent alternative to long-

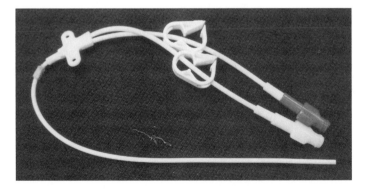

FIGURE 14.2 Hohn catheter.

term tunneled catheters for patients who need an intermediate period of central venous access.

Other options for accomplishing short-term central venous access include modifying temporary catheters for prolonged insertion or simply using tunneled long-term catheters. Modification of a temporary catheter for prolonged insertion largely focuses on the addition of a subcutaneous Vitacuff to the catheter shaft (8). This simple procedure at the time of catheter insertion provides a barrier to catheter infection for up to 6 weeks. The Vitacuff is available as a separately packaged device and is also incorporated into the shaft of a number of commercially available temporary catheters. Though the Vitacuff affords some protection against catheter infection, the disadvantages of using polyurethane catheters for prolonged access remain unchanged. Use of a long-term tunneled catheter addresses this issue, as most popular brands are made of Silastic. The specific characteristics of long-term catheters are noted in the following section. However, use of a small-diameter single-lumen cuffed, tunneled catheter is an acceptable alternative for short-term access.

A final and increasingly popular choice for short-term access is the peripherally inserted central catheter (PICC) (9,10). In many institutions including our own, these central venous catheters are placed by specially trained nurses (11). These PICC lines, as they are called, are small-diameter Silastic or polyurethane catheters inserted into the central venous circulation through a peripheral vein, usually the median antecubital (Figure 14.3). Details of PICC insertion appear later in this chapter. Because of the peripheral site of venous cannulation, compli-

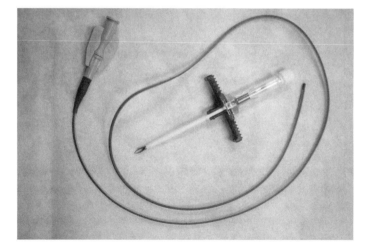

FIGURE 14.3   PICC line.

cations related to placement are usually of no significant consequence and primarily involve peripheral hematomas or superficial thrombophlebitis. This is quite distinct from the known complications of central venous catheter placement, such as pneumothorax and major vascular injury. Though infection rates of PICC lines are less than with CVCs in general, the potential exists for catastrophic thrombophlebitis of the central venous system and endocarditis despite the peripheral origin of these devices (10). These advantages of PICCs over traditional CVCs make them an attractive selection for short-term intravenous access.

Long-Term Catheters

Patients in need of central venous access for periods in excess of 6 weeks require placement of a long-term CVC. Common indications for placement of this type of CVC include prolonged chemotherapy for malignancies, prolonged parenteral nutrition for short-gut syndrome, and absence of peripheral venous access in a chronically ill patient. This category of catheters can be further subdivided into three components: (a) tunneled, cuffed, external CVCs; (b) implanted CVCs with subcutaneous reservoirs; and (c) peripherally inserted CVCs with subcutaneous reservoirs. The characteristics, advantages, and disadvantages of these access options are outlined below.

In selecting a long-term catheter for an individual patient, key considerations in catheter selection include the anticipated duration of therapy, the number and types of infusions required, the availability of resources for catheter care, cosmetic concerns of the patient to have an exposed or concealed device, the patient's activity level, and his or her tolerance or intolerance of repeated needle sticks. In general, implanted ports are favored over external catheters for prolonged infusions of single agents in active patients, patients who desire concealed devices, or those who lack the resources required for regular catheter care necessary with external devices. Peripheral ports are acceptable for low-viscosity single infusions requiring infrequent access. Examples of this include single-agent chemotherapy in patients with solid tumors or prolonged antibiotic infusions. Multilumen centrally placed ports are available and can be used, but they carry a higher risk of infectious complications compared with single-lumen ports. In patients with the anticipated need for multiple infusions and multiple blood samplings, such as leukemia and bone-marrow transplant patients, tunneled, cuffed, external catheters are a better alternative to implanted ports. Large-diameter multiple-lumen external catheters meet the needs of these often very ill patients far better than the implanted reservoirs.

Tunneled, Cuffed, and External CVCs

The introduction of the Broviac and subsequently the Hickman catheters ushered in the modern era of long-term central venous access (12,13). These devices were made of silicone rubber or Silastic and were intended to be a less thrombogenic alternative to the polyvinyl chloride catheters that preceded them. Catheters that share the basic design of the Broviac and Hickman are now the mainstays of long-term venous access devices. These tunneled catheters are available in a vast array of sizes and lumen configurations. A Dacron cuff is incorporated into the shaft of the catheter and positioned in the subcutaneous tissue 1 to 2 cm from the catheter exit site. Over a period of 4 to 6 weeks, the cuff becomes incorporated into the subcutaneous tissue through fibrous ingrowth. Once the cuff becomes well healed into the subcutaneous tissues, a barrier to bacterial migration along the catheter is established to minimize catheter infection. Moreover, the scarred-in cuff provides some protection against accidental catheter removal.

Recently, Vitacuffs have been added to a number of these tunneled catheters to provide additional protection against infection in the first 4 to 6 weeks when tissue incorporation of the Dacron cuff proceeds. During this early phase of healing, the biodegradable collagen Vitacuff discharges a continuous supply of silver ions and provides some antibacterial activity near the catheter exit site (8).

One increasingly popular modification of tunneled, cuffed external CVCs is the Groshong catheter. This catheter is unique in its design by the presence of a slit-valve at its tip. The construction of the slit-valve allows it to function as a two-way valve compatible with both aspiration and injection (Figure 14.4).

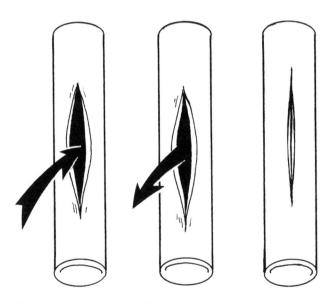

FIGURE 14.4 Drawing of Groshong tip.

However, without these forces applied to the valve, it rests in a neutral, closed position and prevents reflux of blood into the catheter lumen. Thus, the catheter does not require daily flushing with heparinized solutions, or require placement of a concentrated heparin dwell. The care recommended is weekly flushing with normal saline. This innovation greatly reduces the cost and amount of care required to maintain catheter patency. Like other tunneled, cuffed, external CVCs, the Groshong is made of Silastic. Moreover, use of a thin-walled arrangement allows the Groshong catheter to provide similar lumen sizes as its Hickman counterparts packaged in a smaller outside diameter. The disadvantage of this design is a much more fragile catheter that, in our own experience, is prone to fracture. In addition, removal of Hickman catheters often requires only gentle traction to disengage the subcutaneous cuff, whereas similar traction applied to the thin-walled Groshong may result in catheter disruption. Therefore removal of a Groshong often requires a limited cutdown procedure over the subcutaneous cuff.

Most of the available tunneled, cuffed, external catheters are provided as self-contained insertion trays containing all the equipment necessary for percutaneous insertion. Tunneled external CVCs have a durability limited only by material strength, patency, and avoidance of infection. With the exception of the Groshong catheter noted above, a regular maintenance schedule is required to include flushing of all lumens with heparin and scrupulous cleansing of the exit site with application of sterile dressings (14). The need for regular care and maintenance of external catheters must be factored into the decision as to what type of long-term device to place for an individual patient. These care considerations may prove prohibitive for patients who do not have access to professional ambulatory care agencies or who lack either the personal ability or family support to ensure that meticulous catheter care is achieved. In these types of patients, the lower maintenance required of an implanted reservoir may influence the access device selected.

Implanted CVCs with Subcutaneous Reservoirs

Implanted venous access ports combine the attributes of a CVC with the ease of management and cosmetic acceptability of a completely implanted device. Most available implantable venous ports comprise a Silastic catheter with an implantable reservoir. A number of manufacturers have devices available with either a preassembled catheter and port or a detached catheter (Figure 14.5). Subtle differences in placement technique are required, depending upon the configuration of the device, and are described below, under ''Common Placement Techniques.'' The reservoir generally consists of a plastic or titanium housing with a silicone diaphragm. When noncoring needles are used for access, a multitude of punctures can be achieved without extravasation. Titanium or plastic housings are used to reduce the likelihood of image scatter when subjected to computed

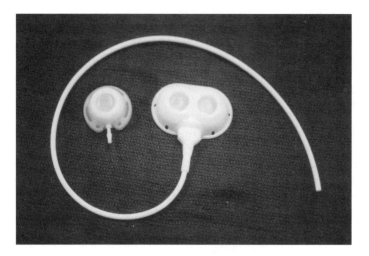

FIGURE 14.5   Port with and without attached catheters.

tomography. The implantable ports are available from a number of manufacturers as double or single-lumen designs as well as multiple housing sizes to accommodate pediatric patients and adults with limited subcutaneous tissue.

Because the catheter and reservoir are completely sealed beneath the skin, implanted ports offer a cosmetic appeal to patients expected to need prolonged intravenous therapy. Furthermore, active patients may resume regular physical activity, including swimming, with an implantable port, unlike the case with external catheters, which have activity restrictions associated with their use by nature of their location (15). The disadvantage of this arrangement is that the patient must endure the pain of a needle puncture when the port is cannulated, in contrast to the external catheters, which may be accessed without discomfort to the patient. This difference between tunneled catheters and implanted ports brings to light the fact that patient concerns and tolerance of needle sticks is yet another factor in determining the most appropriate access device.

Peripherally Inserted CVCs with Subcutaneous Reservoirs

A final option for long-term venous access evolved from both implanted venous ports and PIC lines. The P.A.S. Port (Pharmacia Deltec, Inc., St. Paul, MN) is an example of a CVC inserted through a peripheral vein and is attached to a subcutaneous reservoir implanted in the upper extremity (Figure 14.6) (16). Like the PIC line, the P.A.S. Port has a peripheral entry site that minimizes the chance for significant placement complications without compromising the advantage of tip placement in a large central vein. A small-profile implanted reservoir is placed

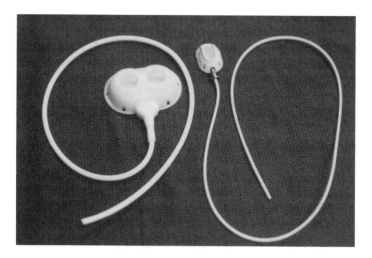

FIGURE 14.6   PAS port compared with regular port.

in the subcutaneous tissue of the arm, as described in detail below. The P.A.S. Port and related devices offer cosmetic advantages similar to those of centrally placed implanted ports and also permit resumption of normal physical activity once the site is completely healed. As in the case of centrally placed ports, each time the peripheral port is accessed, the patient must submit to a needle puncture. However, the reduced reservoir size of peripheral ports limits the recommended size of the cannulation needle to a 22-gauge and also confines the septum area available for rotation of access sites. These attributes exclude patients who may need multiple infusions from having peripheral ports as an access alternative.

COMMON PLACEMENT TECHNIQUES

Basic Techniques and Components

Central venous access devices may be placed in a number of environments. Principles of sterile technique should be strictly adhered to regardless of whether the CVC is placed at the bedside or in a specialized suite such as an operating room or angiography unit. Important components of the placement environment include adequate lighting, an adjustable bed or stretcher, and the availability of personnel to provide assistance to the individual performing the placement procedure. These components are independent of the type of CVC to be inserted. For bedside temporary CVC placement, the need for continuous electrocardiographic (ECG) and/or pulse oximetry monitoring is unclear. Our own approach is to use either the operating room patient prep area or the postanesthesia care unit for all catheter insertions on inpatients not already in an intensive care setting. By virtue of the usual care provided at these sites, ECG is readily available and is routinely employed. We do not routinely use conscious sedation when placing bedside CVCs; however, use of this technique would mandate the need for noninvasive monitoring in most institutions today.

The expedience of having the patient in an adjustable bed cannot be overstated. Not only does a fully adjustable bed or stretcher facilitate patient positioning to enhance venous distention, but the ability to adjust the patient's height to an optimal level for the operator has immeasurable benefit in avoiding prolonged periods in a hunched position over a patient for whom the bed height is not adjustable. Exposure of the important anatomical landmarks is also of universal importance for insertion of all CVCs. For most of our CVC placements, exposure, along with sterile prepping and draping, includes the area bounded by the mandibles, nipples, and shoulders. This provides excellent visualization of the critical landmarks and also affords the availability of a multiple of contingency placement sites if we are unable to successfully access our primary site. With the generous preparation we describe, secondary sites may be accessed without the need for repositioning, reprepping, and redraping. As a minimum, sterile gloves, a mask, and protective eyewear are used for all catheter insertions. Use of a cap and sterile gown has not been clearly shown to reduce catheter infection rates for bedside insertion except for placement of dedicated CVCs for total parenteral nutrition. When CVCs are inserted in the operating room or angiography suite, standard techniques for surgical scrub as well as cap, mask, gown, and glove utilization are applied.

Most CVCs designed for bedside placement are available as self-contained placement trays. These kits usually include the catheter and the necessary accessories for insertion such as needles, syringes, an allotment of 1% lidocaine, guidewire, suture, drapes, dressing, povodine-iodine solution, and even sterile gloves. Though unnecessary for uncomplicated insertions, we recommend having replacement parts readily available for the common difficulties likely to be encountered during CVC placement. A plethora of situations may arise during CVC insertion that require replacement of an individual component of an insertion tray. A simple example of this is dropping the guidewire on the floor before its role is completed. Replacement components may be as simple as extra syringes and sutures or may be as specialized as a replacement catheter or guidewire (Figure 14.7). Often another complete insertion tray must be opened for a simple component that could be readily available on an individual basis with the appropriate forethought. Opening complete trays to retrieve individual pieces is wasteful and expensive. With the exception of the catheters themselves, individually packaged replacement components are readily available. To this end, individual

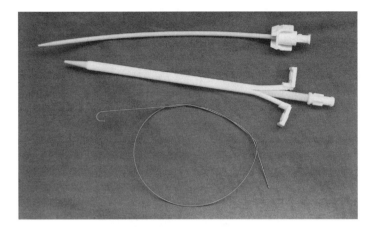

FIGURE 14.7   Spare parts available, including dilator, guidewire, and sheath.

packaged catheters are available for a number of the temporary hemodialysis catheters.

Aside from the availability of replacement parts, adjunctive devices that may facilitate catheter insertion should be accessible. These may include an assortment of guidewires and peel-away sheaths. Previously, we alluded to our use of a peel-away sheath to facilitate Hohn catheter insertion at the bedside. Based upon our experience, we now make sure to have the appropriately sized sheath available for all Hohn placements. Finally, an adequate quantity of injectable normal saline, heparin flush, and local anesthetic should be easily accessible to the operator.

For bedside catheter placement, one of the keys to an uneventful insertion is organization. Once the patient has been positioned and the skin prepared, it is the authors' preference to organize the components to be used in catheter placement on either a Mayo stand or the patient's tray table prior to beginning the invasive part of the procedure. This avoids inadvertent loss of a portion or all of the tray should patient movement occur—a problem associated with resting the insertion tray on the patient's chest. Subtle points that can expedite catheter insertion include assembling selected needles and syringes, disengaging the guidewire introducer tip from the guidewire housing sheath, unsheathing the knife blade, unpacking the suture, and having the catheter and dilator readily available for immediate use (Figure 14.8). Once the components are organized on the stand, the procedure commences.

The operating room or angiography suite is more likely to be the site of placement of long-term catheters. In general, these catheters are larger in diameter

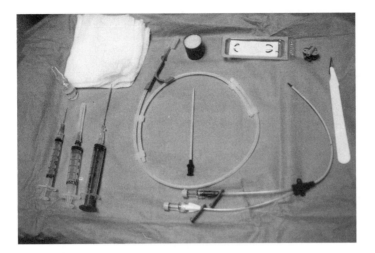

FIGURE 14.8   CVL kit laid out on Mayo stand.

and have a variable length compared with temporary catheters. These two characteristics of long-term catheters escalate the risks associated with CVC placement. Fortunately, most long-term catheters are placed with fluoroscopic guidance in environments with an abundance of personnel and resources to assist with placement should difficulties be encountered. With this in mind, it is optimal to have an assortment of guidewires and peel-away sheaths readily available during catheter insertion. This is in addition to the array of replacement components describe above for bedside CVC placement.

Percutaneous Insertion

By far the most common method used today for the introduction of catheters into the vascular system is the percutaneous method. The single most important historical landmark in percutaneous catheter insertion is the introduction of the over-the-wire technique first described by Seldinger in 1953 (17). Aside from minor modifications in component construct, the Seldinger technique has been modified little since its first description. The basic Seldinger technique comprises the cannulation of the chosen vessel with a needle followed by the passage of a guidewire through the needle into the vascular system. The guidewire, which remains in place until the procedure is completed, functions as a rail over which catheters or devices are safely introduced into the vascular system.

Percutaneous placement of CVCs requires an absolute familiarity with regional anatomy as well as an understanding of potential anomalies and pathological conditions that may either contraindicate or complicate percutaneous insertion. The specific anatomy for a number of access sites is discussed in subsequent sections. Specific details of the patient's history and physical should be noted including prior catheter insertion: a history of bleeding abnormalities; history of trauma or surgery to the neck, chest, extremities, and/or pelvis; and any signs or symptoms of active infection. The physical assessment prior to CVC insertion should pay special attention to any swelling in the extremities, areas of venous engorgement, areas of active phlebitis, and scars from previous CVCs. Informed consent should be obtained from each patient, with a detailed discussion of the risks of catheter placement regardless of the technique chosen for catheter insertion. Although no absolute contraindications for percutaneous placement of catheters exist, the presence of certain conditions may prompt the operator to restrict access to certain sites or evaluate the patient with more intensive testing prior to CVC placement. For example, patients with a history of multiple previous CVC placements and physical signs of central venous obstruction such as extremity swelling or engorgement of subcutaneous veins should undergo assessment with either duplex scanning or venography to document patency of selected central venous sites. As another example, CVC placement in a patient with an active bleeding diathesis might be limited to percutaneous access of the femoral vessels only, since bleeding complications at this site may be more easy to control and have less impact on the patient's overall condition as compared with bleeding complications at the jugular or subclavian locations.

Percutaneous insertion begins with an assessment of the typical landmarks for placement at a chosen site. It is the authors' preference to use a surgical marker and draw anatomical landmarks on the patient's skin, as palpable and visual landmarks may become obscured by infiltration anesthesia, prepping, and draping. Preparation of the skin with a bactericidal agent followed by draping with sterile towels or prefabricated drapes should provide adequate sterile field protection without limiting access to multiple sites if possible. The selected access vein is then cannulated with a large bore introducer needle (usually 16-gauge). Some operators prefer to use a smaller needle (22-gauge) as a "finder" needle to verify the position and depth of the vein prior to using the larger needle. Once the vein is accessed, the syringe is disconnected from the needle and the guidewire passed into position through the back of the introducer needle. The authors prefers to use a nonlocking Luer syringe to avoid over manipulation and misplacement of the needle when disconnecting the syringe, which may occur with a locking Luer syringe. This specific concern is addressed by the Arrow safety syringe (Figure 14.9). This system is constructed such that the guidewire is introduced through the back of the plunger on the syringe, avoiding the task of disconnecting the needle from the syringe, with its attendant risk of needle movement. Unfortunately, the Arrow safety syringe is available only in certain CVC kits and has not been universally well received by physicians.

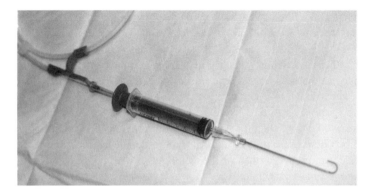

FIGURE **14.9**   Arrow safety syringe.

An assessment of the color and flow of blood through the introducer needle should take place prior to passage of the guidewire. Bright red, pulsatile flow emanating from the introducer needle implies an arterial puncture. When this complication occurs, we recommend removing the needle, halting the procedure, and applying direct pressure to the puncture site for 10 min prior to resuming the placement procedure. Unless the patient has a coagulopathy or severe thrombocytopenia, these maneuvers will prevent the development of a significant hematoma and allow further attempts at placement at the same site. Patience on the part of the operator in achieving adequate hemostasis of an unintentional arterial puncture is usually rewarded with few major bleeding complications requiring surgical intervention. This is true even of the subclavian artery, which can be tamponaded through the simultaneous application of direct pressure from both above the clavicle and below the clavicle. Andros et al. demonstrated that even larger (7 to 9F) arterial punctures of the subclavian artery can be safely controlled with this method in their series of 569 direct puncture subclavian artery arterial interventions (18).

If there is any doubt as to the nature of the blood flow from the introducer needle—i.e., arterial versus venous—a simple method to resolve this dilemma prior to attempting guidewire passage is to connect the introducer needle to a pressure transducer system and measure the blood pressure. The applicability of this technique requires the availability of hemodynamic monitoring equipment with sterile pressure tubing. An argument further in favor of placing all CVCs in a critical care environment. The guidewire should pass through the introducer needle without any resistance. This point cannot be overstated. Any resistance encountered during passage of the guidewire suggests malposition and should signal the operator to reassess needle location. Most temporary catheters are stiff enough that they can be passed directly over the guidewire into the desired position. The exception to this is the Hohn catheter, described above.

The soft Silastic long-term catheters present different challenges for percutaneous placement inherent to their design. Recently, adjunctive components have been developed to facilitate passage of very large diameter, soft, Silastic catheters into the venous system, since the catheters are innately too compliant to traverse the skin and subcutaneous tissue. The most common addition is the peel-away sheath introducer which when combined with a dilator provides a rigid system to pass through the skin and subcutaneous tissue and develop a large pathway for placement of large-diameter pliable devices (19). Removal of the dilator portion then leaves a large sheath to introduce the device into position. Once the catheter is positioned, the sheath "peels away," leaving the catheter in proper position. The dilator is tapered to gradually open these tissues and provide for resistance-free passage of the sheath. Absolute care must be exercised in introducing the dilator/sheath complex over the guidewire to provide resistance-free passage. We recommend a push-pull technique to ensure that the guidewire continues to slide easily through the device during insertion (Figure 14.10). One hand pushes the dilator over the guidewire while the other pulls the guidewire through the dilator. After an interval advancement of the device, the guidewire is subsequently pushed back into place prior to the next push-pull maneuver. As long as the guidewire is moving freely through the dilator, the dilator cannot advance ahead of the guidewire—a condition that can result in vessel perforation. When a hang-up is encountered where the wire will not pass easily through the device during its introduction, the device should not be advanced further and imaging should be used to guide the remainder of the insertion. Often a kink will be seen in the guidewire when the device was advancing ahead of and off the course of the guidewire (Figure 14.11). We also recommend the use of fluoroscopy in placing large-diameter sheaths and dilators, so that the entire insertion can be visualized. In this way, the course of the dilator/wire complex is well visualized and uncontrolled dilator or catheter tip advancement can be avoided.

Once the sheath is positioned and this is confirmed with fluoroscopy, the soft catheter can be placed through the sheath. We do not peel away the sheath until we have confirmed catheter position. Occasionally, upon peeling away the sheath, the catheter tip is withdrawn out of the desired location. When this occurs, we use a hydrophilic glidewire passed through the catheter under fluoroscopy to manipulate the catheter tip back into position. This technique is also useful for placement of catheters through very tortuous brachiocephalic venous systems. In this circumstance, the dilator/sheath complex cannot be safely advanced into the superior vena cava. To overcome this problem, we remove the short guidewire provided with the catheter kit from the dilator and we replace it with a Teflon-coated glidewire 150 cm in length, placing the guidewire through the right atrium and into the inferior vena cava. Rather than removing the dilator and guidewire

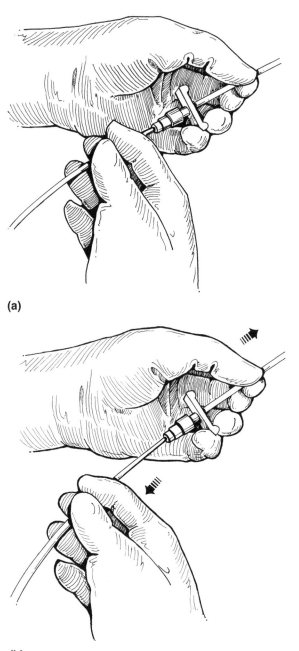

(a)

(b)

FIGURE 14.10 Drawing of (a) push (b) pull technique for dilator over guidewire.

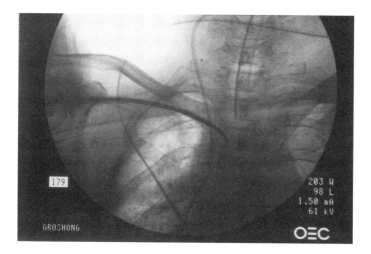

FIGURE 14.11 Kinked guidewire from device advancing ahead of guidewire.

to pass the catheter through the sheath, we remove only the dilator. In addition, we thread the glidewire through the catheter to facilitate the passage into the superior vena cava. The glidewire provides enough length to course through a tortuous brachiocephalic system, yet its hydrophilic coating permits easy passage through the Silastic catheters. Stenting the catheter with a guidewire can also overcome the occasional problem of the sheath is kinking at the costoclavicular ligament (20). The soft Silastic catheter cannot pass through the kinked sheath in this circumstance; however, removing the sheath as the catheter is advanced allows the catheter to enter the proximal subclavian vein. Without a guidewire through the catheter to maintain access to the central circulation, this maneuver often results in loss of venous access. An alternative technique comprises the passage of serially sized dilators over the guidewire to dilate the ligament beyond the size of the sheath.

With the availability of fluoroscopy and adjuncts such as accessory guide-wires, extra sheaths, and intravenous contrast agents, most catheters at the authors' institutions are placed using percutaneous methods. Along with published series, we believe that percutaneous insertion may even be more hemostatic compared with cutdown techniques through the sparing of the subcutaneous tissue butress normally in place around vessels with percutaneous insertion (21). This may make this method more appealing for the patient with a mild coagulopathy. The use of fluoroscopy not only allows visualization of the passage of guidewires and devices but also provides a means to immediately interrogate venous anatomy with venography should difficulties in placement be encountered. All procedures involving long-term catheter placement conclude with an extensive fluoroscopic survey of the catheter course, making note of catheter tip location. We strive to place all upper body long-term catheter tips within the superior vena cava (SVC) such that a portion of the catheter is parallel to the SVC to avoid catheter tip obstruction from oblique placement in the brachiocephalic veins (Figure 14.12). An additional adjunct used in the authors' institutions for long-term catheter insertions is an iodine-impregnated occlusive plastic drape placed with the draping procedure. Use of this occlusive drape prevents the catheters from coming into contact with the patient's skin—a detail that may reduce catheter infection.

Final details of catheter placement revolve around the type of CVC inserted. For temporary-access catheters, the length is usually fixed and the catheter is inserted to a defined point, such as a suture wing or mark on the catheter. Care must be exercised in selecting an appropriately sized catheter, depending upon the insertion site selected, with increasing catheter lengths required for right internal jugular, left internal jugular, and left subclavian positions, respectively. For tunneled long-term catheters and implantable ports, catheter length depends upon tip configuration. Tunneled catheters with specialized lumen configurations such as those used for dialysis do not permit trimming the catheter length, therefore care must be exercised in determining the appropriate exit site so as to position the Dacron cuff about 2 cm from the skin exit. Some tunneled catheters have squared-off tips and are sized by simply cutting the catheter to the appropriate length once an exit site has been selected. Many of the implantable ports come equipped with a specialized tip that may be tapered or have a Groshong valve incorporated. These ports come unassembled and the catheter is sized by trimming excess material from the end of the catheter, which is inserted into the reservoir itself once an appropriate length has been estimated. Catheter sizing may seem a trivial exercise, but precise catheter positioning cannot be overemphasized. Correct catheter positioning in the SVC for upper body catheters is a prerequisite for proper, uninterrupted catheter function. Moreover, for tunneled catheters, choosing an exit site that allows for easy catheter care and lets the patient conceal the catheter comfortably under clothing requires little effort on the part of the operator but yields tremendous appreciation from both the patient and the infusion team. Accurately sizing catheter length is pivotal in making sure these needs are met and that the Dacron cuff is safely positioned for maximal function.

Most tunneled catheters are supplied with a tunneling trocar that functions adequately. Other instruments that have found utility in catheter tunneling are a number of reusable and disposable shunt tunnelers. Regardless of the instrument employed, care must be exercised to avoid damaging the catheter tip or stretching and weakening the catheter shaft during the tunneling procedure. For implantable ports, extreme care must be used in suturing the port to the subcutaneous tissue in such a fashion that the port is prevented from flipping over in the pocket. Furthermore, meticulous hemostasis of the subcutaneous pocket for port place-

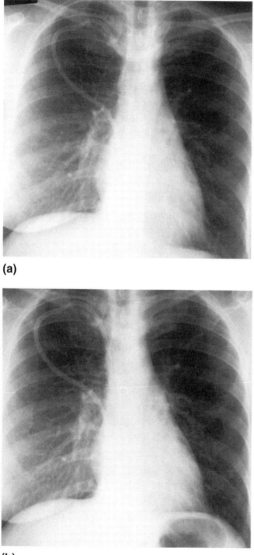

(a)

(b)

FIGURE **14.12** CVL tip in brachiocephalic trunk (a). Repositioned to appropriate location in the SVC (b).

ment should be practiced to prevent hematomas. This point is particularly emphasized in patients at risk for bleeding, such as those with thrombocytopenia from either prior chemotherapy or inherent due to their disease process, such as leukemia. Port-pocket hematomas not only limit the utility of the device but predispose to pocket infections. In addition to being careful with hemostasis, we often make a practice of accessing implantable ports with a noncoring needle at the time of placement in any patient for whom the port will need to be used within 72 h. The needle, with its attached segment of tubing, is left in place and secured with occlusive dressings. This practice spares the patient the pain associated with accessing the port in the immediate postoperative period and also avoids manipulation of the site in the early postoperative course. Catheter function should be confirmed prior to completion of the procedure. All lumens should be verified to aspirate and flush without resistance. The catheter course should be inspected fluoroscopically to confirm tip location and make sure there are no kinks in the course of the catheter. We strongly advocate the judicious use of contrast injection through the catheter should there be any question as to function or position. At the conclusion of the procedure, all catheters should be flushed with heparinized saline solution and filled with a dwell. The concentration of the heparin dwell is not well defined but ranges from 100 to 10,000 U/mL. Finally, all access procedures conclude with a portable upright chest x-ray to verify catheter positions and assess for any cardiopulmonary complications.

Cutdown

Catheters can be introduced into the central venous circulation using a cutdown technique. In general, this technique is reserved for tunneled, cuffed, long-term catheters to avoid the infection and bleeding risks associated with nontunneled, short-term catheters if placed using these methods. Unlike the percutaneous techniques, which are based upon a relatively blind puncture of the selected vein using anatomical landmarks as guides, cutdown methods are based upon the direct visual placement of the catheter into a central vein or through one of its tributaries. Access to the SVC can be gained via a direct cutdown on the internal jugular vein or through the subclavian vein using a cutdown on the cephalic vein as the pathway. In the lower extremity, the inferior vena cava can be accessed through a cutdown on the saphenous vein in the groin. Specific mention of the anatomic relationships and exposure for cutdown placement appear in the sections below describing access sites.

As in the case of percutaneous methods, an utmost familiarity with regional anatomy is required to be proficient at CVC placement using cutdown techniques. The general method is summarized as follows: The selected anatomical region for access is prepared with a bactericidal skin preparatory agent and sterile drapes. An incision is made over the selected access site and the vessel is gently dissected and circumferentially controlled with Silastic vessel tapes. A purse-string suture is placed on the anterior wall of the selected access vein using either fine mono-filament vascular suture or fine absorbable suture. For access via the cephalic or saphenous veins, some authors recommend ligating the vein distally to avoid bleeding around the catheter. In the jugular position, care must be taken to avoid ligating the vein with the purse-string suture. Once the catheter has been tunneled from the chosen exit site to the insertion site, a small venotomy is made in the center of the purse string. The vessel loops provide for proximal and distal hemostasis while a vein pick is introduced into the venotomy. With the vein pick in position, the catheter is threaded into place through the venotomy and into the chosen vein. Fluoroscopy is utilized to guide catheter tip placement. Occasionally, tortuous central veins require the use of a guidewire threaded through the catheter to properly position the tip in the SVC. After the wounds are closed and the catheter secured at its exit site, a completion chest x-ray is obtained to confirm tip placement and to assess for cardiopulmonary complications.

The cutdown technique is an important component in the armamentarium of the vascular access surgeon. It finds particular application in patients who have had multiple prior CVCs, have multiple sites of venous thrombosis, and for whom percutaneous access of a central vein is unsuccessful. Whether the presence of a bleeding diathesis connotes an absolute contraindication to percutaneous CVC placement is not clear. However, for those patients in dire need of long-term access with complicating coagulopathies, the cutdown method offers a mechanism for catheter placement that provides direct visualization and control of the large peripheral access veins. Although the complications traditionally associated with percutaneous placement—such as pneumothorax, hemothorax, arterial injury, or thoracic duct damage—are less common using the cutdown technique, these complications may also occur due to the proximity of these structures to the central veins (22). In experienced hands, the incidence of these complications is quite low (<1%), regardless of the insertion technique chosen (23).

Adjunctive Measures

Fluoroscopy

A detailed discussion regarding the use of intraoperative fluoroscopic imaging during CVC placement appears in Chapter 15. Though fluoroscopy is not universally required for all CVC insertions, it can be a useful adjunct for placement of all long-term catheters. One reason for this lies in the design differences between temporary and long-term CVCs. In general, temporary CVCs are fabricated of a fixed length, which is not easily alterable at the time of insertion. Most temporary catheters are constructed to be inserted to a fixed point of the device, such as a hub or suture wing. By this design, the catheter tip usually lies in the SVC when the device is inserted to its fullest length. By contrast, most long-term CVCs are of a variable length. Depending upon the site chosen for insertion as well as the exit site, the catheter is either trimmed to the appropriate length or manipulated into the correct position. Since long-term catheters are designed to have their lengths altered at the time of insertion, confirmation of tip location is more critical. Moreover, owing to the inherent pliability of long-term CVCs, more manipulation is often required to steer the catheter into position. For many patients receiving long-term CVCs, these devices become a lifeline for extended treatment. A poorly function CVC may become a source of severe morbidity; therefore we strive to achieve perfection in placement and function for every long-term CVC. As part of this, we believe that intraoperative fluoroscopy provides a mechanism to confirm an accurate catheter tip position and an unobstructed catheter course in a setting where minor adjustments can be undertaken without the need to bring the patient back for catheter revision or replacement at a future time, with its attendant disruption to the patient's therapy.

The use of fluoroscopy at the time of long-term CVC insertion enables the operator to visually follow the path of insertion of guidewires, dilators, and introducer sheaths. Intraoperative imaging provides a source of confirmation of resistance-free passage of these devices into the desired location. This may reduce the chance of perforation of either a great vessel or the heart by blind placement. Moreover, the availability of fluoroscopy at the time of CVC insertion also provides a means of defining variant or unexpected pathological anatomy with the use of intravenous contrast agents. When resistance to passage of a guidewire is encountered in an otherwise uneventful cannulation, venography may reveal an occult venous obstruction, segmental venous stenosis, or severe tortuosity as a cause. Using the image capture ferature of most modern portable imaging equipment, a ''road map'' is provided that may guide the operator in placing the catheter using adjunctive methods, such as the glidewire technique mentioned above. Alternatively, if an occult venous occlusion is unmasked, this information will not only assist the operator in promptly aborting the current site, thereby reducing the chance of complications from repeated punctures, but will also provide useful information to guide future access attempts in the same patient. We have found the use of intraoperative fluoroscopy extremely helpful and use this technology for all long-term catheter insertions.

Ultrasound

The traditional method for gaining access to the central venous circulation relies on anatomical landmarks to localize the vein. Although this method is reasonably safe, it is effectively a blind puncture. Since 1984, Doppler and ultrasound techniques have been described to facilitate the localization of central veins for subsequent cannulation (24–26). Only recently, with the availability of relatively inexpensive systems that are ergonomically appealing to the environment in which

CVCs are placed, has ultrasound guidance become a more common adjunct to catheter insertion.

One example of an ultrasound device specifically designed for CVC placement is the Site-Rite (Dymax Corporation, Pittsburgh, PA) (Figure 14.13). The Site-Rite is a compact, portable, battery-operated B-mode ultrasound system with transducers designed to facilitate vessel cannulation. The transducers are available in 7.5- and 9-MHz configurations, which provide real-time imaging at depths of 4 and 2 cm, respectively. The probe also has a needle guide incorporated into its design for concomitant imaging and cannulation of the selected vessel.

Not surprisingly, ultrasound guidance for placement of CVCs found its first advocates in radiology, where these imaging devices were readily available. However, typical ultrasound instrumentation is large, not easily portable, cumbersome to operate, and quite expensive. As a result, limited experience with ultrasound-guided CVC insertion was reported. The availability of a small, inexpensive, and simple to operate ultrasound device specifically designed for the varied environments in which CVCs are placed has kindled significant enthusiasm for the use of this adjunct. A number of reports have demonstrated an overall improvement in efficiency and reduction in complication rates when ultrasound guidance is used for CVC insertion. In a prospective comparison of ultrasound guidance versus landmark techniques for CVC insertion in the internal jugular vein, Denys et al. reported significantly better results in the ultrasound-guided group in regards to success rate, access time, and complication rate (26). Similar

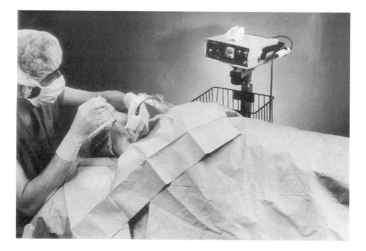

FIGURE 14.13   Site-Rite.

findings were published by Gualtieri et al. in their randomized report of subclavian vein cannulation by inexperienced operators (27). Whether ultrasound guidance is necessary for CVC insertion often depends upon a number of factors: the experience of the operator, the physical characteristics of the patient, and the number of prior CVCs the patient has had that might alter venous anatomy. The reported success and complication rates for CVC insertion by landmark technique cover a broad scope, with successful cannulation ranging from 80 to 99% and complications ranging from <1 to 10% (26). The rates that individual operators achieve are often dependent on the factors mentioned above, with emphasis placed on operator experience. In our own institutions, ultrasound guidance has been adopted for routine use not only in teaching situations but by many operators with varied backgrounds and levels of experience. Its availability has proven useful to the surgical staff in difficult cannulation situations. We commend its accessibility to any institution with a significant volume of CVC placements, particularly if the experience of operators covers a wide range.

Other Adjuncts

In addition to the use of fluoroscopy for catheter positioning and ultrasound for venous access, two other methods have been described for catheter-tip positioning that are intended to avoid the added expense and inconvenience of fluoroscopy. One method relies on the use of ECG monitoring to locate the position of the right atrium (28). The other technique employs a specialized guidewire with a transmitting tip and an external receiver (Cath-Finder, SIMS Deltec, Inc., St. Paul, MN), which allows the operator to monitor tip location as the wire is advanced through the central circulation (29). Both the ECG monitoring and Cath-Finder technologies may reliably locate the catheter tip in the SVC and prevent catheter positioning in the right atrium or other undesirable positions; however, both are limited to tip positioning only and do not address questions of catheter course, thereby, in our opinion, limiting their applicability for any long-term access catheter.

COMMON ACCESS SITES

Subclavian Vein

The subclavian vein (SCV) is a common site for placement of all types of CVCs. Its use is specifically not recommended for placement of temporary or long-term dialysis catheters in any patient for whom an extremity arteriovenous access is a possibility in the future due to the significant incidence of subclavian vein stenosis related to large-diameter CVCs. This concern has been detailed in the earlier chapter devoted to dialysis CVCs. For nondialysis indications, however, the SCV offers a direct route to the SVC from either the right or left approach.

The most common method to access the SCV is through an infraclavicular approach, though supraclavicular and axillary methods have been described and utilized in limited reports (30,31). The SCV is accessed just distal to its exit from the thoracic outlet (Figure 5.15) and lies anterior and slightly inferior to the subclavian artery. Numerous techniques are described for accessing the SCV by both percutaneous and cutdown methods.

Surface anatomy is important in preparing for SCV access. The crucial landmarks include the clavicle, first rib, sternal notch, and deltopectoral groove. With deep palpation under the clavicle in the deltopectoral groove, one can often feel the pulsation of the subclavian artery, particularly in a thin patient. For percutaneous access, the site for venous entry is just under the angle of the clavicle; however, skin puncture should take place a few centimeters lateral to this point. To facilitate passage of the needle under the clavicle in a straight line roughly parallel to a coronal plane, we abduct the shoulders. In some patients, this requires use of a rolled towel in a vertical or transverse position between the shoulders, depending upon body habitus. After prepping and draping, our usual technique is as follows:

1. A 22-gauge needle is used to infiltrate the infraclavicular skin, subcutaneous tissue, area under the clavicle, and into the periosteum of the clavicle to provide analgesia and anesthesia. Often this needle is used to localize the subclavian vein, taking care to avoid an intravascular injection of any anesthetic agent.
2. A 16-gauge needle is used to access the subclavian vein by puncturing the skin a few centimeters lateral to the angle of the clavicle. While one hand advances the needle and applies negative pressure to the syringe, the other is positioned with the index finger in the sternal notch and the thumb applies external pressure over the needle to facilitate its smooth, straight passage under the clavicle.
3. Once an easy-flowing flash of dark blood has been obtained, the guide-wire is passed into position and the procedure continues as described in the earlier section on percutaneous placement.

Some descriptions of SCV cannulation advocate marching the needle down the clavicle to get under it and enter the vein. Though this technique does result in venous cannulation, it also leads to a wire and subsequent catheter course that is angulated. This may result in pinching of the soft Silastic catheters and even catheter fracture over the long term (32). We prefer instead to concentrate on a straight-line access under the clavicle, which is facilitated by entering the skin sufficiently lateral to allow for a straight catheter position and smooth entry point into the vein.

The SCV can be reached both directly and indirectly via the cephalic vein using cutdown techniques as well. For direct access, an infraclavicular incision is made similar to that which appears in Figure 5.14 for an axillo-axillo-arteriove-nous graft. The more common method to reach the SCV using a cutdown takes advantage of the more superficially located cephalic vein, which lies in the delto-pectoral groove and joins the subclavian vein directly. To expose the cephalic vein requires a more laterally placed incision between the angle of the clavicle and the anterior axillary line. The vein is located within the groove and can be encircled with vessel loops or ligatures. Once the vein is localized, we prefer to access it with a 16-gauge angiocath followed by the guide wire and procede as though a percutaneous access was performed. This often precludes the need to ligate the distal vein, as the integrity of the vein wall is preserved around the catheter. Alternatively, once the vein is isolated, a venotomy is performed and the catheter is introduced with the aid of a vein pick and manipulated into posi-tion. We still employ fluoroscopy to aid in the positioning of the catheter tip and for verification of a smooth catheter course. Guidewire aided manipulation of the catheter is still feasible and may be necessary even when a cutdown has been performed for access to the vein. The remainder of the CVC placement procedure is conducted as described above for the individual catheter types. Whether cathe-ter tunneling or port assembly takes place prior to or subsequent to catheter intro-duction into the vein depends upon the construction of the device and requires some forethought on the part of the operator.

Internal Jugular Vein

Like the SCV, the internal jugular vein (IJV) is a common site for CVC placement and can be reached by both percutaneous and cutdown techniques. The right IJV offers the straightest course to the SVC and is consistently reported to have the lowest complication rate for CVC placement. Moreover, the right IJV is our pre-ferred site for placement of all hemodialysis catheters, as described in Chapter 10.

The IJV lies deep to the sternocleidomastoid muscle within the carotid sheath and lateral to the carotid artery. It can be accessed through a number of anatomical approaches based upon the sternocleidomastoid muscle. The anterior approach is based upon the vein's position in the triangle comprising the clavicu-lar and sternal heads of the sternocleidomastoid muscle. In thin patients, this triangle is readily observed by having the patient lift his or her head slightly. Often the small-gauge needle used for infiltration of local anesthesia is also used to identify the position of the IJV. For the anterior approach, needle puncture takes place in the apex of the triangle formed by the heads of the sternocleidomas-toid muscle. Palpation of the carotid artery pulse provides further anatomical information regarding the location of the IJV. The needle is angled toward the ipsilateral nipple at 30 to 45 degrees. The patient's head is rotated slightly away from the chosen side. If the head is rotated to the extreme opposite side, the IJV flattens out and overlies the carotid artery, thereby increasing the risk of carotid puncture. Placing the patient in the Trendelenburg position often dilates the IJV, making access somewhat easier. The posterior approach takes its name from the posterolateral border of the sternocleidomastoid muscle. Needle access occurs at this position and is directed medially toward the sternal notch at 30 to 45 degrees downward. Another anatomical approach is termed the *supraclavicular* and actually achieves access at the junction of the IJV and the SCV (33). Needle puncture occurs just superior to the midpoint of the clavicle and is angled toward the sternoclavicular joint.

Regardless of the access approach chosen, once venous access is heralded by the easy aspiration of dark blood, the guidewire is placed and catheter insertion proceeds as described previously. Cutdown exposure of the IJV usually requires a small transverse incision in the triangle formed by the heads of the sternocleido-mastoid muscle (Figure 14.14). The vein is exposed by bluntly dissecting in this space. Once the vein is exposed, it can be accessed with a 16-gauge angiocath followed by guidewire passage or it can be circumferentially dissected and controlled for placement of an anterior wall purse-string suture. Small-diameter catheters can often be introduced without the need for circumferential control and a

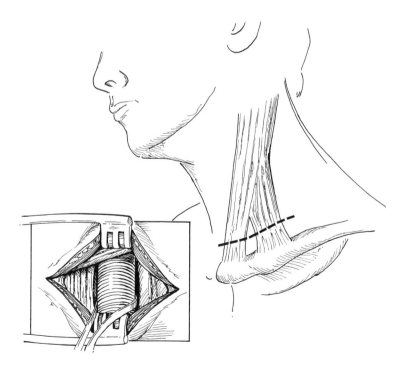

FIGURE 14.14 IJ exposure.

purse-string suture. However, the larger diameter tunneled dialysis catheters often require a purse-string suture to prevent bleeding around the catheter where it enters the vein.

Placement of left-sided IJV CVCs can be tricky due to tortuosity of the brachiocephalic segment that separates the IJV from the SVC. For placement of temporary catheters through largely blind approaches, it is vital to achieve absolutely resistance free passage of the guidewire through the introducer needle and the subsequent resistance-free passage of dilators and catheters over the guidewire. Any resistance encountered to either guidewire, dilator, or catheter advancement should tell the operator that there is a problem and the procedure should be terminated. Resistance to wire, dilator, or catheter advancement can occur for many reasons, such as malposition in the vertebral vein, down the left SCV, or across into the right SCV. More troublesome is the resistance which results when a stiff device cannot traverse a severely tortuous brachiocephalic trunk. All these scenarios can result in either a poorly placed CVC or tearing of the central circulation with resultant mediastinal hemorrhage or cardiac tamponade. Respect for these potential complications should tell the operator to abort the procedure when any resistance to device advancement is encountered with a blind left IJV approach. These problems are less frequently encountered with a right IJ approach, since it has a direct straight-line communication with the SVC.

The concerns raised in the preceding paragraph are less prominent when placing tunneled CVCs or ports, since we use fluoroscopy routinely for these device insertions. Fluoroscopy provides an immediate mechanism to image the guidewire and steer it through a tortuous brachiocephalic system as well as the ability to inject contrast and define the venous anatomy. Moreover, though guidewire passage may occur without resistance, passage of the stiff dilators and sheaths may be prohibited by a severely tortuous brachiocephalic system. Successful CVC placement will demand finess in limiting the depth of placement of the dilator and sheath to the distal most left IJV/proximal brachiocephalic vein and the use of a guidewire within the catheter to manipulate the catheter into final position once the sheath has been cleared. This avoids the dangerous practice of advancing the dilator and sheath through an extremely tortuous central vein, which can result in tearing of the vein wall by the shear forces imposed by straightening the vessel. Whether the left IJV is accessed through a cutdown or percutaneous methods, we advocate the use of fluoroscopy when placing tunneled CVCs and ports to safely and accurately position these devices to minimize complications and maximize function.

Femoral Vein

Access to the femoral vein is commonly required for temporary CVCs. The use of the femoral vein or its saphenous branch for long-term access is limited largely

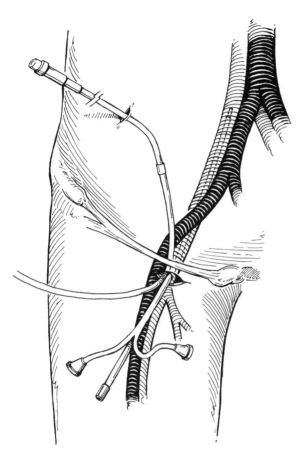

FIGURE 14.15 Femoral vein exposure.

by the higher infection rate seen with devices placed in the groin (34). Access to the femoral vein is easily obtained either percutaneously or through a small cutdown. The femoral vein is one of the neurovascular components in the groin and lies medial to the femoral artery (Figure 14.15). A common method to local-ize the femoral vein is to begin with a needle puncture 2 cm lateral and 2 cm inferior to the pubic tubercle. Alternatively, the pulsation of the femoral artery is easily felt and needle puncture is placed medial to the femoral artery and 2 cm inferior to the inguinal ligament. The course of the needle is cephalad at a 45-degree angle. Once a free-flowing aspiration of venous blood is obtained, the angle of the needle is reduced to 10 to 20 degrees. This flattening of the angle facilitates guidewire passage. A cutdown incision in this same area will provide access directly to the femoral vein or indirectly via the greater saphenous vein, which lies superficial to the femoral vein. Tunneled, cuffed catheters and venous ports are usually positioned on the lower quadrant of the anterior abdominal wall between the belt line and the groin. Catheters placed via a femoral approach should have their tips positioned in the inferior vena cava to minimize the risk of thrombotic complications. Though fluoroscopy is not mandatory for femoral CVC placement, its utility in confirming catheter position cannot be overstated. When a cutdown is necessary, the saphenous may be preferential to the common femoral vein, since it is more superficially located and can be ligated should any complications ensue that mandate catheter removal.

In our practice, femoral vein access is most commonly used in emergency situations for temporary CVC placement for hemodialysis or plasmapheresis when the jugular sites are not available or if the patient has a significant contraindication to jugular or SCV cannulation, such as severe thrombocytopenia or coagulopathy. Occasionally, the femoral site is used for massive fluid resuscitation in patients undergoing repair of a ruptured abdominal aortic aneurysm or other causes of shock. Once the immediate threat to the patient's life has passed, jugular or subclavian CVC placement usually replaces the femoral access. Infrequently, we have placed tunneled dialysis access catheters in this position in patients who have exhausted alternative sites for access (35).

External Jugular Vein

The external jugular vein (EJV) can often be seen distended in the subcutaneous tissue of the neck as it courses from cephalad to caudad, from medial to lateral across the sternocleidomastoid muscle. By emptying into the SCV behind the clavicle, the IJV offers yet another indirect route to the SVC, which is readily accessible through either percutaneous or cutdown methods. Although it is often easy to cannulate the EJV, passage of guidewires and catheters into the SCV through this approach can be difficult owing to the acute angle the IJV assumes at its entry point into the SCV (Figure 14.16). Because of this angle, EJV cannulation is limited to soft, small-diameter, over-the-wire catheters such as the Hohn or multilumen temporary CVCs. Passage of a guidewire from the EJV into the SCV may require manipulation of the shoulder to facilitate traversing the angle into the SCV (36). In our own practice, the difficulty and time required to manipulate a catheter into the SVC through the EJV approach has limited the application of this approach in favor of the IJ and SC vein insertion sites.

LESS COMMON VENOUS ACCESS SITES

The following discussion of unusual venous access sites is limited to placement of soft Silastic catheters for either tunneled cuffed long-term applications or for

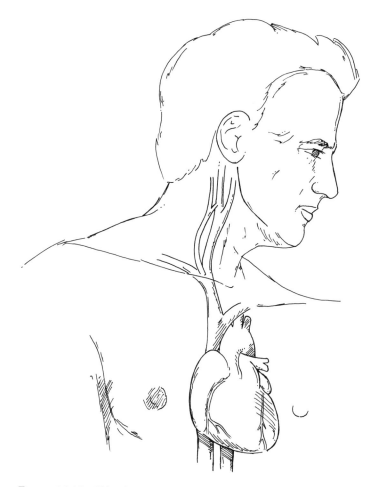

Figure 14.16 EJ vein anatomy.

implantable venous access ports. Due to the remote location of these sites in relation to either the SVC or the inferior vena cava, placement of rigid temporary catheters is not recommended. Published experience with most of these alternative sites is limited to case reports. Moreover, indirect access to the central venous circulation in any patient is limited only by an individual physician's creativity, as many other named venous branches could function as conduits for CVC placement in the appropriate clinical scenario. Our discussion will be limited to the more popular "less common" access sites.

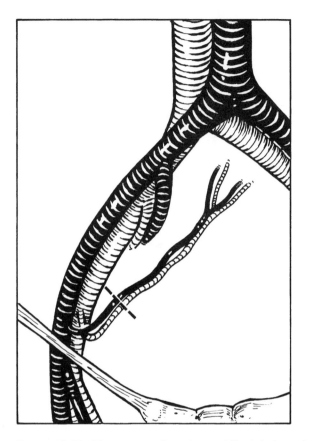

FIGURE 14.17   Exposure and anatomy of the inferior epigastric vein.

Inferior Epigastric Vein

The inferior epigastric vessels are accessed via cutdown. This approach offers the advantage of not transversing the inguinal ligament, thus minimizing the effect of leg motion on catheter position. Though a more common approach in pediatric patients, it is useful in adults as well (37). A transverse incision is made in the lower abdominal wall superior and parallel to the inguinal ligament (Figure 14.17). The external oblique fascia is incised, revealing the inferior epigastric vessels just medial to the spermatic cord or round ligament. Venous control is obtained, a venotomy performed, and a previously tunneled catheter inserted in the vein. Fluoroscopy is used to direct the catheter into the inferior vena cava. Access to the inferior vena cava by the inferior epigastric vein is via the external iliac vein. The small size of the inferior epigastric vein limits the application of this technique to small-diameter cuffed CVCs or venous ports.

Internal Mammary Vein

In contrast to the inferior epigastric vein, the internal mammary vein direct communicates with the SVC and offers another alternative for CVC placement in patients with more distal venous occlusion involving the jugular and subclavian veins (38). Because of its small diameter, use of the internal mammary vein is limited to smaller Silastic CVCs. Access to the internal mammary vein is readily obtained through a limited incision in the second intercostal space. Once the vein is isolated, placement proceeds as previously described for other upper body CVCs. Fluoroscopy aids in positioning the catheter tip in the SVC.

Retroperitoneal Approaches

An alternative to the femoral or epigastric approach to the inferior vena cava is through the retroperitoneum. The gonadal veins, the lumbar veins, and direct access into the inferior vena cava itself have all been described for difficult access situations (39–41). All three of these approaches can be used to gain CVC placement in patients who have sustained iliofemoral venous thrombosis and who have exhausted upper body access sites.

Gonadal Vein

On the right side the gonadal vein empties directly into the inferior vena cava. On the left side, the gonadal vein empties into the left renal vein (Figure 14.18). Access to the gonadal vein is obtained through a limited flank incision with the patient supine with a roll under the flank. A standard muscle splitting incision is used followed by retroperitoneal exposure gained by bluntly sweeping the peritoneum medially. The right side is preferred for a number of reasons (39). First, the gonadal vein provides direct access to the vena cava. Second, the right retroperitoneal exposure provides access to the lumbar veins and the vena cava directly should the gonadal vein be unavailable due to thrombosis. The dissection is carried down to the gonadal vein, which lies anterior to the psoas muscle and near the right ureter. The catheter is tunneled from the anterior abdominal wall and placed via direct cannulation of the gonadal vein. Sufficient slack in the catheter should be left to allow for return of the retracted peritoneal contents and to anticipate patient movement in order to prevent catheter dislodgement.

Lumbar Vein

The lumbar veins can be used for access to the inferior vena cava as well. The patient is positioned as for the gonadal vein approach described above. The retroperitoneal space is entered in a similar fashion, after a flank incision anterior to

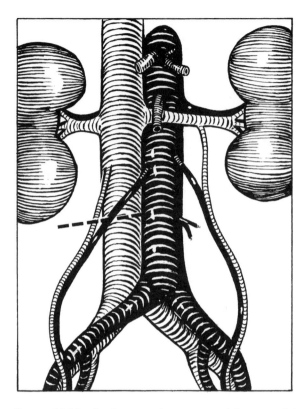

FIGURE 14.18 Anatomy and exposure of the gonadal veins, lumbar veins, and inferior vena cava.

the 12th rib. A suitable lumbar vein should be isolated just above the psoas muscle and vascular control obtained near the inferior vena cava. The catheter is then inserted under direct vision. Intraoperative fluoroscopy is often useful to confirm correct placement of the catheter, as the sharp angle between the lumbar veins and the inferior vena cava can be difficult to transverse. Because the lumbar veins can be extremely fragile, the catheter is secured in place at the venotomy with a vascular nonabsorbable suture. As in the gonadal vein approach, enough laxity in the catheter must remain to allow the peritoneal contents to relax back into the field without causing catheter dislodgement.

Inferior Vena Cava

If the gonadal and lumbar veins are found to be unsuitable at the time of operation, direct cannulation of the inferior vena cava is also possible. Once adequate vascular control is obtained, a purse-string suture is placed in the side of the vein.

The previously tunneled catheter can then be inserted under direct vision with the same proviso regarding catheter length as mentioned above applying in this circumstance.

Thoracic Approaches

Direct access into the azygos system, the right atrium, and the SVC can be accomplished by thoracotomy (Figure 14.19) and tunneling of the catheter from a suitable position on the chest wall (42–44). As these interventions are quite major, they should be reserved for those patients in whom no other vascular access sites exist.

Azygos Vein

Access to the chest is gained through a right posterolateral thoracotomy in the fifth intercostal space. The dissection can be either intrapleural or retropleural. After the azygos vein or one of its large tributaries is isolated, direct cannulation provides access to the SVC. The catheter is secured in place with a purse-string suture and brought out onto the chest wall after traversing over the fifth rib and in the subcutaneous tissues.

Superior Vena Cava

The SVC can be selected at the time of thoracotomy if the azygos vein is not usable due to thrombosis or stenosis. The approach is identical to that for the azygos vein, with the venotomy performed in a more central location. Since complete control of the SVC is difficult with this exposure, two purse-string sutures are placed in the wall of the cava and the CVC is placed through a venotomy in the center of the sutures, similar to cannulation of the aorta during cardiopulmonary bypass. Extra care must be exercised to secure the catheter and prevent dislodgement, which could be met with exsanguinating hemorrhage into the large-volume hemithorax.

Right Atrium

Direct cannulation of the right atrium is as an absolute last option, as no other sites will be usable once a right atrial line fails because of thrombosis or infection. A right anterolateral thoracotomy is performed in the third intercostal space and the pericardium entered. The right atrial appendage is used for the atriotomy, and the previously tunneled catheter is secured in place to the atrium, the pericardium, and the chest wall.

Alternative Approaches

Percutaneous translumbar and transhepatic approaches have been described (45,46). These techniques mandate image guidance to access the inferior vena cava through either approach and require custom-length catheters. These two

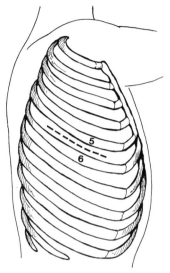

(a)

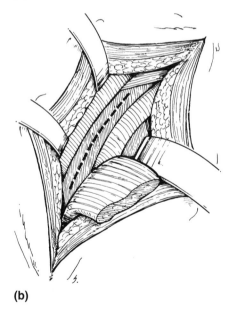

(b)

FIGURE 14.19 Anatomy (a) and exposure (b,c) of the azygos vein and superior vena cava through a posterolateral thoractomy in the fifth interspace.

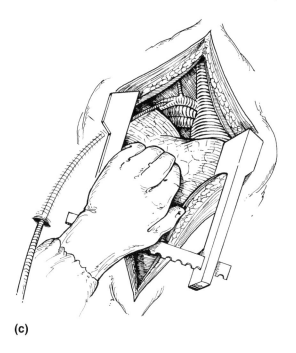

(c)

techniques have largely been relegated to interventional radiologists with an interest in vascular access. Because these two approaches provide direct access to the inferior vena cava, even large-diameter dialysis/pheresis catheters can be placed using these techniques. For translumbar placement, the patient is placed in the prone or left lateral decubitus position. The inferior vena cava is accessed percutaneously just above the iliac crest and lateral to the midline. Once the vena cava is accessed, a guidewire is passed and catheter placement proceeds as previously discussed. Nuances unique to this approach include the need to adequately dilate the track to the IVC prior to passage of the introducer sheath and a need for a long catheter to be tunneled subcutaneously from a site on the anterior abdominal wall to the entry site of the guidewire. For the transhepatic placement, ultrasound is used to guide percutaneous access through the liver into the inferior vena cava. As in the translumber approach, care must be taken to dilate the track through the hepatic substance prior to passage of the introducer sheath.

Both the translumber and transhepatic approaches to CVC placement offer yet two more alternatives to the patient in whom access is difficult. Reports of both techniques for chemotherapy, stem cell harvesting, and hemodialysis suggest that these techniques are safe and effective, with complication rates not dissimilar from those at more traditional access sites in the IJV and SCV. In general, however, experience with translumbar and transhepatic percutaneous catheter placement is limited, since the majority of patients in need of CVC access have other sites available.

PERIPHERALLY INSERTED CENTRAL CATHETERS

With the expansion of outpatient services, including home intravenous antibiotic therapy, chemotherapy, hyperalimentation, analgesics, etc., the need for intermediate and long-term central access has grown immensely. The placement of tunneled central catheters and ports has historically served this role; however, new options now exist that replace these traditional access routes.

Peripheral venous access (i.e., via veins of the upper extremity) to the central venous system has evolved rapidly since the insertion of the first peripherally inserted central catheter (PICC) in 1979. Refinement in access techniques and improved catheter technology have fueled this evolution. Peripheral access catheters as well as peripheral subcutaneous implanted infusion ports are in common use in many centers and are often a preferred route over central venous access sites (SCV, IJV) (47).

PICC Lines

A vast array of PICC lines are available today. Catheters in 2 to 6F diameter with single- or dual-lumen (larger diameter catheters) designs are available. Most catheters are made of silicone; however, polyurethane and Silastic catheters are available. A detailed discussion of current catheter technology is beyond the scope of this chapter and appears in Chapter 10.

Perhaps half of all PICC lines are inserted at the bedside by well-trained nurses, nurse practitioners, or physicians. After accessing an antecubital vein using sterile technique, the catheter is fed "blindly" (without imaging guidance) into central veins. Catheter placement is confirmed only after a chest radiograph reveals the position of the catheter tip. The junction of the SVC and right atrium is ideal, but PICCs placed in this fashion are often improperly positioned. Failure during blind placement may occur in patients with poor peripheral veins in whom access cannot be obtained and in patients with spasm or stenoses that make threading the catheter tip difficult. In general, failure rates average approximately 40%, even when appropriately trained personnel are performing placement. Because these catheters are fed directly into superficial veins, the short tissue tract may lead to higher rates of catheter infection. For these reasons, fluoroscopic guidance for placement is now commonly requested. With fluoroscopic guidance, failure is rare (<3%) (48,49).

Fluoroscopic Technique

A small intravenous (IV) catheter is placed peripherally, usually in the nondominant hand or forearm. The arm is prepped and draped and extremity venography is performed through the peripheral IV catheter with a tourniquet applied at the axilla. The basilic vein is localized under fluoroscopy and the skin overlying the vein is anesthetized. The vein is accessed with a needle (thin-walled) under fluoroscopic control. A hydrophilic guidewire is advanced into the central veins, and a "peel away" sheath is used to insert the catheter over the wire under fluoroscopy. Regions of venous spasm or stenosis can be traversed and the catheter tip position immediately visualized and adjusted if necessary.

The basilic vein is preferred over the cephalic vein. It is larger and follows a more direct course to the subclavian vein. The cephalic vein can be used if necessary; however, it is a smaller vessel and is more tortuous. The brachial vein is generally avoided because of its proximity to the neurovascular bundle. Basilic vein puncture is usually in the distal upper arm just above the antecubital fossa. Access here is well tolerated and avoids catheter stress at the elbow joint, which occurs with placement in the forearm. However, catheters can be placed distal to the antecubital fossa, and this is generally well accepted by patients.

PICC line placement under fluoroscopic guidance is uniformly technically successful, and proper positioning of the catheter is seen in all patients. Catheters placed in this manner can deliver several months of venous access, with service intervals nearly as long as those of the surgically placed catheters. At the conclusion of therapy, PICC removal is easily performed, avoiding the occasional difficulty encountered with tunneled central catheters. Complications (infection, thrombophlebitis, catheters shearing) are low (<2%) and minor compared with surgical complications (pneumothorax, hemothorax, catheter embolization, central thrombosis). Nonetheless, patients undergoing therapy exceeding 6 weeks in duration should be considered potential candidates for an infusion port. Patients often prefer ports because the device is concealed, permits greater choice in clothing, improves self-image, and allows recreational activities including swimming.

Peripheral Infusion Ports

Subcutaneously placed peripheral infusion ports were first implanted about a decade ago (50). The frequency of placement of such ports has increased rapidly. Catheters and ports are constantly being modified. Lower profiles, smaller catheter diameters, more biocompatible materials, and greater ease of placement has greatly increased their popularity.

Most ports are plastic or titanium, with a compressed silicon disc access diaphragm designed for 100 to 2000 noncoring needle accesses. As with PICCs, ports can be placed in either the forearm or in the upper arm; the basilic vein is the preferred site. Veins are localized using the aforementioned technique (PICC lines). Rigorous sterile technique is used during placement, as is done for centrally placed ports, except that placement is generally done in the fluoroscopy suite versus the operating room. After access is obtained, an incision is made from the point of skin entry for approximately 4 cm distally. A subcutaneous pocket is formed by blunt dissection. The catheter is then placed through a peel-away sheath over a wire and into the vena cava. The catheter is cut to an appropriate length to position the tip at the junction of the SVC and right atrium. The catheter can then be attached to the port. The port is buried in the subcutaneous pocket and the subcutaneous tissue and skin are closed.

The experience with these devices has grown rapidly. The U.S. experience now exceeds 100,000 annual implantations. The thrombosis rate is approximately 3% and an infection rate that is generally below 5% can be expected.

Peripherally placed ports are an excellent alternative for chemotherapy, long-term antibiotic administration, and repeated blood draws over an extended period of time. The peripherally placed ports are well tolerated and provide an excellent alternative to centrally placed ports. Peripherally placed ports are less expensive to place, their cost being two-thirds to one-half that of surgical implantation of chest wall ports. The peripherally placed ports cause less morbidity, with no risk of pneumothorax during placement. Additionally, service to patients and requesting physicians is often enhanced by eliminating the need to obtain operating room time and anesthesia support (48,51).

Care and Maintenance of Central Venous Catheters

Up to this point, we have focused on selection and placement issues surrounding CVCs in order to achieve prolonged catheter function and reduce morbidity. Once a catheter has been successfully inserted, its fate is also determined by its subsequent care and maintenance. Furthermore, we are occasionally faced with the problem of dealing with a mechanical breakage of a catheter. Some of these are reparable without the need for replacing the entire device. Finally, whether due to device complication or completion of therapeutic course, CVC removal becomes necessary. This final section addresses each of these important issues encompassing CVCs.

Access of Central Venous Catheters

Appropriate technique applied in accessing CVCs is fundamental to their proper function and avoidance of complications, particularly infectious complications. No well-controlled studies exist which yield "etched in stone" dogma of catheter access and care techniques, as evidenced by the paucity of category II data in the recent Centers for Disease Control (CDC) and Prevention draft guidelines for prevention of intravascular device-related infection (52). Careful attention to basic nursing technique and an understanding of a catheter's application and function should guide most daily interactions.

For all catheters regardless of specific type, absolute adherence to basic hand-washing recommendations is probably the single most important act in terms of reducing infectious complications. For any CVC receiving a continuous infusion, that infusion should be connected directly to the hub of the lumen as opposed to a needle piercing an injection cap. Direct connection to the hub will reduce the likelihood inadvertent disconnection of the infusion. For nondialysis CVCs, the injection caps should be changed on a regular basis if the catheter is in active usage. Prior to accessing a nondialysis CVC, the injection cap should be cleaned with an antimicrobial solution of either alcohol or povodine-alcohol (52). All ports of a nondialysis CVC should be aspirated prior to use to confirm patency and flushed with either heparin or normal saline at the conclusion of a treatment. By virtue of their two-way slit valve, Groshong-tip catheters do not require flushing on a daily basis, since blood cannot leak into the catheter without the application of a negative force. By contrast, non-Groshong-type tunneled CVCs need to be flushed on a regular basis to avoid lumen clotting from fibrin formation. Whether flushing must be done on a daily basis or less often is not clear from the available literature, nor is the need for and concentration of heparin in the flush solution (53–55).

Implanted venous ports must be carefully cleaned with an antimicrobial solution prior to being accessed with a noncoring Huber needle. Prolonged infusions through venous ports should be done using nonsiliconized Huber needles, otherwise the needle may slip out of the septum of the reservoir. Ports require flushing with heparin after each use or on a monthly basis to prevent fibrin buildup within the catheter.

Tunneled and temporary hemodialysis catheters require special care when being accessed. Although there are no well-controlled studies documenting a need for this practice, most hemodialysis and plasmapheresis catheters are filled with a concentrated heparin dwell as high as 10,000 U/mL in each lumen at the conclusion of each treatment session. It is imperative, therefore, that each lumen of a dialysis or plasmapheresis catheter be aspirated of 2 to 5 mL of blood prior to the initiation of and treatment or flushing of the catheter. This will avoid the problem of bolusing a patient with up to 30,000 U of heparin inadvertently, with potentially serious bleeding complications. Moreover, prior to connecting a patient to a dialysis or plasmapheresis machine, the hubs of the catheter are soaked in a povidone-iodine solution. Variations on this theme include filling a hemodialysis with a lytic agent dwell at the conclusion of a session (56). All these measures are intended to reduce the chance of fibrin deposition in the catheter, which leads to catheter failure, and to prevent infection at the connecting sites. Unfortunately, there are no well-controlled studies that compare various antiseptic or anticoagulation regimens.

Exit-Site Care

Unlike the case of access techniques, some attention has been directed to the care of catheter exit sites by a number of studies, mostly centering on catheter dressings and topical antibiotics (57–59). The use of transparent, semipermeable polyurethane dressings has been compared with that of standard gauze and tape dressings, with mixed and confusing results being reported. A large metanalysis suggests that transparent dressing led to a higher risk of infection than did gauze dressings (58). However, this metanalysis suffered from many flaws, chief among them was a rather significant construct change in the type of transparent dressing used in the studies reviewed compared with what was available on the market. The transparent dressing used during the metanalysis did not allow the escape of moisture. Newer dressings that have addressed this issue may reduce skin colonization by allowing moisture to escape from under the dressing. No specific study in the meta review addressed tunneled cuffed CVCs. Amid this confusion, it appears that there is no benefit to one type of dressing over another for CVCs either temporary or tunneled. Similarly, preparation of the skin exit site of a CVC prior to dressing placement has been examined for povidone-iodine, chlorhexidine, alcohol, and antimicrobial ointments (60). Although antiseptics have shown a reduction in infection rates without a clear distinction between agents, antimicrobial ointments have not and may be associated with a higher risk of subsequent fungal infection (61).

The frequency of CVC dressing change is also not well defined. Current recommendations from the CDC suggest catheter site dressing be changed whenever they become damp, soiled, or loose or if inspection of the catheter entry site is necessary (52). The presence of an external tunneled, cuffed CVC does impart some limitations on patient activity. Showering is not recommended until the cuff is well incorporated into the subcutaneous tissue; usually 4 to 6 weeks. Even after that point, showering and getting the catheter wet is not universally endorsed. Dressings need to be left in place over an implanted venous port only until the site heals or when they are accessed. Unlike a tunneled, cuffed CVC, a well-healed venous port site can be left uncovered and the patient can engage in normal activity, including swimming, bathing, and showering.

Catheter Repair

A number of the tunneled, cuffed catheters have repair kits available to address catheter or hub breakage when it occurs in the external portion of the CVC. The repair kits are specific to the actual brand and size catheter in place and must be used specifically for a particular catheter. For catheter breakage, the repair kit usually consists of a new extension with the appropriate number of lumens and ports, a silastic sleeve, and silicone cement (Figure 14.20). Since catheter breakage usually occurs outside the health care setting, patients must be instructed

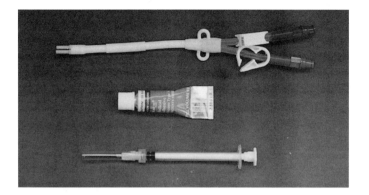

FIGURE 14.20   Catheter repair kit.

how to handle a broken catheter to prevent exsanguination or air embolism. Since most people do not have catheter clamps or hemostats readily available, the simplest way to control the remaining segment of the catheter is to fold it over on itself and tightly wrap it with either tape or a rubber band. Once the patient arrives at the hospital, the catheter can be secured with an atraumatic clamp such as a tubing clamp or rubber-shod hemostat. The catheter is then prepped with an antimicrobial agent and cut to freshen the end. The repair segment usually has a plastic or metal male end which will slip into the catheter remnant. This area is covered with the Silastic sleeve and the silicone cement is injected under the sleeve to completely coat the catheter repair junction. The entire segment is secured with a piece of tongue depressor to give it stability for 24 h while the cement cures. Usually a repaired catheter can be used immediately if absolutely necessary, but ideally one should wait 24 h. It is imperative that whenever tunneled CVCs are placed at an institution, the appropriate number and configuration of repair kits, if available, also be stocked for the catheter. These can save both patient and physician from having to endure another CVC placement procedure.

An easier problem to deal with is breakage of a catheter hub. This also requires a catheter-specific repair kit, but since many of the hub assemblies are secured with simple mechanical pressure, the hassle of gluing and splinting the repaired catheter is avoided and immediate catheter use following the repair is permitted. Similar to the preceding discussion, patient must be educated in controlling the free end of the catheter if the hub assembly breaks. Once the end is secured and the patient arrives at the hospital the catheter is clamped in an atraumatic manner and the edge is trimmed after cleansing with a bactericidal agent. Replacement hubs are generally assembled the same way as they are at the time of catheter placement. One note of caution pertains to hemodialysis tunneled, cuffed catheters: trimming the length of the catheter changes the dwell volume and must be noted and reported to the dialysis staff, so that the appropriate dwell is placed and the patient is not inadvertently anticoagulated.

Catheter Removal

Requests for catheter removal can be received with joy or despair depending on the reason for the request. Satisfaction is felt when a patient presents to have a CVC removed because a course of chemotherapy or antibiotics has been completed or because a native arteriovenous fistula has matured and is functional. Misery is experienced when catheter removal is requested because of poor function or infection. Regardless of the indication for catheter removal, most of these procedures can be done in the office under local anesthesia. The exception is removal of an implanted venous port, which we prefer to do in an operating room. In general, these recommendations for catheter removal apply to upper body tunneled, cuffed CVCs. Removal of CVCs placed in unusual or uncommon lower extremity, thoracic, or retroperitoneal locations will require individualized approaches based upon location and catheter securing procedures.

A temporary CVC is removed simply by cutting the cutaneous suture and removing it with an occlusive dressing in place over the exit site. We generally do this with the patient in the supine or slight Trendelenburg position to avoid any possibility of air embolism. Direct pressure is maintained over the exit site for 10 to 15 min. Prior to removing a temporary dialysis catheter, we aspirate the heparin dwell from the lumens. An occlusive dressing is applied and left in place for 48 h. Most tunneled, cuffed CVCs can be removed with either gentle traction or a limited cutdown incision over the cuff. After infiltrating around the cuff with local anesthesia, slow, steady traction is applied to the catheter. In most instances, either the cuff will disengage from the subcutaneous tissue or the catheter will disengage from the cuff and catheter removal will be accomplished in a simple fashion. Occasionally, the cuff will not release from either the catheter or the subcutaneous tissue without excessive force. In this circumstance a cutdown is performed over the cuff, the cuff is dissected free from the subcutaneous tissue, and the catheter is removed. Periodically, a catheter will break during attempts at removal. Catheter breakage is most likely to occur in this circumstance at the cuff, leaving the cuff and the intravascular portion of the catheter intact. When this occurs, immediate pressure is applied to both the skin tunnel and the catheter entry site (i.e., internal jugular vein or SCV) and a cutdown is performed over the cuff to retrieve the remainder of the catheter. Whenever a cutdown is performed for cuff removal, care must be exercised not to damage the catheter between the cuff and the vein cannulation site, as this could result in catheter breakage and embolization into the central venous circulation. An added note of caution regards catheters that have been placed via a cutdown technique. It is important to know how the catheter was secured to the vein. If a purse-string suture was placed in the vein wall and tied too snugly, the catheter may break if any force is applied to it, resulting in catheter fragment embolization. Unless you specifically placed the catheter, the safest option for catheter removal under this circumstance is in the operating room through a reopening of the cutdown to avoid unexpected problems created by the original catheter insertion technique. Though catheter breakage and embolization is a potentially life-threatening event due to arrhythmias or damage to the pulmonary vasculature, most catheter fragments can be easily removed using modern interventional techniques by percutaneous methods using loop snares, baskets, or biopsy forceps via a jugular or femoral approach (62,63).

Implanted venous ports require a reopening of the subcutaneous pocket. Although this could probably be done in an office setting, we prefer to remove these in an operating room with cautery and suction readily available. After either induction of general anesthesia or infiltration of local anesthesia, the old incision is reopened. The reservoir will have a foreign-body reaction capsule around it, which needs to be incised. The port can then be easily removed from the pocket by cutting the anchoring sutures. We place the patient in a slight Trendelenburg position when withdrawing the catheter from the vein. The pocket is irrigated. Hemostasis is verified and the pocket is closed in layers. If a very thick capsule surrounds the pocket, we excise this and obliterate the dead space with sutures to minimize the risk of seroma formation.

Regardless of the type of CVC or indication for removal, the catheter should be carefully inspected upon removal to make sure its tip is intact. This may be difficult to tell in a Hickman-type catheter with a squared-off edge but more easy to determine if a blunt-tip or Groshong valve is present. Furthermore, if a CVC is being removed due to infection, any pericatheter exudate as well as the catheter tip should be cultured. Finally, retained Dacron cuffs that result from traction removal when the cuff releases from the catheter and not the subcutaneous tissue are left undisturbed unless signs or symptoms of infection develop— an infrequent occurrence (64). In this instance, a limited cutdown over the cuff will both remove the retained foreign body and drain the infection.

REFERENCES

1. Farkas JC, Liu N, Bleriot JP, et al. Single- versus triple-lumen central catheter-related sepsis: A prospective randomized study in a critically ill population. Am J Med 93:277–282, 1992.
2. Pemberton LB, Lyman B, Lander V, Covinsky J. Sepsis from triple- vs single-lumen catheters during total parenteral nutrition in surgical or critically ill patients. Arch Surg 121:591–594, 1986.

3. Early TF, Gregory RT, Wheeler JR, et al. Increased infection rate in double-lumen versus single-lumen Hickman catheters in cancer patients. South Med J 83:34–36, 1990.

4. Modak SM, Sampath L. Development and evaluation of a new polyurethane central venous antiseptic catheter: Reducing central venous catheter infections. Infect Med 23–29, 1992.

5. Bach A, Böhrer H, Motsch J, et al. Prevention of catheter-related infections by antiseptic bonding. J Surg Res 55:640–666, 1993.

6. Welch GW, McKeel DW, Silvestein P, et al. The role of catheter composition in the development of thrombophlebitis. Surg Gynecol Obstet 138:421–424, 1974.

7. Openshaw KL, Picus D, Hicks ME, et al. Interventional radiologic placement of Hohn central venous catheters: Results and complications in 100 consecutive patients. J Vasc Intervent Radiol 5:111–115, 1994.

8. Maki DG, Cobb L, Garman JK, et al. An attachable silver-impregnated cuff for prevention of infection with central venous catheters: A prospective randomized multicenter trial. AM J Med 85:307–314, 1988.

9. Hadaway LC. An overview of vascular access devices inserted via the antecubital area. J Intraven Nurs 13:297–306, 1990.

10. Raad I, Davis S, Becker M, et al. Low infection rate and long durability of nontunneled silastic catheters. A safe cost-effective alternative for long-term venous access. Arch Intern Med 153:1791–1796, 1993.

11. Brown JM. Peripherally inserted central catheters: Use in home care. J Intraven Nurs 12:144–150, 1989.

12. Broviac JW, Cole JJ, Schribner BH. A silicone rubber atrial catheter for prolonged parenteral alimentation. Surg Gynecol Obstet 136:602–606, 1973.

13. Hickman RO, Buckner CD, Clife RA, et al. A modified right atrial catheter for access to the venous system in marrow transplant recipients. Surg Gynecol Obstet 148:871–875, 1979.

14. Handy C. Vascular access devices: hospital to home care. J Intraven Nurs 12:s10–s17, 1989.

15. Shaw JH, Douglas R, Wilson T. Clinical performance of Hickman and Portacath atrial catheters. Aust NZ J Surg 58:657–659, 1988.

16. Hata Y, Morita S, Morita Y, et al. Peripheral insertion of a central venous access device under fluoroscopic guidance using a peripherally accessed system (PAS) port in the forearm. Cardiovasc Intervent Radiol 21:230–330, 1998.

17. Seldinger SI. Catheter replacement of the needle in percutaneous arteriography. Acta Radiol (Stockh) 39:368, 1953.

18. Andros G, Harris RW, Dulawa LB, et al. Subclavian artery catheterization: a new approach for endovascular procedures. J Vasc Surg 20:566–574, 1994.

19. Cohen AM, Wood WC. Simplified technique for placement of long term central venous silicone catheters. Surg Gynecol Obstet 154:721–724, 1982.

20. Atkinson JB, Chamberlin KL, de Csepel J, Srikanth M. Overcoming a kinked peel-away sheath during central line implantation. J Pediatr Surg 29:379–380, 1994.

21. Ahmed Z, Mohyuddin Z. Complications associated with different insertion techniques for Hickman catheters. Postgrad Med J 74:104–107, 1998.

22. Davis SJ, Thompson JS, Edney JA. Insertion of Hickman catheters. A comparison of cutdown and percutaneous techniques. Am Surg 50:673–676, 1984.

23. Shetty PC, Mody MK, Kastan DJ, et al. Outcome of 350 implanted chest ports placed by interventional radiologists. J Vasc Intervent Radiol 8:991–995, 1997.

24. Legler D, Nugent M. Doppler localization of the internal jugular vein facilitates central venous cannulation. Anesthesiology 60:481–482, 1984.

25. Malloy DL, McGee WT, Shawker TH, et al. Ultrasound guidance improves the success rate of internal jugular vein cannulation: A prospective, randomized trial. Chest 98:157–160, 1990.

26. Denys BG, Uretsky BF, Reddy PS. Ultrasound-assisted cannulation of the internal jugular vein. A prospective comparison to the external landmark-guided technique. Circulation 87:1557–1562, 1993.

27. Gualtieri E, Deppe SA, Sipperrly ME, et al. Subclavian venous catheterization: Greater success rate for less experienced operators using ultrasound guidance. Crit Car Med 23:692–697, 1995.

28. Watters VA, Grant JP. Use of electrocardiogram to position right atrial catheters during surgery. Ann Surg 225:165–171, 1997.

29. Carre MC, Lopez Vega JM, Carles J, et al. Central venous brachial catheter (P.A.S. Port) and catheter scanning system (Cath-Finder). J Surg Oncol 55:190–193, 1994.

30. MacDonnell JE, Perez H, Pitts SR, Zaki SA. Supraclavicular subclavian vein catheterization: Modified landmarks for needle insertion. Ann Emerg Med 21:421–424, 1992.

31. Taylor BL, Yellowlees I. Central venous cannulation using the infraclavicular axillary vein. Anesthesiology 72:55–58, 1990.

32. Nostdahl T, Waagsbo NA. Costoclavicular pinching: A complication of long-term central venous catheters. A report of three cases. Acta Anaesthesiol Scand 42:872–875, 1998.

33. Conroy JM, Rajagopalan PR, Baker JD III, Bailey MK. A modification of the supraclavicular approach to the central circulation. South Med J 83:1178–1181, 1990.

34. Goetz AM, Wagener MM, Miller JM, Muder RR. Risk of infection due to central venous catheters: effect of site of placement and catheter type. Infect Control Hosp Epidemiol 19:842–845, 1998.

35. Zaleski GX, Funaki B, Lorenz JM, et al. Experience with tunneled femoral hemodialysis catheters. AJR 172:493–496, 1999.

36. Sparks CJ, McSkimming I, George L. Shoulder manipulation to facilitate central vein catheterization from the external jugular vein. Anaesth Intens Care 19:567–568, 1991.

37. Krog M, Gerdin B. An alternative placement of implantable central venous access systems. JPEN 13:666–667, 1989.

38. Jaime-Solis E, Anaya-Ortega M, Moctezuma-Espinosa J. The internal mammary vein: An alternate route for central venous access with an implantable port. J Pediatr Surg 29:1328–1330, 1994.

39. Coit DG, Turnbull AD. Long term central vascular access through the gonadal vein. Surg Gynecol Obstet 175:362–364, 1992.

40. Boddie AW Jr. Translumbar catheterization of the inferior vena cava for long term angioaccess. Surg Gynecol Obstet 168:54–56, 1989.

41. Williard W, Coit D, Lucas A, Groeger JS. Long-term vascular access via the inferior vena cava. J Surg Oncol 46:162–166, 1991.
42. Birnbaum PL, Michas C, Cohen SE. Direct right atrial catheter insertion with video-assisted thoracic surgery. Ann Thorac Surg 62:1197, 1996.
43. Malt RA, Kempster, M. Direct azygos vein and superior vena cava cannulation for parenteral nutrition. JPEN 7:580–581, 1983.
44. Bahn CH, Kennedy MT. Catheterization of the superior vena cava. Surgery 73:115–117, 1973.
45. Haire WD, Lieberman RP, Lund GB, Kessinger A. Translumbar inferior vena cava catheters. Bone Marrow Transplant 7:389–392, 1991.
46. Kaufman JA, Greenfield AJ, Fitzpatrick GF. Transhepatic cannulation of the inferior vena cava. J Vasc Intervent Radiol 2:331–334, 1991.
47. Duerksen DR, Papineau N, Siemens J, Yaffe C. Peripherally inserted central catheters for parenteral nutrition: A comparison with centrally inserted catheters. JPEN 23:85–89, 1999.
48. Neuman ML, Murphy BD, Rosen MP. Bedside placement of peripherally inserted central catheters: a cost-effectiveness analysis. Radiology 206:423–428, 1998.
49. Cardella JF, Fox PS, Lawler JB. Interventional radiologic placement of peripherally inserted central catheters. J Vasc Intervent Radiol 4:653–660, 1993.
50. Kahn ML, Barboza RB, Kling GA, Heisel JE. Initial experience with percutaneous placement of the PAS port implantable venous access device. J Vasc Intervent Radiol 3:459–461, 1992.
51. Schuman E, Ragsdale J. Peripheral ports are a new option for central venous access. J Am Coll Surg 180:456–460, 1995.
52. Centers for Disease Control and Prevention. Draft guidelines for prevention of intravascular device related infections: Parts 1 and 2. Fed Reg 60:49978–50006, 1995.
53. Hamilton RA, Plis JM, Clay C, Sylvan L. Heparin sodium versus 0.9% sodium chloride injection for maintaining patency of indwelling intermittent infusion devices. Clin Pharm 7:439–443, 1988.
54. Smith S, Dawson S, Hennessey R, Andrew M. Maintenance of the patency of indwelling central venous catheters: is heparin necessary? Am J Pediatr Hematol Oncol 13:141–143, 1991.
55. Kelly C, Dumenko L, McGregor SE, McHutchion ME. A change in flushing protocols of central venous catheters. Oncol Nurs Forum 19:599–605, 1992.
56. Northsea C. Continuous quality improvement: improving hemodialysis catheter patency using urokinase. ANNA J 23:567–615, 1996.
57. Maki DG, Ringer M. Evaluation of dressing regimens for prevention of infection with peripheral intravenous catheters. Gauze, a transparent polyurethane dressing, and an iodophor-transparent dressing. JAMA 258:2396–2403, 1987.
58. Hoffmann KK, Weber DJ, Samsa GP, Rutala WA. Transparent polyurethane film as an intravenous catheter dressing. A meta-analysis of the infection risks. JAMA 267:2072–2076, 1992.
59. Lau CE. Transparent and gauze dessings and their effect on infection rates of central venous catheters: a review of past and current literature. J Intraven Nurs 19:240–245, 1996.
60. Maki DG, Ringer M, Alvarado CJ. Prospective randomized trial of povidone-iodine,

alcohol, and chlorhexidine for prevention of infection associated with central venous and arterial catheters. Lancet 338:339–343, 1991.

61. Maki DG, Band JD. A comparative study of polyantibiotic and iodophor ointments in prevention of vascular catheter-related infection. Am J Med 70:739–744, 1981.

62. Yang FS, Ohta I, Chiang HJ, et al. Non-surgical retrieval of intravascular foreign body: Experience of 12 cases. Eur J Radiol 18:1–5, 1994.

63. Cekirge S, Weiss JP, Foster RG, et al. Percutaneous retrieval of foreign bodies: experience with the nitinol goose neck snare. J Vasc Intervent Radiol 4:805–810, 1993.

64. al-Wali WI, Wilcox MH, Thickett KJ, et al. Retained Hickman catheter cuff as a source of infection. J Infect 26:199–201, 1993.

15

Intraoperative Imaging and Catheter Placement

Thomas Stejskal
Carondelet St. Mary's Hospital, and The Southern Arizona Vascular
Institute, Tucson, Arizona

Scott S. Berman
The University of Arizona, Carondelet St. Mary's Hospital, and
The Southern Arizona Vascular Institute,
Tucson, Arizona

Throughout this text thus far we have emphasized the importance of the availability and utility of fluoroscopy when placing central venous catheters (CVCs). Although a detailed discussion of radiation physics and radiographic techniques is beyond the scope of this text, this chapter is intended to provide a broad overview of some of the important issues regarding the use of imaging in the operating room for catheter placement. The discussion is limited to fluoroscopy and contrast-based methods and is not meant to serve as a substitute for a more comprehensive curriculum or appropriate experience gained in a proctored setting. The use of ultrasound to aid in establishing vascular access appears in Chapter 14 and is not reviewed in the present chapter.

RADIATION SAFETY

Any discussion regarding the use of fluoroscopy and contrast agents should begin with important safety information. Unfortunately, little of this information may be conveyed to operators of radiographic equipment prior to its use. In fact, state regulations vary on the prerequisites to the use of x-ray equipment. Some states require a special license of all physicians who use x-ray imaging, whereas others have little mandate beyond a medical license. Therefore physicians may be working with an extremely dangerous modality with little or no basic education to minimize exposure and protect them their patients, and their support staff.

Exposure to ionizing radiation is an unavoidable consequence of operating any of the presently available fluoroscopic imaging systems. The risk of tissue damage is proportional to the period of exposure to the radiation. Annual limits of radiation exposure have been set and are measured by wearing a dosimeter badge underneath a protective lead apron. The maximum permissible annual dose of radiation for an adult is 5 rems per year. Steps can be taken to minimize all personnel's exposure to radiation in the operating room and can generally be categorized into those that limit contact and those that reduce radiation output by the imaging equipment.

Mechanisms to limit contact between personnel include mechanical barriers and distance. The amount of radiation exposure decreases proportionally to the square of the distance (1). Maximizing the distance between the x-ray tube and personnel whenever possible during an imaging sequence is an important safety measure. Operators of x-ray equipment should be cognizant of this simple act and afford operating room personnel who are not required to be in close proximity to the x-ray tube the opportunity to leave the room prior to any imaging if the patient's condition permits. The most common mechanism to limit exposure to personnel is the use of a protective lead apron. In general, these barriers cover the most radiation-sensitive organs such as the gonads, breasts, and bone marrow. Moreover, since fluoroscopic imaging for vascular procedures often requires that the operator be functioning adjacent to the radiation source, strong consideration should be given to the use of leaded glasses, sterile leaded gloves, and thyroid shields. Despite these measures, a recent study suggests that the single best protection to reduce exposure as measured by dosimeter badges worn under lead aprons is the thickness of the apron itself (2). In that study, the best protection was provided by aprons 1.0 mm thick. A more recent study suggests that aprons 0.5 mm thick provide adequate protection for vascular applications (3).

Radiation output by the imaging equipment can be minimized by attention to some specific details. The single most important and easiest way to reduce radiation output is to minimize the time spent imaging. This may seem intuitive; however, manipulation of guidewires and catheters is somewhat unfamiliar to many surgeons, as the action takes place on the monitor as opposed to being within the surgical field. Because of this, all too often surgeons take their eyes off the monitor and return to the surgical field but fail to take their foot off the fluoroscopy pedal. A simple rule to remember is this: When not looking at the monitor, take your foot off the pedal. With experience in performing catheter and guidewire manipulations, this becomes second nature.

Other methods to reduce radiation output by the imaging equipment require a broader understanding of imaging technology. Radiation exposure is also proportional to the power usage and the amount of scatter produced by the tube. Power usage can be controlled by changing imaging modes. In general, in using fluoroscopic equipment, imaging takes place by a continuous expenditure of energy from the x-ray tube. This allows for live-action imaging without any discontinuity that can be appreciated on the monitor. Some x-ray systems allow this energy mode to be changed from continuous to pulse.

Although this mode displays disjointed imaging on the monitor, it can reduce radiation output significantly and may be satisfactory for survey imaging prior to an intervention. Power output can also be reduced by reducing the frame rate. The frame rate is the number of images generated per second. Higher frame rates result in better image quality and resolution but also cause more radiation exposure. Unlike changing the imaging mode from continuous to pulsed, slowing down the frame rate has only a minimal impact on exposure. Finally, some imaging equipment allows for a process known as *collimation*. In simple terms, collimation prunes undesired areas of the image usually in both the horizontal and vertical directions. When used prior to an imaging sequence, collimation not only reduces scatter and exposure but can also enhance image quality.

Prolonged and excessive radiation exposure can have dire consequences that all operators should be aware of. These include malignancies of the thyroid and hematopoietic systems, sterility, cataracts, and radiation necrosis of the bones in the hand. Beyond the obvious implications of these processes is a frightening potential for career-ending morbidity, which should provide ample motivation for all physicians to acquire and practice radiation safety skills.

IMAGING SYSTEMS

A basic understanding of the available features of imaging equipment is required prior to deciding on which system to use or purchase. Moreover, once a system is selected, it behooves the physician who will be relying on the system's proper function to have at least a cursory understanding of its technical operation. In our own practice, we have often served as the on-site instructor in the operation of our imaging equipment to the second- or third-shift, recently hired, radiology technologist sent to the operating room to run the equipment during off hours. Only through our own knowledge of the equipment and its operation are we able to keep from being stifled in our efforts in these circumstances. Although dedicated equipment and technologists for on-demand vascular imaging would be the ideal, the reality of health care economics and hospital resources does not generally allow for that luxury in most institutions.

The fundamental construct of imaging equipment includes the x-ray tube, the image intensifier, monitors, table, and a computer that integrates and processes the images. The specifics of these components for available systems determine the quality of the images and the costs of the system. Ideally, image quality should be of prime importance; however, some sacrifice of image quality can usually be offered in exchange for significant cost savings without a significant impact on functionality. Specific features that are desirable for vascular applications include an adjustable image intensifier, multiple video monitors, digital subtraction, road mapping, cine loop playback, and an appropriately designed imaging table. Although this list is not complete, it includes pertinent components for intraoperative imaging in vascular procedures.

Adjustable field of view (FOV) image intensifiers permit flexible imaging with two or three field sizes, with higher resolution (and magnification) obtained at smaller FOVs and a large FOV at the higher end. In central venous catheter (CVC) placement for example, it is often desirable to view most of the upper thoracic cavity on scout and diagnostic images and be able to magnify specific areas of interest only when needed.

Since the catheter and guidewire manipulations inherent to CVC placement take place on the video monitor, it is ideal to have at least two monitors to view in a side-by-side configuration. This also becomes critical when contrast injections are used for road mapping or are simply saved and displayed on one monitor for reference while live action is viewed on the adjacent monitor. Digital subtraction technology allows for the computer removal of bony landmarks from the reference image, so that the contrast column becomes the primary feature of the image. The advantages of digital subtraction include the ability to immediately evaluate the results on the monitor, the availability of postacquisition image processing, and use of lower volumes of contrast. However, digital subtraction has its drawbacks, including lower resolution compared with cut-film imaging and a smaller FOV.

Road mapping is a feature that can be indispensable in complex anatomical situations encountered during CVC placement. This feature lets the operator superimpose a previously acquired angiogram on a live-action image. The road map image is acquired first with a contrast injection. It is saved and then superimposed on the next live imaging sequence as long as no movement has occurred in either the system or the patient. With the road map superimposed on the live image, real-time guidewire/catheter manipulations can be performed with an image of the contrast filled vessels as a guide. In trying to traverse a diseased or tortuous vessel, this imaging feature is requisite in avoiding trouble by allowing the operator to visualize impediments and manipulate devices appropriately. Ciné loop playback provides for the immediate viewing of a filming sequence from the digital memory of the computer processor. This feature can expedite interventions by saving time in viewing series of images much faster than other methods, such as videotape or processed film.

Finally, an appropriately designed table completes the imaging package. The table should be easily movable and be of a construct to enhance image acquisition. More detail on table features follows in the discussion of imaging systems.

Two basic types of imaging equipment systems can be utilized for vascular applications: portable and built-in. Both offer advantages and disadvantages for all parties involved, namely the operator, patient, and institution. A brief description and comparison of these two broad categories is provided below.

Portable Imaging Systems

By far the most popular type of imaging in use in operating room environments is the portable C-arm system (Figure 15.1). This offers tremendous advantages over fixed systems for a surgical suite, but imaging purists feel that this comes at the cost of image quality (4,5). First and foremost, portable systems are not restricted to one room and one application, thereby permitting multiple specialties access to the equipment, which can often justify its expense. In any busy operating room, a portable imaging system rarely sits idle for any significant period

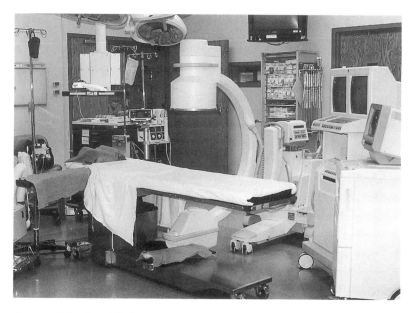

FIGURE 15.1   Portable C-arm system with carbon fiber table and vascular sofware.

of time. This brings us directly to the issue of cost. Even the most sophisticated portable C-arm system outfitted with special software for vascular applications can be acquired for roughly $200,000, far less than the $500,000 to $1.5 million price tag for ceiling-mounted built-in systems. No specific room modifications are required for portable systems, and their operation is usually straightforward and automated.

The portable C-arm systems available today come with many of the essential features found in the more expensive fix-mounted systems, such as digital subtraction, road mapping, adjustable image intensifiers, dual monitors, and ciné loop playback. Portable systems, however, can be limited by their ability to handle the cooling demands needed for prolonged vascular imaging applications. This often results in overheating and system shutdown for periods up to 20 min. This is an unacceptable and potentially risky drawback of portable systems. Portable units have inherently poorer resolution compared with fixed units owing to a basic component of x-ray tube design. However, the differences in resolution between portable and fixed units may be clinically insignificant. Finally, portable fluoroscopy systems make use of whatever table happens to be in the room. Standard operating tables are usually designed for limited imaging but not for panning the entire length of the table. Special end-mounted carbon fiber tables are available for use in conjunction with portable C-arm systems and overcome the limitations of standard operating room tables, but they add roughly $10,000 to the cost of the imaging system.

Built-in Imaging Systems

Built-in systems provide superior image quality and usually incorporate a free-floating table easily controlled by the operator (Figure 15.2). These advantages come at a significant cost for most available units compared with their portable counterparts. Most states require full lead lining of the walls for the suite containing any built-in imaging system. Moreover, reinforced ceilings are usually necessary to support the system.

The essential features required for vascular procedures are readily available for most built-in imaging systems. Digital subtraction, road mapping, multiple monitors, and ciné loop playback are largely standard features of most angiographic suite systems. Placing these systems in an operating room environment requires careful planning, since the system occupies a significant portion of the ceiling space and can make accommodating other essential components of the operating room, such as lighting and anesthesia machines, logistically difficult in all but the largest of rooms.

Ultimately the decision between portable and built-in imaging systems must be settled on an individual operator and institutional basis. Both options offer acceptable image quality for most clinical applications if appropriately outfitted at the time of purchase.

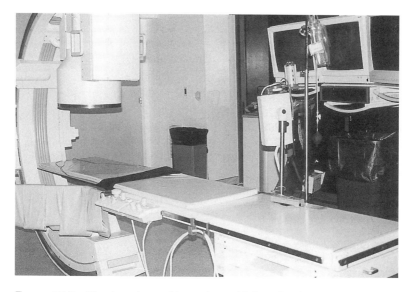

FIGURE 15.2   Fixed angiographic system with free-floating table.

CONTRAST AGENTS

Contrast agents allow visualization of vessels with x-ray imaging upon injection by virtue of their iodine content. There are two basic types of contrast agents: ionic and nonionic. This distinction is based upon whether or not the benzene ring carrier of the iodine dissociates in solution. Ionic contrast agents are typically higher in osmolality (600 to 2200 mOsm) at any given concentration of iodine but markedly less expensive than nonionic agents (300 to 800 mOsm) (Table 15.1). These features are important, as most contrast reactions are related to osmolarity. For most applications related to CVC placement, contrast can be injected by hand. However, if large structures such as the vena cava will be imaged with a small-diameter catheter, a power injector may be necessary to administer an appropriate contrast volume and overcome the resistance of the catheter.

Adverse contrast reactions are usually mild and self-limited. Most commonly, patients experience pain at the site of infusion as well as nausea and vomiting. Some patients experience reactions related to histamine release, which can range from rash and urticaria to cardiopulmonary arrest. Patients at risk for these more profound reactions are those who have a prior history of dye reaction, allergies, asthma, or anxiety. Pretreatment of patients with a history of contrast reactions with antihistamines, H_2 blockers, and steroids can virtually eliminate serious reactions.

One of the most serious complications related to contrast agent administra-

TABLE 15.1   Contrast Agents

Agent	Iodine content (mg/ml)	Osmolality (mosm/kg H_2O)	Cost ($) (50ml)
Ionic			
Conray 60	282	1539	3.75
Conray 325	325	1797	10.56
Renograffin 60	292	1549	8.97
Renograffin 76	370	2188	2.03
Hexabrix	320	600	43.85
Nonionic			
Isovue 128	128	290	31.12
Isovue 370	370	796	50.00
Optiray 320	320	702	31.94
Omnipaque 140	140	322	102.58
Omnipaque 300	300	672	184.30
Omnipaque 350	350	844	49.99

tion is nephrotoxicity. Patients at highest risk for this complication are those with underlying renal dysfunction prior to the contrast injection. Interestingly, in a patient with normal renal function, there is no relationship between the volume of contrast administered and the risk of nephrotoxicity. Unfortunately, a normal serum creatinine does not guarantee normal renal function, particularly in patients with diabetes, hypertension, and/or atherosclerotic cardiovascular disease, so contrast should always be administered judiciously and kept to the minimum necessary to obtain needed diagnostic information. Other patients at risk are those with diabetes and specifically those treated with metformin (Glucophage) (6). Withholding metformin for 48 h after contrast administration can reduce the risk of nephrotoxicity in these patients. The best prophylaxis against nephrotoxicity is making sure the patient is adequately hydrated and maintaining adequate urine output. Preinjection hydration and the use of mannitol and Lasix have all been championed in this effort.

IMAGING TOOLS

This section provides a brief description of the necessary tools to accomplish imaging and access in difficult CVC placement situations. Having a state-of-the-art imaging system at your disposal in the operating room is useless without the appropriate tools necessary to access the circulation, image the anatomy, and treat uncovered lesions.

Catheters

Catheters are available in a broad range of sizes and configurations. This section is limited to a description of diagnostic angiographic catheters. Chapters 10 and 14, respectively, are dedicated to discussions of hemodialysis and nonhemodialysis CVCs. Diagnostic catheters are usually small on the order of 4 or 5F and range in length from 65 to 110 cm. They are constructed of polymers such as polyethylene, polyurethane, nylon, Teflon, or combinations of these. Catheters are available in a multitude of head shapes, depending on their principal application (Figure 15.3). For example, "tennis racket" or "pigtail" catheters are designed for high-volume injections in the aorta, whereas a "cobra" catheter is designed for selective catheterization of branch arteries. A straight catheter or the slightly angled-tipped Berenstein catheter is likely to find utility during difficult CVC placements for diagnostic venography. An assortment of all these designs should be kept readily available in any suite where vascular imaging is performed.

Guidewires

Like catheters, guidewires are available in a range of sizes, lengths, and constructions. A full discussion of guidewire technology is beyond the scope of this book. However, a basic understanding of guidewire features is necessary for any operator placing CVCs. Most CVC kits come with an appropriate sized J wire made of steel with a soft tip. For the majority of CVC placements, this is all that is

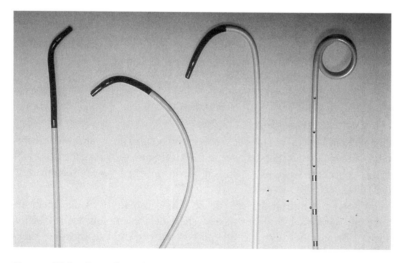

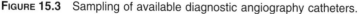

FIGURE 15.3 Sampling of available diagnostic angiography catheters.

necessary. When variant anatomy is encountered which may require complex diagnostic and even therapeutic interventions prior to placing the CVC, a broader selection of guidewires should be available to facilitate completion of the diagnostic and therapeutic interventions.

Guidewire size is the first feature to consider and is comprised of length and diameter. Most CVC applications require a short 50- or 60-cm guidewire to accomplish primary placement. For diagnostic purposes, most off-the-shelf guidewires begin at length of 145 cm and go up to 260 cm. This is important, because the extra length must be handled carefully to avoid contamination during manipulations. Guidewire diameters are also variable depending upon the application. Most CVCs are inserted using 0.035-in. wires. Smaller catheters come with 0.025- or 0.018-in. wires. Large devices such as large sheaths or balloons usually require a wire diameter of 0.038 in.

Guidewires can be constructed to achieve a variable level of stiffness. Stiff guidewires such as the Amplatz are useful in delivering large devices, as they allow the device to negotiate tortuous vessels by virtue of their stiffness. Floppy wires such as the glidewire are therefore pliable and excellent for negotiating tight lesions but need to be exchanged for stiff wires (with or without hydrophilic coating) when deploying devices. Finally, guidewires can have specialized tips, such as soft floppy J's, or stiff, straight tips. Floppy-tips wires and J wires are less like to cause damage, but cannot get through tight lesions. Angled-tip or steerable wires can be used to maneuver through complex lesions or to cannulate branches.

For CVC placement, we have found the most utility in using straight or angle-tipped glidewires. These wires are used to negotiate through a venous stenosis prior to dilation. More commonly, we have used the glidewire to stent a soft Silastic catheter to help maneuver it through a tortuous brachiocephalic venous system or a kinked sheath. Like diagnostic catheters, an assortment of the more commonly used guidewires should be at the operator's disposal when performing CVC placement.

Sheaths

Most tunneled-cuffed CVC and ports come complete with peel-away sheaths specific for the type and size of catheter in the kit (Figure 15.4). As these sheaths can sometimes become wrinkled or kinked, replacement peel-away sheaths need to be available.

Another type of sheath that should be within proximity of the operating room is the angiographic introducer sheath. These devices are thin-walled Teflon sheaths with a hemostatic valve and side port on one end and usually come packaged with a dilator (Figure 15.5). The dilator is about 2 cm longer than the sheath. Sheaths are available in a number of sizes based upon their inner diameter and

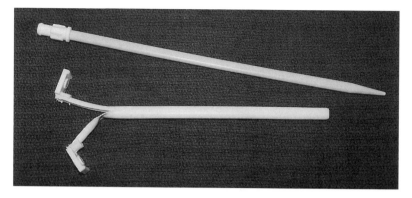

FIGURE 15.4   Peel-away sheath for placement of soft Silastic central venous catheters.

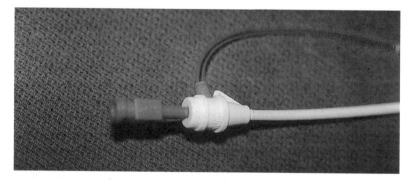

FIGURE 15.5   Introducer sheath with hemostatic valve.

length. Their main function is to provide atraumatic access to the circulatory system for the introduction of other devices, thereby sparing the artery and vein repeated trauma from threading devices over a guidewire. In CVC placement, a sheath would be necessary to dilate a venous lesion uncovered during a difficult catheter insertion, as in the case of a brachiocephalic vein stenosis. Once successful dilation is accomplished, the angiographic sheath is exchanged over the guidewire for the peel-away sheath to complete catheter insertion. For most CVC applications, sheaths ranging in size from 7 to 9F should be adequate and available. More complex interventions such as stenting may require longer and larger sheaths, depending upon the application and the device. Introducer sheaths are

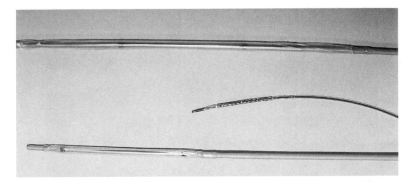

FIGURE 15.6   A sampling of balloon angioplasty catheters.

available with radiopaque markers at the tip of the sheath to avoid deployment
of devices within the sheath proper.

Balloons

The last tool necessary to place a difficult CVC are balloon dilation catheters
(Figure 15.6). Like the other components described above, balloons are available
in a vast array of sizes, materials, and structures. For venous interventions, balloons ranging in size from 7 to 14 mm must be available to dilate lesions in the
jugular, brachiocephalic, or caval positions to facilitate CVC placement. Balloon
catheters come in a variety of balloon and catheter lengths. Balloons of 2- and
4-cm lengths will be adequate for most applications, but longer balloon lengths
may be necessary for specialized applications. For venous applications, high-
pressure balloons of 17 atm are usually required to overcome the resiliency of
venous lesions.

REFERENCES

1. Mehlman CT, DiPasquale TG. Radiation exposure to the orthopaedic surgical team
    during fluoroscopy: "how far away is far enough?" J Orthop Trauma 6:392–398,
    1997.
2. Marx MV, Niklason L, Mauger EA. Occupational radiation exposure to interventional
    radiologists: A prospective study. J Vasc Interv Radiol 3:597–606, 1992.
3. Kicken PJ, Bos AJ. Effectiveness of lead aprons in vascular radiology: results of
    clinical measurements. Radiology 2:473–478, 1995.
4. Carosio G, Taverna G, Ballestrero G, Reale M, Molendi V. Portable fluoroscopic X-
    ray systems and traditional fixed angiographic systems: a comparison in the detection
    of coronary stenosis. G Ital Cardiol 9:979–983, 1998.

5. Aliabadi D, Pica MC, McCullough PA, Grines CL, Safian RD, O'Neill WW, Goldstein JA. Rapid bedside coronary angiography with a portable fluoroscopic imaging system. Cathet Cardiovasc Diagn 14:449–455, 1997.

6. Nawaz S, Cleveland T, Gaines PA, Chan P. Clinical risk associated with contrast angiography in metformin treated patients: a clinical review. Clin Radiol 5:342–344, 1998.

16

Catheter Related Complications: Their Prophylaxis and Management

John M. Marek
University of New Mexico School of Medicine,
Albuquerque, New Mexico

Scott S. Berman
The University of Arizona, Carondelet St. Mary's Hospital, and
The Southern Arizona Vascular Institute,
Tucson, Arizona

Access to the venous circulation for infusion of medications was first described by Sir Christopher Wren, who, in 1657, using a cannula made from a goose quill, injected drugs into the veins of dogs (1). The central venous circulation, however, was not successfully accessed until 1929, when Forssmann (2), a German surgeon and urologist, introduced a catheter from a peripheral vein into his own right atrium and confirmed the catheter position by radiograph. With advances in areas such as total parenteral nutrition (TPN), hemodialysis, critical care, and chemotherapy that emerged in the 1960s, a need was created for a more durable central venous catheter. Subsequent progress in materials technology has resulted in a wide array of external and implantable devices with improved compliance, decreased thrombogenicity, and better resistance to infection, making long-term venous access a lasting alternative. With the current widespread use of these devices in a variety of patients in both the hospital and the home-care setting, it becomes important for health care practitioners to understand the potential complications that may be encountered during and after placement of these catheters. This chapter discusses these complications—their management and prevention. Certain aspects of hemodialysis and long-term catheters are discussed separately, as the incidence, prevention, and management of complications in these separate patient populations may differ significantly.

HEMODIALYSIS CATHETERS

A complete discussion of catheter design and selection criteria appears in Chapter 10. Intravenous double-lumen catheters are commonly used as vascular access for hemodialysis. Central venous cannulation is primarily indicated in patients with acute renal failure requiring temporary dialysis or in chronic end-stage renal disease (ESRD) patients awaiting placement, maturation, or revision of their permanent access. A subset of ESRD patients, including young children and adults who have exhausted permanent fistula options, may be entirely dependent on these catheters for hemodialysis access. Indeed, due to the many inherent problems with prosthetic arteriovenous fistulae, some authors have advocated use of these catheters as an alternative when autogenous fistula construction is not an option (3). These large diameter double-lumen catheters may also be used for plasmapheresis or for stem cell harvest for bone marrow transplantation. While these double-lumen catheters provide an effective and safe method of access to the venous circulation, they are not without potential complications.

Transcatheter venous access for hemodialysis was first described by Shaldon et al. (4) using separate venous and arterial cannulas placed through a femoral approach. Many changes in catheter placement techniques and design have occurred since the introduction of the central venous dialysis catheter by Erben et al. in 1969 (5). Catheter construction using silicone rubber (Silastic; Dow Corning Corp., Midland, MI), polytetrafluoroethylene (Teflon), or polyurethane materials has been discussed in Chapter 10. The majority of catheters presently in use for long-term hemodialysis access are constructed of soft silicone rubber, are usually placed in the operating room, and are tunneled. A Dacron felt cuff is bonded to the catheter and is designed to prevent infection by promoting tissue ingrowth, thus forming an anatomical barrier to organisms ascending along the outer aspect of the catheter. A recent modification to enhance infection resistance is the incorporation of a second cuff constructed of silver ions bound to a collagen matrix (Vitacuff) to form an antimicrobial barrier for 4 to 6 weeks until the Dacron cuff becomes well incorporated (6).

LONG-TERM VENOUS ACCESS CATHETERS

The development of TPN in the late 1960s created the need for a long-term central venous catheter, since the highly concentrated, hyperosmolar glucose solutions led to chemical phlebitis when infused peripherally. This was first addressed by Broviac et al. (7), who reported on a new type of venous access device specifically designed for prolonged TPN infusion in children. The Hickman and Broviac catheters (Bard Access Systems, Salt Lake City, UT) are nearly identical in construction but were originally designed for different purposes. While the original Broviac catheter was designed for prolonged TPN infusion in children, the original Hickman catheter was a larger-diameter device designed for adult patients undergoing bone marrow transplantation, who usually require multiple blood tests, transfusions, and chemotherapy along with TPN (8). Over the past two decades—with the expanding use of TPN, multiagent chemotherapy, antibiotics and blood products—maintaining venous access has become of primary importance in the care of complex patients. The central venous route remains the preferred method of sustaining circulatory access for long-term use in both the inpatient and outpatient setting.

A detailed discussion of the various types of long-term external catheters that have been developed—including the Broviac, Hickman, and Groshong types of catheters as well as the totally implantable devices—appears in Chapter 14. Early central venous catheters were developed for acute care situations such as the resuscitation and monitoring of trauma and critically ill patients. Like temporary catheters in use today, these catheters were made of firm biomaterials such as polyvinyl chloride, polyurethane, and polyethylene. In contrast, the Broviac and Hickman catheters are made of the more pliable silicone rubber and are more comfortable for the patient while being less traumatic to the venous endothelium. They are also designed with an attached Dacron cuff; therefore they need to be tunneled and are usually placed in a surgical suite. Implantable ports such as the Portacath are available from a variety of manufacturers and include a titanium or plastic reservoir, a silicone access septum, and an attached central venous catheter. These reservoirs and their attached catheters are placed completely beneath the skin and are accessed percutaneously with a special noncoring needle that, despite repeated use, avoids destruction to the silicone septum.

The Hohn catheter (Bard Access Systems, Salt Lake City, UT) is a unique device deserving of special mention. It is available as a single- or double-lumen catheter (5 or 7F) made of soft Silastic. It is unique in that its small size and over-the-wire insertion make it amenable to bedside placement, thereby reducing the expense related to catheter placement. The incorporation of a Vitacuff provides antibacterial resistance for up to 6 weeks. These features have led the Hohn catheter to assume a role as an intermediary to long-term use catheter when central venous access is needed for a limited time. Examples of indications for Hohn catheter placement include patients who need central venous access for antibiotics (e.g., osteomyelitis) or for TPN while recovering from extensive bowel surgery or ischemic colitis. Occasionally difficulty is encountered in introducing the catheter into the proximal vein even with the guidewire in place. This problem can easily be overcome by using a 7 or 9F peel-away introducer, which should be readily available at the time of placement.

Peripherally inserted central venous silicone catheters (PICC lines) were first reported in 1975 by Horshal (9). There has been a recent resurgence in the popularity of the PICC catheter. The catheter can now be placed by nurses after a short training period without many of the potential complications of central venous approaches. A novel modification of the PICC catheter is the peripheral implantable port (PAS Port, Pharmacia Deltec Inc., St. Paul, MN). The PAS port is smaller than other central venous implantable reservoirs and is designed for a periperal location in the arm (usually the inner aspect of the upper arm) (10). Interested readers are referred to the detailed discussion of the PICC lines and PAS ports included in Chapter 14.

INTRAOPERATIVE COMPLICATIONS

The delineation of complications related to venous access devices varies between studies but can be generally divided into the intraoperative and postoperative. Intraoperative complications such as pneumothorax, hemothorax, hemomediastinum, air embolism, and cardiac tamponade account for less than 3% of catheter-related complications. They can, however, easily be fatal if not recognized and managed expeditiously. Distinct complications such as exit site hematomas, arterial puncture, adjacent nerve injury, and chylothorax must also be properly managed but are usually not of a life-threatening nature. The wide spectrum of complications described following central venous access procedures reflects the complexity of the anatomy of the neck and thoracic inlet.

The prevention of intraoperative complications begins with a careful preoperative evaluation. Patients should have a history and physical focusing on prior central venous line placements, evidence of central venous thrombosis (prior line infection or malfunction, arm edema), body habitus, local anatomical abnormalities, or prior surgery in the area to be accessed. Mansfield et al. (11) prospectively evaluated 821 patients undergoing elective placement of subclavian vein catheters. They noted that failed attempts and complications during line placement were associated with prior surgery in the region ($p = 0.002$), a body-mass index (the weight in kilograms divided by the square of the height in meters) higher than 30 or lower than 20 ($p = 0.009$), and prior catheterizations ($p = 0.043$). Years of postgraduate training of the physician also correlated with inability to access the subclavian vein ($p = 0.003$). Several other studies have shown that physician experience is a dominant factor in determining the risk associated with the placement of venous access devices. Experienced physicians have complication rates of less than 2%, whereas inexperienced physicians have complication rates as high as 12% (12). Bernard and Stahl (13) found that individuals who had performed less than 50 central venous catheterizations had a far greater complication rate, suggesting that this was a minimum number to attain proficiency.

Central venous catheter placement techniques as well as the use of intraoperative imaging have been discussed in prior chapters. Briefly, venous access devices may be inserted by a cutdown approach or percutaneously. A cutdown method may be preferred over the percutaneous method for patients with obesity, severe coagulopathy, or in small children. The majority of devices placed today, however, are via a percutaneous approach. Use of fluoroscopy is recommended to confirm proper guidewire placement and final catheter position. Use of other imaging techniques during catheter placement, such as duplex ultrasonography, is controversial and has failed to improve results obtained by experienced clinicians (11). In select groups of patients, notably those with prior subclavian catheter placement, the incidence of subclavian vein thrombosis or stenosis may be as high as 50% (14,15). Preoperative duplex scanning or venography can identify these abnormalities and may prevent access attempts of thrombosed vessels, with their attendant complications (16).

Patients may require the use of femoral vein catheters for venous access while hospitalized and infrequently for long-term access. The femoral approach maybe used for venous access while infection at a subclavian or jugular catheter site is resolving or in patients for whom the risk for pneumothorax or hemothorax is high and either complication would prove to be catastrophic due to severe underlying pulmonary compromise. We have rarely had to use this approach in patients with complete upper extremity and jugular venous thrombosis. Catheters placed in the femoral vein have several disadvantages, including decreased patient mobility and a higher risk of infection (17). In addition, the combination of patient immobility and an indwelling foreign body increases the risk for deep venous thrombosis (Figure 16.1) (18).

Some authors have advocated the use of a percutaneous translumbar approach for catheter placement in the inferior vena cava (IVC) for long-term access or stem cell harvest. This option may be selected in patients for whom jugular or subclavian vein access is not an option, but in several studies IVC catheters were associated with both IVC thrombosis and a high rate of catheter malposition and malfunction (19,20). Overall, while this technique remains an option, we have rarely found it to be indicated.

Pneumothorax

Smith et al. (21) have pointed out that the pleura is only 5 mm posterior to the subclavian vein beyond the edge of the first rib. Therefore it is not surprising that a common complication of central venous catheter placement is pneumothorax with a reported incidence varying from 0 to 12% (12,22). Of 1000 percutane-

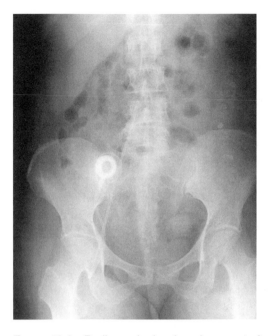

Figure 16.1 Radiograph showing placement of a venous port through a femoral approach. Catheter lies in the inferior vena cava.

ous subclavian catheters placed by a single operator, Defalque (23) reported a 0.3% incidence of pneumothorax. A similiar experience was reported in a series of 1000 internal jugular catheter placements with a 0.2% incidence of pneumothorax (24). All studies stress the importance of thoroughly understanding the anatomy of the region, with operator experience being a major factor. In experienced hands, the risk of pneumothorax should be less than 1%. The site of placement (jugular vs. subclavian) does not clearly affect the rate of pneumothorax as long as the physician is experienced with that particular approach. The risk of pneumothorax may be eliminated by placing the catheter through a cutdown approach or by using a peripheral route (PICC line or arm port).

The patient who develops a pneumothorax may be asymptomatic and require no treatment or may develop a life-threatening tension pneumothorax requiring prompt intervention. Symptomatic patients often complain of chest pain, dyspnea, and coughing and on examination may have diminished breath sounds. With a tension pneumothorax, patients may have jugular venous distention and hypotension. All patients should have a chest x-ray (CXR) performed after an attempted central line placement even if the attempt is unsuccessful. The decision

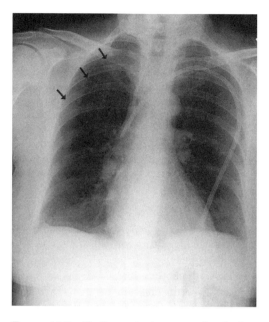

FIGURE 16.2   Radiograph shows small apical pneumothorax (arrows) following attempt at right-sided central venous line placement.

between placement of a chest tube versus observation can be difficult. Small, asymptomatic pneumothoraces (<25%) may be observed with serial CXRs and oxygen therapy (25,26). If the pneumothorax remains stable for 12 h, it will likely be reabsorbed without the need for decompressive therapy (Figure 16.2). Larger or symptomatic pneumothoraces should be managed with tube thoracostomy. If a chest tube is placed, complete reexpansion of the collapsed lung should be documented on repeat CXR. Excellent results may be obtained with a small-diameter chest tube (9F) with an attached one-way valve if no significant air leak is present. These tubes are much less painful than a full-sized chest tube and are equally effective for uncomplicated pneumothoraces related to central venous catheter placement.

Hemothorax, Hemomediastinum, Cardiac Tamponade

Bleeding related to placement of a central venous access device can be local, mediastinal, intrapleural, or pericardial. Local hemorrhage or exit site hematoma generally occurs in patients with coagulopathy and is managed with manual pressure and, if necessary, correction of the underlying coagulation abnormalities (primarily thrombocytopenia). Even in patients with coagulopathy, this complication is rare, occurring in less than 1% (24,27). Thrombocytopenia is not an absolute contraindication to central venous catheter insertion because patients can undergo platelet transfusion during or immediately prior to catheter placement. We recommend platelet transfusion for patients with platelet counts less than 50,000/mL (1 U single-donor or 6 U random-donor platelets) within 2 h of catheter insertion.

Hemorrhage into the thoracic space is the most feared complication of central venous catheter placement and is the leading cause of procedure-related deaths (28–33). Hemorrhage can occur at the time of insertion, from operative trauma, or after the catheter has been in place, from erosion through the vein wall. Guidewire insertion may cause venous perforation if the wire is too stiff or a non-"J"-tipped wire is used. More commonly, significant venous injury occurs during placement of the stiffer percutaneous introducer sheath and dilator. As the sheath is inserted, it may fail to negotiate the path of the venous system and impinge on the vein wall. Perforation usually occurs contralateral to the side of insertion. Constantly ensuring that the guidewire slides freely through the dilator/sheath complex and placement of the introducer sheath under direct flouroscopy are the most effective ways of avoiding this complication. Placement of catheters by the right internal jugular or left subclavian approach may be associated with a decreased risk due to a straighter path into the superior vena cava. Use of a cutdown technique may also decrease the incidence of significant intrathoracic bleeding (34). Intrapleural hemorrhage may manifest as sudden chest pain or hemodynamic collapse. Prompt recognition and treatment are essential. Initial therapy includes placement of a tube thoracostomy and, when necessary, thoracotomy in the unstable patient.

Mediastinal hemorrhage occurs in less than 1% of insertions and is usually manifest by mediastinal widening on postoperative radiography, although symptoms of chest pain and respiratory difficulties may occur. Usually this situation is self-limited as long as the catheter remains in the venous system. Failure to recognize mediastinal placement followed by infusion of TPN or other agents carries a high mortality rate (31). If there is any question of the placement, venography through the catheter should be performed to document placement in the venous system. If the catheter is in the mediastinum, it should be removed under controlled conditions with personnel prepared to explore the patient should hemorrhage ensue. Although there are no large series of studies on mediastinal perforations, our own limited experience offers some understanding of the treatment options. If the patient remains hemodynamically stable upon withdrawal of the catheter, he or she may be observed in an intensive care unit with serial echocardiograms and CXRs. The low-pressure venous system may allow these injuries to be self-limited. Small pericardial effusions can be managed expectantly with pericardiocentesis as needed. Surgical intervention is reserved for hemodynamic collapse or recurrent hemopericardium causing tamponade.

Catheter-induced cardiac tamponade is a highly lethal complication, with reported mortality rates exceeding 90%. Cardiac tamponade may occur at the time of catheter placement from perforation of the right atrium or in a delayed fashion from erosion of the catheter tip through the myocardium followed by instillation of fluid into the pericardial sac. The mechanical error that precedes this complication is probably improper positioning of the catheter tip in the right atrium. Most early reports of this complication were related to stiff polyurethane catheters, whereas this complication is uncommon when soft Silastic catheters are used for long-term access. While prior reports stressed the dangers of leaving the catheter tip in the right atrium, more recent reports question the significance of this finding, with some authors now advocating placement in the right atrium to prevent catheter malfunction or venous thrombosis (35,36). Once a problem is recognized, prompt therapy to relieve the tamponade must be undertaken. Pericardiocentesis may be attempted in relatively stable patients. An unstable patient requires emergency pericardial window or median sternotomy as their clinical course dictates.

Arterial Injury

Inadvertent subclavian or carotid artery puncture, laceration, or cannulation may be a serious complication. If an arterial puncture is recognized before the guidewire is passed into the artery, this may be managed simply with removal of the needle and holding pressure for 5 to 10 min. If the arterial injury goes unrecognized until a large-bore catheter or dilator has been passed into the artery, it would be unwise to remove the catheter unless one were prepared to explore the patient emergently should hemorrhage ensue. Catheters as large as 13 F may be removed from the carotid or subclavian artery and serious complications avoided by holding pressure for 30 to 45 min, but this should be performed in the operating room (37). Traumatic arteriovenous fistula has been described following misplaced subclavian or internal jugular catheter insertion (Figure 16.3), but this complication is rare (38).

Air Embolism

Air embolism may be a lethal complication of central venous catheterization. Kashuk and Penn (39) demonstrated a 50% mortality and a 42% incidence of transient or permanent neurological deficits among survivors of this complication. When the normal negative intrathoracic pressure is transmitted to the venous system, air may enter the venous circulation whenever it is open to the surrounding atmosphere. Air embolism may occur at any time from catheter placement to after the catheter has been removed. Ordway (40) extrapolated from animal experiments and estimated that a lethal embolism requires the introduction of 70 to 100 mL/s of air.

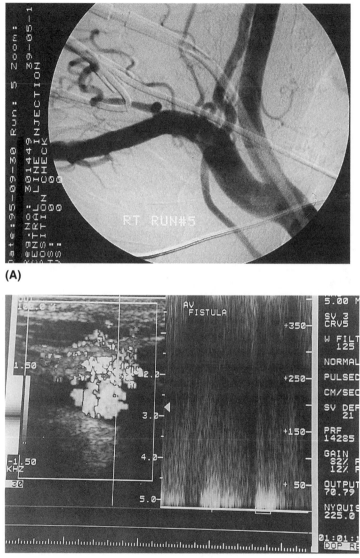

(A)

(B)

FIGURE 16.3   (A) Arch angiogram demonstrating inadvertent catheter placement into the right common carotid artery through the internal jugular vein. Catheter was removed without incident or need for operative intervention. (B) Duplex scan months later confirming presence of an asymptomatic posttraumatic arteriovenous fistula between the carotid artery and jugular vein in the same patient.

The diagnosis of a significant air embolus is primarily clinical. The syndrome of tachypnea or apnea, hypotension, pulmonary wheezes, and characteristic "mill wheel" heart murmur is considered classic for air embolism (41). Any suspicion of air embolism should prompt emergency treatment, which consists of turning the patient onto his or her left side and placement in the Trendelenburg position. Because death may be due to an airlock that obstructs the pulmonary outflow tract, this maneuver keeps the air within the apex of the right ventricle. If the patient is unstable, attempts at air aspiration by percutaneous transthoracic puncture of the right ventricle with a spinal needle have been suggested by Feliciano et al. (42).

Introduction of a significant air embolus during catheter placement may be prevented by ensuring adequate patient hydration and by placing the patient in the Trendelenburg position. Equally important in preventing the introduction of a significant air embolus into the central venous circulation is education of other health care providers on the hazards of air embolization during manipulation of the catheter tubing. Finally, the placement of an air-occlusive dressing over the insertion site after removal of the central venous catheter can minimize the occurrence of this unusual but potentially lethal complication. This dressing should stay in place for a minimum of 24 h after catheter removal to allow adequate closure of any chronic sinus tracts that may from during the interval in which the catheter is in place. Particularly when managing large-diameter temporary dialysis catheters that have been in place for up to 2 weeks, the residual tract communicates directly with the internal jugular vein and may be of a significant size (13.5F), therefore easily allowing the passage of air if prescribed maneuvers are not followed.

Chylothorax/Hydrothorax

Chylothorax may result from direct injury to the thoracic duct as it enters the left jugulosublclavian venous junction. It may be recognized immediately by clear lymph drainage from the insertion site or may present in a delayed fashion with ipsilateral or contralateral pleural effusion (43). Treatment includes removal of the venous catheter, maintenance of a low-fat oral or parenteral diet, and continuous pleural drainage until the leak seals spontaneously, which may take as long as 6 weeks.

Hydrothorax results from the intrapleural instillation of fluid through a malpositioned catheter with an extravascular tip. The appearance of hydrothorax may be immediate, as soon as an infusion is begun through the catheter. Hydrothorax may also present in a delayed fashion thought to be due to erosion of the catheter through the vessel wall into the pleural cavity. Treatment revolves around prompt catheter removal. Rarely, this complication may progress to fibrothorax from chemical irritation or empyema requiring open drainage or decortication.

Nerve Injury

Injuries to the brachial plexus or phrenic nerve and Horner's syndrome have all been described as a result of central venous cannulation (21,24,44). This is not surprising considering the proximity of these structures to the central veins. Phrenic nerve injury has been noted to result in paralysis of the diaphragm. The majority of these injuries recover completely and may be due to direct injury or pressure from a hematoma. These complications have been noted as high as 0.5% but should be rare in experienced hands.

Retained Catheter Fragments

Portions of central venous catheters or guidewires may be broken off by improper insertion techniques or occasionally during removal of the catheter. This is rare with today's catheter design, which relies upon the Seldinger over-the-guidewire technique and avoids the earlier practice of passing the catheter through the sharp bevel of the access needle. Intravascular catheter fragment emboli demand immediate removal (Figure 16.4). Richardson et al. (45) reviewed 202 cases in the literature and documented a 24% mortality without removal and an additional 21% morbidity from endocarditis, pulmonary embolism, myocardial perforation, and superior vena cava syndrome. Fortunately, the majority of retained catheter fragments can be removed percutaneously by employing an intravascular loop snare or wire basket, thus minimizing the need for thoracotomy or median sternotomy (46).

POSTOPERATIVE COMPLICATIONS

Intraoperative complications are usually due to errors in technique and consequently are largely avoidable, while many postoperative complications are inevitable with a prolonged intravascular device in place. Postoperative complications include catheter malfunction, venous thrombosis, and infection. The incidence of these complications varies widely among reports in the literature, depending on the patients' diagnoses, level of nursing care, treatment schedule, and the enthusiasm with which the diagnoses are pursued.

Hemodialysis Catheter Malfunction

The effectiveness of hemodialysis is dependent on the delivery of a high blood flow rate and the avoidance of recirculation of blood. Hemodialysis catheter malfunction may be defined several ways but in general is an inability to consistently maintain a blood flow rate of greater than 200 mL/min (47). Traditionally, blood flow rates of 200 to 300 mL/min have been prescribed when double-lumen catheters have been used for hemodialysis access. In addition to blood flow rates, other

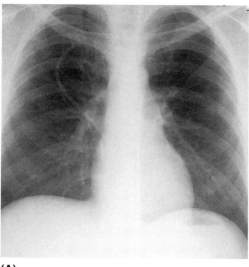

(A)

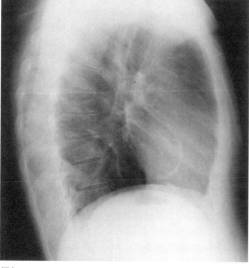

(B)

FIGURE 16.4   PA (A) and lateral (B) chest x-rays demonstrating broken catheter at subclavian entry site with catheter fragment retained within the right atrium.

studies have examined criteria for recirculation rates and excessive venous or arterial pressures (48,49). Bregman and colleagues looked at a small number of double-lumen dialysis catheters (Vas-Cath SC-4000) (47). They recommended minimum performance standards for double-lumen catheters at a flow rate of 200 mL/min: cannula inlet arterial pressure (CIAP) of -100 mmHg maximum; venous pressure of less than 150 mmHg; and recirculation of less than 5%. The CIAP is the negative pressure applied by the dialysis machine and reflects the maximum flow rate one can obtain before risking blood hemolysis. High CIAP may vary with catheter design or may indicate cannula abutment against the wall of the vena cava. Excessive venous pressure will produce high ultrafiltration and may limit attainable flow rates. The average recirculation percentages achieved using hemodialysis catheters range from 2 to 8% with blood flows of 200 to 250 mL/min, and no significant increase in this recirculation rate occurs with flow rates up to 400 mL/min (47–49) (Table 16.1).

TABLE 16.1 Treatment of Tunneled Cuffed Catheter Dysfunction

Catheter dysfunction is defined as failure to attain and maintain an extracorporeal blood flow sufficient to perform hemodialysis without significantly lengthening the hemodialysis treatment. The Work Group considered sufficient extracorporeal blood flow to be 300mL/min. (opinion) Urokinase is currently not available on the U.S. market. Preliminary studies using thromboplastin activator (TPA) and recombinant urokinase (rUK) in the treatment of hemodialysis catheter dysfunction are under way and appear promising. At this time neither agent has sufficient evidence for the guidelines to recommend wholesale adoption.

A. A dysfunctional catheter should be treated in the hemodialysis unit using the protocol for intraluminal urkinase administration. (evidence)
B. If urokinase treatment fails, a radiographic study using catheter contrast injection should be performed. Further treatment should then be performed based on the radiographic findings. Appropriate treatments include:
   1. Fibrin sheath stripping using a snare if a fibrin sheath is present (evidence)
   2. Exchanging the thrombosed catheter over a guidewire if a fibrin sheath is present, or if the catheter is malpositioned, or of inadequate length (evidence)
   3. Intracatheter urokinase infusion (e.g., 20,000 U/lumen/h) for 6 h if a fibrin sheath is present or a luminal thrombosis remains (evidence)
   4. Performing embolectomy on the catheter if the lumens show residual thrombus (opinion)
   5. Repositioning a malpositioned catheter using a snare (evidence)

Source: Modified from Ref. 50. Guideline 23.

Vanholder et al. (51) performed a retrospective evaluation of the morbidity and mortality of hemodialysis catheters including 786 catheters over a 10-year period at their own institution. They reviewed 11 published series of hemodialysis catheters (1542 catheterizations) and performed a questionnaire-based survey of 16 dialysis centers (approximately 4000 catheterizations). Catheter malfunction requiring replacement due to insufficient flow occurred in 7.6% of catheters placed. Moss et al. (3) presented a review of their experience with 168 silicone dialysis catheters with a Dacron cuff inserted over a 4-year period. Their estimated 1- and 2-year catheter survival was 65 and 30%, respectively. Median catheter survival was 18.5 months, with reported average blood flow rates of 243 mL/min and recirculation of 7.5%.

Bour et al. (52) evaluated their experience with 53 double-lumen silastic PermCath (Quinton Instrument Co., Bothell, WA) catheters placed in 49 patients. Using the jugular approach for access, they found no catheters that failed to function over the period of review. Catheter thrombosis occurred 40 times in 10 patients, all of which were successfully treated with infusion of streptokinase or urokinase. Catheters remained in place an average of 84 days (range 1 to 573 days). Arterial flow rates ranged from 100 to 250 mL/min (average 212 mL/min). Recirculation rates reported for 9 patients in their series averaged 5.6% with a range of 0 to 11%.

Proper catheter function must be assured before the patient leaves the operating room and is tested by the ability to rapidly withdraw through both ports of the catheter. The catheter should also be tested with the patient in an upright sitting position to make sure that the expected movement in the catheter tip that occurs with patient positioning does not adversely affect catheter function. The use of image intensification during catheter placement is important to verify the absence of any kinks in the catheter course and confirm catheter tip placement. If a catheter fails to provide adequate flow rates from its first use, it will likely require replacement. There has been a recent stance assumed by the interventional radiology community advocating that all tunneled catheters be placed by that specialty. A single series by Lund et al. (53) has reported 100% catheter function and a 0% complication rate in catheters placed by radiologists. Whether this high standard can be duplicated by others awaits further published experience. Catheters that develop thrombosis or low blood-flow rates may be salvaged with lytic therapy or possibly removal of the fibrin sheath surrounding the catheter tip. This problem is discussed in more detail in the following section.

Long-Term Venous Access Catheter Malfunction

The function of long-term venous access devices can be divided into two components: withdrawal and infusion. The first catheter function to fail is usually withdrawal, manifest by progressive inability to aspirate blood for testing. This has been ascribed to the adherence of fibrin or thrombus to the tip of the catheter, forming a one-way valve. Before the development of effective therapy, this complication led to removal of up to 25% of catheters (54). While this remains one of the most common complications today, it can often be treated successfully with lytic agent infusion and results in catheter removal in less than 5% of cases (3,54,55).

If a venous access device initially functions well but acutely develops withdrawal dysfunction or complete occlusion, it should be treated with urokinase, 5000 U (Open-Cath, Abbott Laboratories, Abbott Park, IL). The urokinase is instilled into the access device and left in place for 20 to 30 min before it is withdrawn and another attempt made to use the catheter. This process may be repeated several times. Catheters resistant to bolus urokinase have been salvaged with a regimen of 6-h infusion of urokinase at a rate of 40,000 U/h (56). The recent withdrawal of urokinase from the U.S. market has necessitated the use of tissue plasminogen activator (TPA) as a substitute lytic agent for catheter clearing. Since protocols using TPA for catheter clearance are evolving, recommended dosages are not yet available.

Catheters may also be occluded by precipitation of poorly soluble fluid components such as calcium or magnesium salts, drugs (phenytoin, vancomycin, amikacin, and others), or lipid accumulation in patients receiving total parenteral nutrition. These occlusions generally do not respond well to thrombolytic therapy. Catheter occlusions of this nature may be treated with infusion of 0.1 N hydrochloric acid (HCl) for mineral or drug precipitation or 70% ethanol for lipid accumulation (57,58). Werlin et al. (58) have recommended using tuberculin syringes to inject 0.5 mL of either 0.1 N HCl or 70% ethanol with maximum doses of 3 mL (1 mL for infants between 1 and 3 kg). Hydrochloric acid administration is safe at this concentration even in infants, and the risk of inducing metabolic acidosis is negligible. Using this regimen, Werlin et al. (58) were able to restore patency in 34 of 39 occluded catheters in pediatric patients, the majority of whom had failed urokinase therapy. Because of their safety and low cost (especially compared with catheter replacement), HCL or ethanol should be considered adjunctive agents for clearing obstructions of unknown etiology.

Should initial treatment with thrombolytic or chemical agents fail to restore proper catheter function, percutaneous removal of the fibrin sheath encasing the catheter has been described. Early reports with this technique have shown good success in restoring function in hemodialysis catheters with a 98% success rate. Unfortunately continued patency may require multiple stripping procedures (59). We have experienced limited success with this technique in also restoring patency to long-term catheters placed for chemotherapy and stem cell harvesting.

Thrombotic occlusion of the catheter to withdrawal or infusion is frequent but is not considered by some authors to be a significant event because of the effectiveness of lytic agents in treating this complication. However, in some patients, thrombotic occlusion of the catheter may be a sign of complete vascular thrombosis. Lokich et al. (60), in a series of 92 patients with totally implanted venous access devices, noted that nearly half the patients with withdrawal occlusion (6 of 13) were noted to have vascular thrombosis.

Central Venous Stenosis and Thrombosis

Central venous thrombosis following catheterization was first reported by McDonough and Altemeier (61) in 1971. The incidence of clinically apparent thrombi associated with central venous catheterization has been reported to range from 3 to 5%; however, these figures underestimate the actual occurrence of thrombosis. Prospective studies utilizing venography have documented an incidence of 30 to 50% occurring primarily in asymptomatic patients (14,15,62,63). Venous thrombosis may be nonocclusive and therefore asymptomatic or may result in complete thrombosis of the superior vena cava and even right atrial thrombus formation (64). Life-threatening complications such as pulmonary embolism and suppurative thrombophlebitis of the central veins may be more common than once believed, and their actual incidence may be related to the intensity with which the diagnosis is pursued (65).

Several mechanisms may contribute to the formation of thrombosis and stenosis of the venous system in patients with a central venous catheter; however, few of these factors have been studied in a prospective fashion (66). The first mechanism is the obvious intimal disruption by the catheter itself as it enters the vein. A fibrin sheath forms on virtually all plastic catheters, and this has been proposed as the nidus for thrombus formation. In addition, the function of the catheter—such as infusion of acidic, hyperosmolar TPN, toxic chemotherapeutic agents, or high-flow dialysis—may continually act to injure the venous endothelium. Other factors may include the site of placement (jugular vs. subclavian), size of the catheter, catheter material, and hypercoagulable states such as malignancy. Bozzetti et al. (62) demonstrated venographically a 46% incidence of thrombosis with the use of a polyvinyl chloride catheter versus a 11.5% incidence with a silicone rubber catheter. Pithie et al. (36) have shown that use of TPN solutions containing higher lipid concentrations decreased the incidence of central venous thrombosis and suggested that placement of the catheter tip in the right atrium may further decrease the incidence of thrombosis.

Although the majority of catheter-related venous thromboses are clinically silent, multiple presentations are possible. Venous thrombosis should be considered in any patient presenting with swelling, pain in the arm, shoulder, or neck ipsilateral to the side of catheter placement. Patients may present with signs and symptoms of pulmonary emboli. Simple withdrawal occlusion of the catheter may be a sign of venous thrombosis in an otherwise asymptomatic patient. Diagnosis of central venous thrombosis is made by upper extremity venography with contrast injection into a peripheral vein (60,65). Injection of contrast through the catheter is not adequate to document proximal venous thrombosis. Duplex ultrasonography or computed tomography have been suggested as alternative diagnostic methods. Diagnosis of pulmonary embolism requires a high index of suspicion, as many of its common symptoms—such as chest pain, dyspnea, tachycardia, or fever—may frequently be present in cancer or dialysis patients. Monreal et al. (67) prospectively studied 86 consecutive patients with catheter-related deep venous thrombosis (DVT) and noted a 15% incidence of pulmonary emboli, with a 2% incidence of fatal pulmonary embolism (PE) despite anticoagulation. Overall, despite some controversy in the literature, the incidence of clinically significant pulmonary emboli from upper extremity DVT appears to be less than 15% (68).

The traditional subclavian approach has been reported to cause subclavian vein stenosis or occlusion in up to 50% of dialysis patients. This may result in venous obstruction and arm edema as well as the loss of the arm for future construction of permanent access with an AV fistula or graft. Many of these stenoses or occlusions remain asymptomatic until a fistula is placed in the ipsilateral arm and subsequent arm edema and high venous pressures result (69). Placement of the catheter in the jugular system via the right internal or external jugular approach has a lower incidence of stenosis and has become the preferred method in renal failure patients.

Schillinger et al. (15) prospectively studied the subclavian-brachiocephalic vein in 100 renal failure patients with venography. Fifty patients had been dialyzed using a subclavian catheter while the remaining fifty had been dialyzed using an internal jugular catheter. Both groups were similar in patient demographics, duration of catheter insertion, type of catheter, and frequency of removal of catheters for malfunction or infection. Venography revealed a dramatic difference in the incidence of subclavian stenosis: 42% in the subclavian catheter group and 10% in the internal jugular catheter group. Similarly, Cimochowski et al. (14) studied the subclavian-brachiocephalic vein in 52 dialysis patients 1 to 27 months after insertion of hemodialysis catheters: 32 subclavian and 20 jugular. No stenoses were noted in the internal jugular group compared to a 50% incidence of mild to severe stenosis in the subclavian group, with 90% of these being severe 70 to 100% stenosis or occlusion. Of the 32 patients, 6 had bilateral severe strictures rendering neither upper extremity available for fistula placement. In several of these patients, attempts were made to treat the catheter-induced stenoses with balloon angioplasty; however, this intervention was universally unsuccessful.

Prevention of Central Venous Stenosis

Measures available to prevent the development of thrombophlebitis and thrombosis include maintenance of adequate intravascular volume, use of less thrombogenic silicone catheters, and placement of the catheter tip in the superior vena cava (SVC) or right atrium. In dialysis patients, use of the right internal jugular vein is clearly beneficial in preventing subclavian vein stenosis, which has a high incidence and renders the ipsilateral arm useless for future dialysis fistulae. Bern et al. (70), in a small, randomized, prospective trial, looked at the question of whether low-dose warfarin decreases the incidence of catheter-associated venous thrombosis. Chemotherapy patients undergoing placement of chronic central venous catheters were randomized to receive low-dose warfarin (1 mg/day) or placebo. Warfarin was started 3 days before catheter insertion and continued for 90 days. In the group of 42 patients on warfarin, 4 (9.5%) had venogram-proven thrombosis and all 4 had symptoms from the thrombosis. By contrast, in the 40 patients not receiving warfarin, 15 (37.5%) had venogram-proven thrombosis, and 10 (25%) had symptoms ($p < 0.001$). There were no appreciable coagulation abnormalities or thrombotic complications from low-dose warfarin therapy. The authors concluded that this protocol can protect against catheter thrombosis without inducing a hemorrhagic state. Currently, at the University of Arizona Health Sciences Center, all bone marrow transplant patients receive low-dose warfarin by this regimen for prophylaxis of venous thrombosis.

Management of Central Venous Stenosis and Thrombosis

Any patient with symptoms suggestive of venous thrombosis should undergo diagnostic studies: duplex scanning and/or venography. The decision of anticoagulation with heparin and warfarin versus thrombolytic therapy should be tailored to the specific patient. Patients with newly discovered venous thrombosis who no longer need their catheter should have it removed and anticoagulation instituted with heparin and warfarin for 3 months. Asymptomatic patients with a functional catheter may have the catheter left in place, but anticoagulation should be started to prevent further propagation of thrombus and pulmonary embolism. Patients who are symptomatic despite catheter removal or in whom an attempt to salvage the catheter is indicated have been treated with thrombolytic therapy followed by chronic anticoagulation with variable success (71).

Schwab et al. (72) evaluated 47 patients with fistula dysfunction with venography and demonstrated subclavian vein stenosis in 12 patients. Percutaneous transluminal angioplasty (PTA) was performed in 11 of 12 patients with initial success in all cases noted by a decrease in venous pressure, improvement in arm edema, and restoration of a functional access site. Lesions recurred in 2 of 11 patients and were successfully retreated with PTA with an average follow-up period of 12.7 months. However, these encouraging results are not universal. Kovalik et al. (73) demonstrated a 30% initial failure rate in 30 patients with central venous stenosis treated with PTA. Moreover, the same authors reported a recurrence rate of 81% in those patients with initial treatment success at a mean follow-up of 7.6 months. Similarly, Lund et al. (74) reported an initial failure rate of 15% and a recurrence rate of 74% at a mean follow-up of 4 months in their experience of 27 subclavian or innominate vein stenoses. Like other authors, they observed that these central venous stenoses related to dialysis access fistulae and grafts are highly elastic and suggested a possible role for adjunctive stenting to maintain patency (Figure 16.5). This specific issue was addressed by Criado et al. (75), who applied a combination of PTA and stent placement for central venous stenoses with disappointing results. These authors were successful in treating only 8 of 17 (47%) patients and, moreover, were largely unsuccessful treating subclavian occlusions with this technology. Encouraging results have been reported by Schoenfeld et al. (76) in their treatment of central vein stenosis, with an initial success rate of 68%; however, follow-up in this series is too limited to mitigate significantly the overall pessimism regarding PTA in treating these difficult lesions.

Bypass of subclavian vein strictures using large-caliber ePTFE grafts (10- to 12-mm) or jugular transposition in an attempt to salvage failing fistulae caused by central venous stenosis or occlusion has been reported in a few instances (75,77). Extension of the fistula to the ipsilateral internal jugular vein as an outflow conduit remains a final option for salvaging an access with subclavian vein outflow occlusion.

Catheter Infection

In addition to venous thrombosis, the most prevalent problem with long-term venous access devices remains infection and sepsis. Catheter-related infections have been reported to occur in 10 to 50% of catheters (1 to 6 per 1000 catheter days) and necessitates removal of 5 to 30% of catheters despite use of appropriate antibiotics (78–84). In recent reviews of the literature, including nearly 4000 catheters placed, the incidence of catheter infection was 22% (1.9 per 1000 catheter days), with 7.7% of catheters removed for suspected infection (83,84). The rate of catheter infection varies with patient diagnosis, frequency of catheter use, diligence of aseptic technique, and type of catheter placed. Debate still surrounds the treatment of catheter-related infections, including the duration of antibiotic treatment and whether the catheter or device should be removed.

Defining Catheter Infection

Unfortunately, the terms *catheter-related sepsis* and *infected catheter* have often been used by authors in many different ways to explain a fever or bacteremia of undetermined origin in a patient with an indwelling vascular access catheter. This inconsistency in terminology has resulted in confusion. Infections can be local, systemic, or both in presentation. *Exit site infections* present with erythema, mild induration, tenderness, and purulent drainage around the catheter's cutaneous exit site or the implanted port's surface needle access site. This classification comprises 20 to 45% of device infections. While most patients do not have systemic

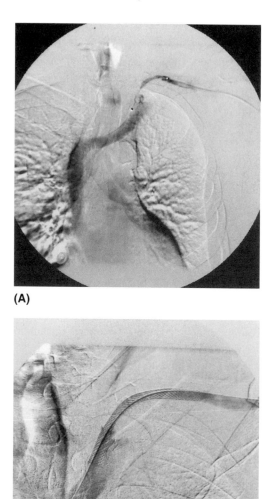

(A)

(B)

FIGURE 16.5 (A) Venogram of the left brachiocephalic vein demonstrating complex stenotic lesion. (B) Successful treatment with balloon angioplasty and Wallstent deployment in the brachiocephalic vein.

complaints, exit site infections may be associated with symptoms of sepsis and bacteremia in 50% or more of cases. *Catheter tunnel infections* present with more severe erythema, induration, and tenderness extending at least 1 cm from the catheter exit site and tracking proximally along the catheter tract (80). The exit site may or may not be involved in the process. A tunnel infection involves a more severe soft tissue infectious process and patients generally have systemic signs of sepsis. Implantable ports may develop a similar process called a port-pocket infection. Catheter tunnel or port pocket infections constitute 2 to 14% of device-related infections.

   Catheter-related sepsis may be defined as an episode of clinical sepsis in a patient with a central venous catheter who has no other apparent source for the sepsis and no external evidence of catheter infection. In many patients it may be difficult to separate sepsis related to catheter infection from that due to another source. Indeed, many patients who have central venous access devices placed, especially cancer patients receiving chemotherapy and other immunosuppressed patients, are predisposed to febrile episodes without culture-proven bacteremia or may have multiple potential sources of infection. In some studies *sepsis of unknown origin* occurred twice as frequently as sepsis attributable to the catheter (82,83). Unfortunately, the only definitive test for catheter-related sepsis is removal and culture of the catheter combined with the patient's complete resolution of clinical signs of sepsis. Catheter removal and subsequent replacement, however, is not without morbidity and cost. In an attempt to differentiate catheter-related sepsis from septicemia of unknown origin, many institutions have used either quantitative or qualitative blood cultures drawn simultaneously from the periphery and from the venous device. Using qualitative cultures, the highest likelihood of device infection occurs when cultures are positive from the device and negative from the peripheral venous culture. Using quantitative catheter-tip cultures and blood cultures drawn from the device and peripherally, device-related bacteremia or fungemia is defined using the criteria listed in Table 16.2 (80,82,85,86). For evaluation of potentially infected subcutaneous ports, cultures

TABLE 16.2 Criteria for Device-Related Bacteremia or Fungemia

1. A 10-fold or greater increase in colony-forming units (cfu) of organism per milliliter of blood obtained through the device compared with simultaneous peripheral blood cultures
2. In the absence of peripheral blood cultures, more than 1000 cfu of organism obtained through the device.
3. A positive result of catheter tip culture (>15 cfu per plate) when the device was removed specifically for suspected device-related infection in the absence of cultures, as stated above

of the particulate matter from within the port has also been shown to correlate well with device infection (87).

The most common organism isolated from indwelling venous access devices is *Staphylococcus epidermidis* (50 to 60%). Other organisms frequently cultured include *Staphylococcus aureus* (20%), *Escherichia coli* (10%), *Pseudomonas* species (5 to 20%), *Streptococcus* species (3%), *Bacillus* species (7%), Enterobacteriaceae (25%), and *Candida* species (2 to 7%) (78–83). Because the majority of catheter infections are due to *Staphylococcus* species (60 to 70%) it was initially postulated that catheter infections were caused by skin contaminants traveling along the catheter from the entrance site or contamination during catheter placement. This led to the development of fibrous or antibiotic-impregnated cuffs attached to the catheter designed to prevent infection by forming a barrier to organisms ascending along the catheter from the skin. This mechanism of catheter-related sepsis, however, has been challenged. Investigators who have examined phage types of coagulase-negative staphylococci have documented little correlation between phage types from skin around the catheter site and those recovered from the blood or catheter tip (88). In a prospective study of 135 patients, Linares et al. (89) demonstrated a high proportion of infections resulting from colonized hubs and proposed that colonization of the inner surface of the catheter hub was followed by intraluminal progression, tip infection, and sepsis. Other investigators have demonstrated a correlation between isolates from the catheter hub and those from blood cultures (90). Recent studies have also shown that the tunneling of catheters may not decrease catheter sepsis as much as previously thought, suggesting that proper sterile technique of the port or catheter hub may play a larger role (91,92).

Several other factors—including the type of venous access device placed, the number of catheter lumens, use of the catheter for TPN, and patient factors such as type of malignancy, neutropenia, or diabetes—have been evaluated regarding incidence of device infection. Recent experience suggests that patients who have completely implanted ports may be less prone to device-related infection. Groeger et al. (80) prospectively evaluated cancer patients who received either a Hickman-type tunneled Silastic catheter or a completely implanted subcutaneous port. At least one device-related infection occurred in 341 of 788 (43%) catheters as compared with 57 of 680 (8%) completely implanted ports ($p < 0.001$). Device-related bacteremia or fungemia was the predominant infection occurring with catheters, whereas implanted ports had a more equal distribution of pocket, site, and device-related bacteremia. The prevailing organisms isolated in catheter-related bacteremia were gram-negative bacilli (55%), compared with gram-positive cocci (65.5%) in port-related bacteremia. The number of infections per 1000 device days was 2.77 for catheters versus 0.21 for ports. Implantable ports lasted longer than catheters (mean 408 days versus 210 days), and this difference persisted across all patient subgroups. The study by Groeger et al. (80)

was not, however, a randomized study. Typically, external catheter lumens are flushed daily with heparinized saline, often at home by patients, whereas ports are flushed only after use and every 4 to 6 weeks, usually by experienced personnel. The only prospective *randomized* trial to date did not show a difference in infection rates between subcutaneous ports and catheters implying that the above-noted findings of Groeger et al. (80) may be related more to the frequency of device usage and device care techniques rather than to the type of device itself (93). Overall, if a venous access device is required for intermittent therapy for more than several months, a subcutaneous implantable port would likely be superior to an external catheter owing to decreased infection rates, less home maintenance, and normal patient activity.

In addition to the type of device, the number of lumens required must also be tailored to the patient's needs. Henriques et al. (94), in a nonrandomized study of 355 lines placed for long-term venous access, demonstrated an increase in infectious complications in patients with an abnormal white blood cell count (<2000 mm^3 or $>20,000$ mm^3 in leukemia) and with the use of double-lumen compared with single-lumen catheters (double-lumen catheter sepsis = 18.4%, single-lumen = 4.4%, $p < 0.01$). An increase in the number of catheter lumens may simply reflect a need for more frequent use and manipulation of the catheter hub, thereby resulting in the increase risk of infection. In contrast, Moosa et al. (95), in a study of 123 bone marrow transplant patients, noted no increase in infection risk comparing triple-lumen to single-lumen catheters in these patients, who require multiple lumens following their transplants. However, based on the fact that additional catheter hubs add potential sites of infection and a number of studies reporting increased thrombosis rates with larger catheters, we recommend placing a catheter with the least number of lumens necessary to suit the specific patient's need.

Placement methods and a history of diabetes may affect infection risk. Moss et al. (3), in their study of 168 tunneled hemodialysis catheters in ESRD patients, noted that catheters placed by a percutaneous method had significantly fewer exit-site infections than those placed by the cutdown method (10.6 vs. 31%). Overall, exit-site infections occurred in 21% of patients and bacteremia in 12%. There where significantly more exit-site infections in diabetics than nondiabetics (33 vs. 11%). Exit-site infections resolved with parenteral antibiotic therapy in 90% of cases and bacteremia in 25% without catheter removal. Unresolved bacteremia was the most common cause of catheter removal and led to the loss of 7% of catheters. The authors noted that bacteremia resolved in 50% (4 of 8) nondiabetic patients with parenteral antibiotics alone but that bacteremia never resolved in diabetic patients (0 of 8) without catheter removal (3).

The use of TPN appears to increase the risk of catheter infection as compared with catheters used strictly for chemotherapy or other infusions. In 310 pediatric patients with cancer, Christensen et al. (96) showed an overall infection rate of 0.06 infections per 100 days. During the period of TPN administration, the rate increased to 0.5 infections per 100 days. In evaluating the entire study population, infection was more likely to occur with the use of Hickman/Broviac catheters than with subcutaneous ports ($p < 0.01$) in patients with acute non-lymphocytic leukemia ($p < 0.01$), or in those who received parenteral nutrition ($p < 0.02$). There was no relationship between infection and catheter duration, days hospitalized, or days neutropenic (96).

Ranson et al. (97) noted that patients undergoing chemotherapy for leukemia or bone marrow transplantion (BMT) had a higher incidence of catheter sepsis than patients being treated for solid tumors (57 vs. 16%) as well as a higher percentage of catheters requiring removal for sepsis (17 vs. 0%) (98). Other studies have verified this increase infectious risk in patients with hematological malignancies and those undergoing BMT compared with those having solid malignancies (80).

Several small series have suggested that venous access devices can be placed in other immunosuppressed patients [human immunodeficiency virus (HIV)–positive or acquired immune deficiency syndrome (AIDS)] without an increase in infectious complications (98,99). Raviglione et al. (100), however, demonstrated an increased risk of Hickman catheter infection in 44 patients with AIDS compared with control patients (36 vs. 8%). Seven AIDS patients developed catheter-related septicemia in the first week following catheter placement, and two of these episodes were fatal. *Staphylococcus aureus* was responsible for 87% of the infections in the AIDS patients. The authors stressed avoiding the use of Hickman catheters in AIDS patients unless absolutely necessary (100).

Prevention of Catheter Infection

Many studies have investigated potential methods of preventing the infection of venous access devices. These studies have evaluated placement techniques, catheter design, use of antibiotics at the time of placement, and, most importantly, catheter care protocols.

Ranson et al. (97) performed a randomized controlled study to address the question of the value of antibiotic prophylaxis at the time of catheter placement. They randomized 98 cancer patients to receive vancomycin prior to and following placement of long-term venous catheters. They found that the incidence of catheter-related sepsis was greater in patients with more severe and prolonged immunosuppression; however, there was no improvement in infection rate with antibiotic prophylaxis (97). This study supported the findings of a smaller study by McKee et al. (88). Neither of these studies involved subcutaneous ports, which require a larger incision and in our opinion deserve a single dose of prophylactic antibiotics at time of placement. Skin preparation with antiseptics during device placement does not remove all skin bacteria, and it has been reported that catheter-tip contamination may occur in almost one-quarter of patients at the time of insertion (88). Our specific protocol employs application of an iodine-impregnated occlusive drape after the prep to completely exclude any skin from the operative field.

Maki et al. (101) demonstrated decreased infection rates with temporary central venous catheters that have attached subcutaneous silver-impregnated collagen cuffs (catheters in place 7 to 9 days total). The Vitacuff is a cuff of collagen impregnated with bactericidal silver ion. There is immediate bactericidal activity with the silver ion, which last for a few weeks while subsequent tissue ingrowth occurs into the collagen, forming a physical barrier. Because most long-term catheter infections occur on average 3 months following placement, it would be unlikely for this cuff alone to play a significant role in reducing catheter infections (80). Studies judging the value of these cuffs in long-term catheters have failed to demonstrate a significant benefit (102).

Several studies have recently questioned the value of tunneling catheters. Nontunneled catheters may be placed outside of the operating room with an obvious decrease in cost. Two recent studies have demonstrated no clear benefit of subcutaneous tunnel insertion even in immunocompromised patients (91,92). These studies primarily involved silicone catheters with or without an attached cuff. Fueled by potential cost savings, nontunneled catheters will likely constitute an increased percentage of catheters used in the future.

In regard to prevention of infection of temporary central venous catheters or pulmonary artery catheters (polyurethane or polyvinyl chloride), multiple studies have examined the question of how often catheters should be changed and whether a new venipuncture is necessary (103,104). Overall, no increase in infection rates has been demonstrated for catheters changed over guidewires at the same site as compared with new venipunctures. The incidence of mechanical complications as well as patient discomfort is decreased with a protocol of changing catheters intermittently (approximately every 7 days) over a guidewire. Catheter tips should be sent for semiquantitative culture and, if positive, the catheter should be removed, as there is a 70% incidence of the new catheter becoming infected in this instance.

Present evidence suggests that meticulous adherence to catheter care by trained staff may be the single most important factor in minimizing the incidence and morbidity arising from catheter-related sepsis. Studies have shown that when breaks in aseptic protocol for catheter care occurred, the rate of catheter sepsis increased from 3 to 20% (105). Because the infectious focus is usually found at the level of the hub, there should be strict rules concerning its use. It has been clearly shown that when TPN solutions are used, the same line must not be used for taking blood samples or for any other purpose. Manipulation of the needle and hub should be kept to a minimum and strict protocols for dressing and tubing changes should be followed (90). Semipermeable transparent dressings are widely used, but evidence is accumulating that they increase the risk of infection as compared to using simple dry sterile gauze dressings (106).

Treatment of Catheter Infection

The treatment of catheter-related infection should take into account the patient's diagnosis and condition, type of device infection, and future need for the venous access device. The dialysis outcome quality initiative (DOQI) guidelines appears in Table 16.3. While in many situations catheter-related infections may be treated without catheter removal, it should be remembered that an infection may progress from a minor clinical problem to a life-threatening situation. Particularly in immunocompromised patients, catheters should be removed if the patient's condition fails to improve following 48 h of treatment, recurs following treatment, infection involves pseudomonal or fungal species, or if the device is no longer needed. Because the most common infecting organisms are *Staphylococcus* species, initial treatment should include vancomycin (25). Immunocompromised patients should also be treated with gram-negative coverage, including antipseudomonal antibiotics (25). Fungemia represents a life-threatening condition, with mortality rates approaching 50%. Most clinicians would recommend removal of a venous access device without a trial of treatment, since early catheter removal is associated with improved outcome in pediatric patients with this specific type of infection (107).

Exit-site infections can usually be treated with local care and antibiotics while leaving the catheter in place in approximately 90% of cases (80,83). Results of swab culture of any discharge should be used to guide antibiotic therapy. The patient's clinical status and any associated signs of sepsis will dictate whether intravenous or oral antibiotics will suffice for treatment. Most patients who respond to initial empiric parenteral antibiotics may be switched to oral antibiotics and managed on an outpatient basis, with therapy continuing for 10 to 14 days.

Tunnel or port-pocket infections are treated with administration of empiric parenteral antibiotics until cultures are available. If symptoms resolve rapidly, within 24 to 48 h, the antibiotics may be continued with the device left in place. In general these infections require removal of the device (16 of 17 tunnel and 12 of 13 port-pocket infections requiring removal in one large series) (80). Occasionally, patients will require more extensive debridement of soft tissue infections in addition to removal of the access device. After removal of grossly infected implanted ports, the wound should be left open and allowed to heal by secondary intention. Antibiotic therapy should last 10 to 14 days for tunnel infections regardless of whether the device is removed. Infections due to *Pseudomonas* species generally fail conservative treatment and require catheter removal (in one series 12 of 15 catheters requiring removal were infected with *Pseudomonas*) (82).

The treatment of catheter-related bacteremia remains controversial, primarily concerning whether the device can remain in place. Successful treatment has

TABLE 16.3   Treatment of Infection in Tunneled Cuffed Catheters

Tunneled cuffed catheter infection is a serious problem. Appropriate treatment is dependent upon the nature of the infection:

A. Catheter exit site infections—characterized by redness, crusting, and exudate at the exit site in the absence of systemic symptoms and negative blood cultures—should be treated as follows:

1. Apply topical antibiotics, ensuring proper local exit site care; do not remove the catheter (opinion).

2. If there is tunnel drainage, treat with parenteral antibiotics (antistaphylococcal, antistreptococcal therapy pending exit site cultures) in addition to following appropriate local measures. Definitive therapy should be based on culture results. Do not remove the catheter unless the infection fails to respond to therapy. If the infection fails to respond to therapy, remove the catheter and replace it using a different tunnel and exit site (evidence/opinion).

B. Catheter-related bacteremia, with or without systemic signs or symptoms of illness, should be treated by initiating parenteral treatment with an antibiotic(s) appropriate for the organism(s) suspected, usually *Staphylococcus* and *Streptococcus* (evidence).

Definitive therapy should be based on the organism(s) isolated (evidence).

1. The catheter should be removed in all instances if the patient remains symptomatic more than 36 h (evidence).

2. Preliminary reports suggest that after obtaining a bactericidal level of the antibiotic in the blood, stable asymptomatic patients without exit site or catheter tunnel tract involvement may be treated by changing the catheter over a guidewire plus a minimum of 3 weeks of systemic antibiotic therapy. Blood cultures should be repeated periodically during and immediately after this treatment to monitor its effectiveness. The catheter should also be removed in any clinically unstable patient (opinion).

3. A new permanent access should not be placed until blood cultures, performed after cessation of antibiotic treatment, have been negative for at least 48 h (opinion).

Source: Modified from Ref. 50, Guideline 26.

been shown to be possible in 60 to 90% of patients without device removal (78–80,89,108). Patients with evidence of septic emboli or septic thrombophlebitis, persistent sepsis despite appropriate antibiotics, recurrence of infection following treatment, or those who no longer require the device should have it removed. As with other types of device infection, initial coverage pending culture results should include vancomycin with gram-negative coverage for immunocompromised patients. Prior to the extensive use of central venous catheters, *Staphylococcus aureus* bacteremia gave rise to a 64% incidence of infective endocarditis (109). More recent studies, however, have noted a much lower incidence of deep-seated infections such as endocarditis associated with *S. aureus* bacteremia, particularly when bacteremias are associated with intravascular catheters (110,111). Duration of antibiotic treatment for *S. aureus* bacteremia is generally recommended as a 10- to 15-day course of parenteral antibiotics; however, in some of these studies, all catheters were removed at the time of diagnosis (110). It may still be preferable to use longer courses of therapy in patients considered at higher risk for complications, such as those who do not rapidly improve with therapy, those who are severely immunocompromised, or patients with known valvular heart disease. Moss et al. (3) in their study of hemodialysis catheters recommended completion of 4 weeks of appropriate antibiotic therapy with catheters removed for recurrence of bacteremia with the same organism. They also noted failure of antibiotic therapy in diabetic patients without catheter removal. Following removal of an infected catheter, if another access device is required, it can be safely placed on the contralateral side within 1 to 3 days provided that the bacteremia has resolved clinically (83).

In 1980, Glynn et al. (112) reported clearance of an occluded and septic catheter with the use of urokinase and antibiotics. They postulated that the thrombolytic agent lysed the clot and fibrin adherent to the catheter which may have harbored the bacteria and prevented the immune system from adequately clearing the infection. Since that time, others have shown clearance of resistant catheter infections with the combined use of antibiotics and thrombolytic therapy in upward of 100% of patients (79,108,113). This usually involves a bolus of 1 to 2 mL of urokinase (5000 U/mL) into the catheter, being repeated 24 h later. However, the only randomized, prospective study of the use of urokinase in catheter infection did not demonstrate a benefit for this approach, leaving the role of thrombolytics in catheter infection uncertain (114).

REFERENCES

1. Garrison FH. An Introduction to the History of Medicine, 4th ed. Philadelphia: Saunders; 1929:273.
2. Formann W. Die Sondierung des rechten Herzens. Klin Wochenschr 8:2085, 1929.
3. Moss AH, Vasilakis BS, Holley JL, et al. Use of a silicone dual-lumen catheter with a Dacron cuff as a long-term vascular access for hemodialysis patients. Am J Kidney Dis 16:211–215, 1990.
4. Shaldon S, Chiandusi L, Higgs B. Hemodialysis by percutaneous catheterization of femoral artery and vein with regional heparinization. Lancet 2:857–859, 1961.
5. Erben J, Kvasnicka J, Bastecky J, et al. Experience with routine use of subclavian vein cannulation in haemodialysis. Proc Eur Dial Transplant Assoc 6:59–64, 1969.

6. Maki DG, Cobb L, Garmen JK, et al. An attachable silver-impregnated cuff for prevention of infection with central venous catheters: A prospective randomized multicenter trial. Am J Med 85:307–314, 1988.

7. Broviac JW, Cole JJ, Scribner BH. A silicone rubber atrial catheter for prolonged parenteral alimentation. Surg Gynecol Obstet 136:602–606, 1973.

8. Hickman RO, Buckner CD, Clift RA, et al. A modified right atrial catheter for access to the venous system in marrow transplant recipients. Surg Gynecol Obstet 148:871–875, 1979.

9. Horshal VL. Total intravenous nutrition with peripherally inserted silicone elastomer central venous catheters. Arch Surg 110:644–646, 1975.

10. Kahn ML, Barboza RB, Kling GA, Meiser TE. Initial experience with the percutaneous placement of the PAS-port implantable venous access device. J Vasc Intervent Radiol 3:459–461, 1992.

11. Mansfield PF, Hohn DC, Fornage BD, et al. Complications and failures of subclavian-vein catheterization. N Engl J Med 331:1735–1738, 1994.

12. Lockwood A. Percutaneous subclavian vein catheterization: Too much of a good thing? Arch Intern Med 144:1407–1408, 1984.

13. Bernard RW, Stahl WM. Subclavian vein catheterizations: A prospective study. I. Noninfectious complications. Ann Surg 173:184–190, 1971.

14. Cimochowski GE, Worley E, Rutherford WE, et al. Superiority of the internal jugular over the subclavian access for temporary dialysis. Nephron 54:154–161, 1990.

15. Schillinger F, Schillinger D, Montagnac R, Milcent T. Post catheterization vein stenosis in haemodialysis: Comparative angiographic study of 50 subclavian and 50 internal jugular accesses. Nephrol Dial Transplant 6:722–724, 1991.

16. Haire WD, Lynch TG, Lieberman RP, Edney JA. Duplex scans before subclavian vein catheterization predict unsuccessful catheter placement. Arch Surg 127:229–230, 1992.

17. Harden JL, Kemp L, Mirtallo J. Femoral catheters increase risk of infection in total parenteral nutrition patients. Nutr Clin Pract 10:60–66, 1995.

18. Trottier SJ, Veremakis C, O'Brien J, Auer AI. Femoral deep vein thrombosis associated with central venous catheterization: Results from a prospective, randomized trial. Crit Care Med 23:52–59, 1995.

19. Lund GB, Lieberman RP, Haire WD, et al. Translumbar inferior vena cava catheters for long-term venous access. Radiology 174:31–35, 1990.

20. Haire WD, Lieberman RP, Lund GB, Kessinger A. Translumbar inferior vena cava catheters. Bone Marrow Transplant 7:389–392, 1991.

21. Smith BE, Modell JH, Gaub ML, Moya F. Complications of subclavian vein catheterization. Arch Surg 90:228–229, 1965.

22. Voegele LD. Subclavian vein catheterization in abdominal surgical practice. Am J Surg 131:178–180, 1976.

23. Defalque RJ. Subclavian venipuncture. A review. Anesth Analg 47:677–682, 1968.

24. Goldfarb G, Lebrec D. Percutaneous cannulation of the internal jugular vein in patients with coagulopathies: An experience based on 1,000 attempts. Anesthesiology 56:321–333, 1982.

25. Whitman ED. Complications associated with the use of central venous access devices. Curr Probl Surg 33:312–378, 1996.

26. Morton JE, Jan-Mohamed RMI, Barker HF, et al. Percutaneous insertion of subclavian Hickman catheters. Bone Marrow Transplant 7:39–41, 1991.

27. Foster PF, Moore LR, Sankary HN, et al. Central venous catheterization in patients with coagulopathy. Arch Surg 127:273–275, 1992.

28. Barton BR, Hermann G, Weil R. Cardiothoracic emergencies associated with subclavian hemodialysis catheters. JAMA 250:2660–2662, 1983.

29. Fine A, Churchill D, Gault H, Mathieson G. Fatality due to subclavian dialysis catheter. Nephron 29:99–100, 1981.

30. Merrill RH, Raab SO. Dialysis catheter-induced pericardial tamponade. Arch Intern Med 142:1751–1753, 1982.

31. Sheep RE, Guiney WB. Fatal cardiac tamponade: Occurrence with other complications after left internal jugular vein catheterization. JAMA 248:1632–1635, 1982.

32. Vaziri ND, Maksy M, Lewis M, et al. Massive mediastinal hematoma caused by a double-lumen subclavian catheter. Artif Organs 8:223–226, 1984.

33. Brandt RL, Foley WJ, Fink GH, et al. Mechanism of perforation of the heart with production of hydropericardium by a venous catheter and its prevention. Am J Surg 119:311–316, 1970.

34. Raff JH. Results from use of 826 vascular access devices in cancer patients. Cancer 55:1312–1321, 1985.

35. McGee WT, Ackerman BL, Rouben LR, et al. Accurate placement of central venous catheters: A prospective, randomized multicenter trial. Crit Care Med 21: 1118–1123, 1993.

36. Pithie A, Soutar JS, Pennington CR. Catheter tip position in central vein thrombosis. J Parenter Enter Nutr 12:613–614, 1988.

37. Andros G, Harris RW, Dulawa LB, et al. Subclavian artery catheterization: A new approach for endovascular procedures. J Vasc Surg 20:566–576, 1994.

38. Hansbrough JF, Narrod JA, Rutherford R. Arteriovenous fistulas following central venous catheterization. Intens Care Med 9:287, 1983.

39. Kashuk JL, Penn I. Air embolism after central venous catheterization. Surg Gynecol Obstet 159:249, 1984.

40. Ordway CB. Air embolus via CVP catheter without positive pressure: Presentation of a case and review. Ann Surg 179:479, 1974.

41. Lippman M. Air embolism. Int Anesthesiol Clin 10:93, 1972.

42. Feliciano DV, Mattox KL, Graham JM, et al. Major complications of percutaneous subclavian vein catheters. Am J Surg 138:869, 1979.

43. Ryan JA. Complications of total parenteral nutrition. In Fischer JE, ed. Total Parenteral Nutrition. Boston: Little, Brown; 1976:68–69.

44. Epstein EJ, Querski MSA, Wright JS. Diaphragmatic paralysis after supraclavicular puncture of subclavian vein. Br Med J 1:693, 1976.

45. Richardson JD, Grover FL, Trinkle JK. Intravenous catheter emboli. Experience with twenty cases and collective review. Am J Surg 128:722, 1974.

46. Aldridge HE, Lee J. Transvascular removal of catheter fragments from the great vessels and heart. Can Med Assoc J 117:1300–1304, 1977.

47. Bregman H, Miller K, Berry L. Minimum performance standards for double-lumen subclavian cannulas for hemodialysis. ASAIO Trans 32:500–502, 1986.

48. Angeles A, Lerner AL, Goldstein SJ, et al. Comparison of coaxial and side-by-

side double lumen subclavian catheters with single lumen catheters. Am J Kidney Dis 7:221–224, 1986.

49. Kelber J, Delmez JA, Windus DW. Factors affecting delivery of high-efficiency dialysis using temporary vascular access. Am J Kidney Dis 22:24–29, 1993.

50. NKF-DOQI. Clinical Practice Guidelines for Vascular Access. New York: National Kidney Foundation, 1997:61, 64.

51. Vanholder R, Hoenich N, Ringoir S. Morbidity and mortality of central venous catheter hemodialysis: A review of 10 years experience. Nephron 47:274–279, 1987.

52. Bour ES, Weaver AS, Yang HC, Gifford RM. Experience with the double lumen silastic catheter for hemoaccess. Surg Gynecol Obstet 171:33–39, 1990.

53. Lund GB, Trerotola SO, Scheel PF, et al. Outcome of tunneled hemodialysis catheters placed by radiologists. Radiology 198:467–472, 1996.

54. Hurtibise MR, Bottino JC, Lawson M, McCredie KB. Restoring patency of occluded central venous catheters. Arch Surg 115:212–213, 1980.

55. Lawson M, Bottino JC, Hurtibise MR, McCredie KB. The use of urokinase to restore patency of occluded central venous catheters. Am J Intrav Ther Clin Nutr 9:29–32, 1982.

56. Haire WD, Lieberman RP. Thrombosed central venous catheters: Restoring function with a 6-hour urokinase infusion after failure of bolus urokinase. J Parenter Enter Nutr 16:129–132, 1992.

57. Shulman RJ, Reed T, Pitre D, Laine L. Use of hydrochloric acid to clear obstructed central venous catheters. J Parenter Enter Nutr 12:509–510, 1988.

58. Werlin SL, Lausten T, Jessen S, et al. Treatment of central venous catheter occlusions with ethanol and hydrochloric acid. J Parenter Enter Nutr 19:416–418, 1995.

59. Crain MR, Mewissen MW, Ostrowski GJ, et al. Fibrin sleeve stripping for salvage of failing hemodialysis catheters: Technique and initial results. Radiology 198:41–44, 1996.

60. Lokich JJ, Bothe A, Benotti P, Moore C. Complications and management of implanted venous access catheters. J Clin Oncol 3:710–717, 1985.

61. McDonough JJ, Altemeier WA. Subclavian venous thrombosis secondary to indwelling catheters. Surg Gynecol Obstet 133:397–400, 1971.

62. Bozzetti F, Scarpa D, Terno G, et al. Subclavian vein thrombosis due to indwelling catheters: A prospective study on fifty-two patients. J Parenter Enter Nutr 7:560–562, 1983.

63. Fabri PF, Mirtallo JM, Ruberg RL, et al. Incidence and prevention of thrombosis of the subclavian vein during total parenteral nutrition. Surg Gynecol Obstet 155: 238, 1982.

64. Fincher ME, Caruana RJ, Humphries A, et al. Right atrial thrombus formation following central venous dialysis catheter placement. Am Surg 54:652–654, 1988.

65. Leiby JM, Purcell H, DeMaria JJ, et al. Pulmonary embolism as a result of Hickman catheter-related thrombosis. Am J Med 86:228–231, 1989.

66. Didisheim P. Current concepts of thrombosis and infection in artificial organs. ASAIO 40:230–234, 1993.

67. Monreal M, Raventos A, Lerma R, et al. Pulmonary embolism in patients with

upper extremity DVT associated to venous central lines: A prospective study. Thromb Haemost 72:548–550, 1994.

68. Horattas MC, Wright DJ, Fenton AH, et al. Changing concepts of deep venous thrombosis of the upper extremity: Report of a series and review of the literature. Surgery 104:561–567, 1988.

69. Clark DD, Albina JE, Chazan JA. Subclavian vein stenosis and thrombosis: A potential serious complication in chronic hemodialysis patients. Am J Kidney Dis 15: 265–268, 1990.

70. Bern MM, Lokich JJ, Wallach SR, et al. Very low doses of warfarin can prevent thrombosis in central venous catheters. Ann Intern Med 112:423–428, 1990.

71. Siegel EL, Jew AC, Delcore R, et al. Thrombolytic therapy for catheter-related thrombosis. Am J Surg 166:716–719, 1993.

72. Schwab SJ, Quarles D, Middleton JP, et al. Hemodialysis-associated subclavian vein stenosis. Kidney Int 33:1156–1159, 1988.

73. Kovalik EC, Newman GE, Suhocki P, et al. Correction of central venous stenoses: Use of angioplasty and vascular Wallstents. Kidney Int 45:1177–1181, 1994.

74. Lund GB, Trerotola SO, Metchell SE, et al. Central venous angioplasty: An exercise in futility in hemodialysis patients? Radiology 189:198–199, 1993.

75. Criado E, Marston WA, Jaques PF, et al. Proximal venous outflow obstruction in patients with upper extremity arteriovenous dialysis access. Ann Vasc Surg 8:530–535, 1994.

76. Shoenfeld R, Hermans H, Novick A, et al. Stenting of proximal venous obstructions to maintain hemodialysis access. J Vasc Surg 19:532–538, 1994.

77. Brown L, Mclaren JT. Subclavian to jugular bypass for relief of intractable venous hypertension and salvage of hemodialysis access J Vasc Surg 18:537, 1993.

78. Rotstein C, Brock L, Roberts RS. The incidence of first Hickman catheter-related infection and predictors of catheter removal in cancer patients. Infect Control Hosp Epidemiol 16:451–458, 1995.

79. Schuman ES, Winters V, Gross GF, Hayes JF. Management of Hickman catheter sepsis. Am J Surg 149:627–628, 1985.

80. Groeger JS, Lucas AB, Thaler HT, et al. Infectious morbidity associated with long-term use of venous access devices in patients with cancer. Ann Intern Med 119: 1168–1174, 1993.

81. McDowell DE, Moss AH, Vasilakis C, et al. Percutaneously placed dual-lumen silicone catheters for long-term hemodialysis. Am Surg 59:569–575, 1993.

82. Benezra D, Kiehn TE, Gold JW, et al. Prospective study of infections in indwelling central venous catheters using quantitative blood cultures. Am J Med 85:495–498, 1988.

83. Press OW, Ramsey PG, Larson EB, et al. Hickman catheter infections in patients with malignancies. Medicine 63:189–200, 1984.

84. Howell PB, Walters PE, Donowitz GR, Farr BM. Risk factors for infection of adult patients with cancer who have tunneled central venous catheters. Cancer 75:1367–1375, 1995.

85. Whimbey E, Wong B, Kiehn TE, Armstrong D. Clinical correlations of serial quantitative blood cultures determined by lysis-centrifugation in patients with persistent septicemia. J Clin Microbiol 19:766–771, 1984.

86. Maki DG, Weise CE, Sarafin HW. A semiquantitative culture method for identifying intravenous-catheter-related infections. N Engl J Med 296:1305–1309, 1977.
87. Whitman ED, Boatman AM. Comparison of diagnostic specimens and methods to evaluate infected venous access ports. Am J Surg 170:665–670, 1995.
88. McKee R, Dunsmuir R, Whithy M, Garden OJ. Does antibiotic prophylaxis at time of catheter insertion reduce the incidence of catheter related sepsis in intravenous nutrition. J Hosp Infect 6:419–425, 1985.
89. Linares J, Sitges-Serra A, Garau J, et al. Pathogenesis of catheter sepsis: A prospective study with quantitative and semi-quantitative cultures of catheter hubs and segments. J Clin Microbiol 21:357, 1985.
90. Weightman NC, Simpson EM, Speller DC, et al. Bacteraemia related to indwelling central venous catheters: Prevention, diagnosis and treatment. Eur J Clin Microbiol Infect Dis 7:125–129, 1988.
91. Raad I, Davis S, Becker M, et al. Low infection rate and long durability of nontunneled silastic catheters. A safe and cost-effective alternative for long-term venous access. Arch Intern Med 153:1791–1796, 1993.
92. Andrivet P, Bacquer A, Vu Ngoc C, et al. Lack of clinical benefit from subcutaneous tunnel insertion of central venous catheters in immunocompromised patients. Clin Infect Dis 18:199–206, 1994.
93. Mueller BU, Skelton J, Callender DPE, et al. A prospective randomized trial comparing the infectious and noninfectious complications of an externalized catheter versus a subcutaneously implanted device in cancer patients. J Clin Oncol 10:1943–1948, 1992.
94. Henriques HF, Karmy-Jones R, Knoll SM, et al. Avoiding complications of long-term venous access. Am Surg 59:555–558, 1993.
95. Moosa HH, Julian TB, Rosenfeld CS, Shadduck RK. Complications of indwelling central venous catheters in bone marrow transplant recipients. Surg Gynecol Obstet 172:275–279, 1991.
96. Christensen ML, Hancock ML, Gattuso J, et al. Parenteral nutrition associated with increased infection rate in children with cancer. Cancer 72:2732–2738, 1993.
97. Ranson MR, Oppenheim BA, Jackson A, et al. Double-blind placebo controlled study of vancomycin prophylaxis for central venous catheter insertion in cancer patients. J Hosp Infect 15:95–102, 1990.
98. Dick L, Mauro MA, Jaques PF, Buckingham P. Radiologic insertion of Hickman catheters in HIV-positive patients: Infectious complications. J Vasc Interv Radiol 2:327–329, 1991.
99. Dionigi P, Cebrelli T, Jemos V, et al. Use of subcutaneous implantable infusion systems in neoplastic and AIDS patients requiring long-term venous access. Eur J Surg 161:137–142, 1995.
100. Raviglione MC, Battan R, Pablos-Mendez A, et al. Infections associated with Hickman catheters in patients with acquired immunodeficiency syndrome. Am J Med 86:780–786, 1989.
101. Maki DG, Cobb L, Garman JK. An attachable silver-impregnated cuff for prevention of infection with central venous catheters: A prospective randomized multicenter trial. Am J Med 85:307, 1988.
102. Groeger JS, Lucas AB, Coit D, et al. A prospective, randomized evaluation of the

effect of silver impregnated subcutaneous cuffs for preventing tunneled chronic venous access infections in cancer patients. Ann Surg 218:206–210, 1993.

103. Hagley MT, Martin B, Gast P, Traeger SM. Infectious and mechanical complications of central venous catheters placed by percutaneous venipuncture and over guidewires. Crit Care Med 20:1426–1430, 1992.

104. Armstrong CW, Mayhall CG, Miller KB, et al. Prospective study of catheter replacement and other risk factors for infection of hyperalimentation catheters. J Infect Dis 154:808–816, 1986.

105. Ryan JA, Abel RM, Abbott WM, et al. Catheter complications in total parenteral nutrition. A prospective study of 200 consecutive patients. N Engl J Med 290:757–767, 1974.

106. Fitchie C. Central venous catheter-related infection and dressing type. Intens Crit Care Nurs 8:199–202, 1992.

107. Eppes SC, Troutman JL, Gutman LT. Outcome of treatment of candidemia in children whose central catheters were removed or retained. Pediatr Infect Dis J 8:99–104, 1989.

108. Flynn PM, Shenep JL, Stokes DC, Barrett FF. In situ management of confirmed central venous catheter-related bacteremia. Pediatr Infect Dis J 6:729–734, 1987.

109. Wilson W, Hamburger M. Fifteen years experience with Staphylococcus septicemia in a large city hospital. Am J Med 22:437–457, 1957.

110. Malanoski GJ, Samore MH, Pefanis A, Karchmer AW. Staphylococcus aureus catheter-associated bacteremia. Arch Intern Med 155:1161–1166, 1995.

111. Ehni WF, Reller LB. Short course therapy for catheter-associated Staphylococcus aureus bacteremia. Arch Intern Med 149:533–536, 1989.

112. Glynn MFX, Langer B, Jeejeebhoy KN. Therapy for thrombolyic occlusion of long-term intravenous alimentation catheters. J Parenter Enter Nutr 4:387–390, 1980.

113. Jones GR, Konsler GK, Dunaway RP, et al. Prospective analysis of urokinase in the treatment of catheter sepsis in pediatric hematology-oncology patients. J Pediatr Surg 28:350–357, 1993.

114. LaQuaglia MP, Caldwell C, Lucas A, et al. A prospective randomized double-blind trial of bolus urokinase in the treatment of established Hickman catheter sepsis in children. J Pediatr Surg 29:742–745, 1994.

IV

Peritoneal Dialysis

17

Overview of Peritoneal Dialysis

Dan Ihnat
The University of Arizona,
Tucson, Arizona

Sam H. James and
Stephen J. Ruffenach
The University of Arizona Health Sciences Center,
Tucson, Arizona

HISTORY

The concept of peritoneal lavage was first described over 250 years ago. At that time, Christopher Warrick, a surgeon, had developed a new technique of treating persistent ascites; he performed paracentesis and replaced the "ascitic lymph" with a solution composed of Bristol water and cohore claret (a Bordeaux wine) (1). Since this sclerosing procedure was painful to the patient, the Reverend Stephen Hales proposed the simultaneous infusion and drainage of the medicinal agent in order to produce less discomfort (2). This first description of continuous peritoneal lavage was essentially identical to the method later used for the treatment of uremia.

The next publication on peritoneal lavage waited until 1877, when Wegener, a German physiologist, reported the results of a series of animal experiments in which the effluent fluid volume increased following the infusion of hypertonic saline, sugar, or glycerin solutions into the peritoneal cavity (3). Several years later, Orlow described a series of experiments using solutions of various tonicity to effect volume transfers (4). Other investigators including Starling and Tubby (5) and Putnam (6) began studying the peritoneum as a viable membrane for the transfer of solutes from the blood to the peritoneal cavity and raised the possibility of clinical application. The fact that scientists rather than clinicians performed most of these studies, and the advent of World War I, delayed the development of clinical applications for peritoneal lavage.

The German physician Gantner is traditionally credited with the first attempts at peritoneal dialysis in humans (7). In 1918, he noted clinical improvement in a uremic patient after performing thoracentesis followed by an infusion of isosmolar sodium chloride. Subsequently, he performed intermittent peritoneal irrigation in rabbits and guinea pigs made uremic by bilateral ureteral ligation. In 1923 he reported these results and those of a uremic patient with bilateral ureteral obstruction from a uterine carcinoma. Intermittently instilling physiological saline into the peritoneal cavity of his patient, he noticed clinical improvement. He appreciated that the transient improvement in symptoms of toxicity was directly related to the exchange phases and observed that the undrained fluid may be absorbed. Finally, Gantner noticed the association of peritoneal lavage with peritoneal contamination. Gantner felt that his inability to quantify the uremic changes precluded conclusions regarding clinical applicability.

During the ensuing decade, other groups attempted peritoneal dialysis with variable success. In the mid 1940s, Fine, Frank, and Seligman (8–11) participated in a government-sponsored project studying the scientific needs of the United States in the war effort. Convinced that the peritoneum was an efficient dialysis membrane, the group determined the optimal solution and flow rates so that, in 1946, they were able to report the successful management of uremia by using continuous peritoneal irrigation in a patient with sulfathiazole-induced anuria.

In the 1950s, peritoneal dialysis was still an experimental procedure, and patients frequently developed fatal complications such as pulmonary edema or peritonitis. High sodium and chloride concentrations in peritoneal dialysis solutions were largely responsible for the pulmonary edema seen in these early patients. Maxwell (12) and Doolan (13) determined the optimal solution composition and began using a closed system to instill commercially prepared dialysis solutions. In addition to simplifying peritoneal dialysis, these commercial solutions diminished the rates of pulmonary edema through improved electrolyte composition. Through the use of a closed system, the risk of peritonitis was reduced. High rates of peritonitis were also associated with the continuous peritoneal dialysis technique, which required two catheters. Since these early catheters frequently leaked, the introduction of intermittent peritoneal dialysis, which required only one catheter, helped to further lessen the rate of peritonitis (12–17). The development of improved catheters (12–14) subsequently reduced the incidence of peritonitis yet more.

Stimulated by a desire to expand the number of patients who could benefit from dialysis as well as to diminish the rate of peritonitis, Boen and Scribner devised an automated system by which patients could receive overnight peritoneal dialysis at home (17). The automated system minimized the frequency of opening the closed sterile fluid administration circuit. Furthermore, they utilized an intermittent puncture method to overcome the peritonitis that complicated the use of indwelling catheters (18). This technique was not openly received by the medical community, however, because of the bulky equipment, the length of time required, and the difficulty of abdominal cannulation.

After the successful application of intermittent peritoneal dialysis for acute renal failure, Scribner and associates described the periodic peritoneal dialysis guided by blood creatinine levels of a patient with end-stage renal disease. The original catheter lasted 3 months before requiring replacement, and the patient survived 6 months on peritoneal dialysis before refusing further treatment (unpublished). Spurred by this success, many centers attempted periodic peritoneal dialysis using implanted devices for repeated access to the abdominal cavity. Unfortunately, these attempts were fraught with episodes of recurrent peritonitis from either the catheter site or from manually changing the dialysis bottles. Repeated episodes of peritonitis led to adhesions, obliterating portions of the abdominal cavity and decreasing the efficiency of the dialysis process.

During this time, it became apparent that patients would need more frequent dialysis in order to control their uremia. Consequently, Henry Tenckhoff and George Shilipetar (19) constructed a miniature still that could purify water in the patient's house. This system allowed the patient to dialyze overnight essentially unattended. Additionally, Tenckhoff straightened the Palmer catheter and added a Dacron cuff to the exit site, which made long-term indwelling peritoneal catheters feasible (20). Subsequently, the introduction of reverse osmosis water treatment by Tenckhoff provided a more compact and efficient system (21). These modifications were adapted by a number of hospitals and the Tenckhoff catheter became the standard for peritoneal dialysis.

Milestone legislation in 1972 provided for funding of all patients in the United States who required dialysis. One of the centers subsequently opened was the Austin Diagnostic Center, led by Jack Moncrief. One of the patients at this center was unable to undergo standard hemodialysis because his arteriovenous fistulae repeatedly clotted. In order to be successfully dialyzed by peritoneal dialysis, patients required 60 h of treatment per week. Expanding upon the work of Boen (22), Robert Popovich worked out the kinetics of long-dwell equilibrated peritoneal dialysis, which allowed for the instillation of dialysate followed by 4-h dwell times. They determined that it would take five exchanges of 2 L each day to achieve the desired blood chemistries. This was the beginnings of continuous ambulatory peritoneal dialysis (CAPD). Curiously, this technique (23) was first reported as an abstract in 1976; the manuscript was initially rejected before its publication in 1978 (24). Oreopoulos improved upon this technique by introducing peritoneal dialysis solutions in polyvinylchloride (PVC) bags (25). During the dwell time, the PVC bags could be rolled up under clothing and then unrolled at the end of the dwell time. This reduced the frequency of disconnects and significantly reduced the incidence of peritonitis from 1 in 10 patient-weeks to 1 in 8 patient-months (26).

These advances in peritoneal dialysis provided a safe and convenient alternative to hemodialysis for patients with chronic end-stage renal disease. Further research led to the introduction of a modified CAPD technique called *continuous cycler*, which is programmed to deliver three or four 2-L exchanges overnight with 2 L left in the abdomen for 12 to 14 h during the daytime (27–30). This permitted comparable efficiency to CAPD and required only a single connection/disconnection.

ANATOMY AND PHYSIOLOGY

Peritoneal dialysis partially replaces some of the functions performed by healthy kidneys. It removes solutes such as urea nitrogen, creatinine, phosphate, and potassium; corrects acidosis; and removes excess free water. This process occurs when blood in the interstitial capillaries equilibrates across the peritoneal membrane with infused dialysate in the peritoneal cavity.

Lined by a continuous monolayer of squamous mesothelium, the peritoneal cavity normally contains less than 100 mL of fluid. In the average adult, however, 2 L or more can be instilled into the abdomen for the purpose of dialysis. The surface area of the peritoneal cavity has been estimated to be between 1 and 2 m^2 (31–33). The mesothelial cells are flattened, elongated cells with thickness between 0.6 and 2 µm (34,35) and have numerous microvilli or cytoplasmic extensions that increase the effective peritoneal surface area to an estimated 40 m^2 (36,37). The mesothelial cells are joined by tight junctions (36,38,39) as well as gap junctions and desmosomes (40) and rest on a basement membrane. Their nuclei are oval in shape, while the cellular organelles include a prominent rough endoplasmic reticulum, well developed Golgi apparatus, mitochondria, and lamellar bodies (41). The lamellar bodies contain primarily phosphatidylcholine, which is released by exocytosis to lubricate the peritoneal surface (42).

Deep to the basement membrane lie the interstitium and capillaries. The interstium is a layer of loose areolar tissue composed of reticular collagen bundles and elastic fibers (35,43) embedded in a matrix of mucopolysaccharides such as hyaluronan and chondroitin sulfate (44). Interstitial fluid is entrapped in the gel-like matrix. Probably the most important restriction barrier of solute transport in peritoneal dialysis is the capillary wall. The vascular endothelial cells are coated with a glycocalix that imparts an electronegative charge to the luminal surface (45–47). These surface modifications contribute to the regulation of the transport of small and large molecules across the vascular wall, acting as a size, shape, and charge barrier (48,49). Numerous studies in both animals and humans have demonstrated vasoactive substances that increase mesenteric blood flow will also increase creatinine and urea clearance during peritoneal dialysis (50).

The parietal peritoneum is supplied by the intercostal, epigastric, and lumbar arteries, while venous drainage is via the inferior vena cava. The visceral peritoneum is supplied by the superior mesenteric artery and drained by the portal vein. Thus, intraperitoneally administered drugs will be partially subjected to a higher first-pass hepatic clearance. Lymphatic drainage of the peritoneal cavity occurs mainly along the diaphragmatic surface through stomata, originally described by Von Recklinghausen using silver stain preparations in 1871 (51). The function of these lymphatic openings was not completely accepted until they were confirmed with electron microscopy (52,53) and particles were demonstrated to pass from the peritoneal cavity into the subdiaphragmatic lymphatics (54,55). Augmented by respiration (56,57), the majority of these lymphatics accompany the internal mammary vessels to the anterior mediastinal lymph nodes and drain into the right lymphatic duct (58,59). The second major lymphatic drainage pathway of the peritoneal cavity is via the omental lymphatics, which drain into the thoracic duct through the cysterna chyli (60). The lymphatics draining the mesentery primarily drain the gastrointestinal tract and do not contribute to drainage of the peritoneal cavity.

During peritoneal dialysis, the mesothelial cells develop a cuboidal appearance and increase in density. The rough endoplasmic reticulum, Golgi apparatus, and lamellar bodies undergo hyperplasia while a diminution occurs in the number of microvilli. In addition, abnormal surface protuberances such as blebs and blisters develop on the peritoneal surface (35,43,61–63). Reduplication of the basement membrane of stromal blood vessels is seen, similar to the vascular changes seen in diabetic patients (64–66), and hyalinization of the superficial stromal collagen occurs in patients on long-term CAPD. These changes may ultimately impair efficient exchange across the peritoneal membrane, making the process inefficient.

The peritoneal membrane functions as an imperfect semipermeable membrane. Osmotic pressure is generated when a gradient of a poorly permeable substance exists across the peritoneal membrane and accounts for the bulk flow of water during peritoneal dialysis. This process is called osmotic ultrafiltration. Solutes will exert an effective osmotic pressure gradient proportional to the ratio of the molecular radius of the solute and the radius of the water-filled membrane pores. In a perfect system, the effective and theoretical osmotic pressures are equal. For an imperfect semipermeable membrane like the peritoneum, the effective osmotic pressure is less than the theoretical pressure. The solute reflection coefficient is the ratio of the effective osmotic pressure divided by the theoretical osmotic pressure.

Diffusion and convection are the major mechanisms of solute transport during peritoneal dialysis. Diffusion is the most important transport mechanism for low-molecular-weight solutes such as urea, creatinine, and uric acid. The net diffusion rate of a substance between the capillary and peritoneal cavity is directly proportional to the permeability of the solute, the solute concentration gradient, the pressure difference across the membrane, the membrane surface area, and the temperature. There is a negative correlation between diffusion rate and the square root of the solute molecular weight and the peritoneal membrane thickness.

Convective flow or solute drag is a process whereby molecules are transported across a membrane, with fluid as part of the total fluid transport. This is in contradistinction to the random movement seen in pure diffusion. The rate of convective transport is proportional to the water flux, the solute concentration, and the solute reflection coefficient. It remains controversial whether the main transport mechanism of larger molecules during peritoneal dialysis is by convection (67,68), restricted diffusion (69–72), or both (73).

Solutes of sizes greater than the pore size and macromolecules such as proteins are transported from the capillaries into the peritoneal cavity via pinocytosis or vesicular transport. Small amounts of plasma proteins may leak through pores in the capillary wall into the interstitium of the peritoneum. The return of macromolecules from the peritoneum and interstitium back into the capillaries, however, likely occurs via the lymphatics.

Net removal of sodium and potassium is usually far below their respective concentrations in the extracellular fluid during convective flow. This is due to a sieving effect from either a membrane feature or an interaction between molecules within the membrane channels. The sieving coefficient for a solute is given by the ratio of the solute concentration in the ultrafiltrate to that in the plasma water. Charged substances in the endothelial and mesothelial gap junctions or in the interstitial gel matrix may also impede ultrafiltration forces.

Overall, peritoneal dialysis is a function of capillary flow rate, dialysis flow rate, and a coefficient that reflects the peritoneal membrane surface area and membrane resistance to transfer (74). Clinically, these variables translate into blood pressure, cardiac output, intraperitoneal volume of dialysate, and the physiologic characteristics of the peritoneal membrane.

The advantages of CAPD include a lack of expensive equipment and ready availablity for in-home use following a brief training period. It is less efficient for the removal of small molecules such as urea, although it is more efficient for the removal of middle-sized molecules. Several major disadvantages of CAPD exist, however, including a protein loss of 5 to 15 g/day and the cumbersome, time-consuming nature of the technique, hypertrigyceridemia, hyperglycemia, and weight gain secondary to the absorption of dextrose, which generates up to approximately 850 calories per day (75).

REFERENCES

1. Warwick C. An improvement of the practice of tapping, whereby that operation instead for relief of symptoms, becomes an absolute cure for ascites, exemplified in the case of Jane Roman. Philosoph Trans R Soc 43:12–19, 1744.

2. Hale S. A method of conveying liquors into the abdomen during the operation of tapping. Philosoph Trans R Soc 43:20–21, 1744.

3. Wegener G. Chirugische Bemerkungen über die Peritonealhohle, mit besonderer Berucksichtigung der Ovariotome. Arch Klin Cher 20:51–147, 1877.

4. Orlow WN. Einige Versuche über die Resorption in der Bauchhole. Arch Phys Pfluger 59:170–200, 1895.

5. Starling EH, Tubby AH. The influence of mechanical factors on lymph production. J Physiol 46:140–148, 1894.

6. Putnam J. The living peritoneum as a dialyzing membrane. Am J Physiol 63:548–565, 1923.

7. Ganter G. Ueber die Beseitigung giftger Stoffe aus dem Blute durch Dialyse. Munch Med Wochenschr 70-II;1478–1480, 1923.

8. Fine JH, Frank HA, Seligman AM. The treatment of acute renal failure by peritoneal irrigation. Ann Surg 124:857–875, 1946.

9. Frank HA, Seligman AM, Fine J. Treatment of uraemia after acute renal failure by peritoneal irrigation. JAMA 130:703, 1946.

10. Seligman AM, Frank HA, Fine J. Treatment of experimental uremia by peritoneal irrigation for acute renal failure. J Clin Invest 25:211, 1946.

11. Fine JH, Frank HA, Seligman AM. Further experiences with peritoneal irrigation for acute renal failure. Ann Surg 128:561, 1948.

12. Maxwell MH, Rockney RE, Kleeman CR, Twiss MR. Peritoneal dialysis. JAMA 170:917–924, 1959.

13. Doolan PD, Murphy WP, Wiggins RA, et al. An evaluation of intermittent peritoneal lavage. Am J Med 26:831–844, 1959.

14. Grollman A, Turner LB, McLean JA. Intermittent peritoneal lavage in nephrectomized dogs and its application to the human being. Arch Intern Med 87:379–390, 1951.

15. Reid R, Penfold JB, Jones RN. Anuria treated by renal encapsulation and peritoneal dialysis. Lancet 2:791–751, 1946.

16. Abbott WE, Shea P. Treatment of temporary renal insufficiency (uremia) by peritoneal lavage. Am J Med Sci 211:312–319, 1946.

17. Boen ST, Mulmari AS, Dillard DH, Scribner BH. Periodic peritoneal dialysis in the management of chronic uraemia. Trans Am Soc Artif Intern Organs 8:256–262, 1962.

18. Boen ST, Mion C, Curtis FK, Shilipetar G. Periodic peritoneal dialysis using the repeated puncture technique and an automatic cycling machine. Trans Am Soc Artif Intern Organs 10:409–413, 1964.

19. Tenckhoff H, Shiplipeter G, van Paaschen WH, Swanson E. A home peritoneal dialysis delivery system. Trans Am Soc Artif Intern Organs 15:103–107, 1969.

20. Tenckhoff H, Schechter HS. A bacteriologically safe peritoneal access device. Trans Am Soc Artif Intern Organs 14:181–186, 1973.

21. Tenckhoff H, Meston B, Shiplipeter G. A simplified automatic peritoneal dialysis system. Trans Am Soc Artif Intern Organs 18:436–439, 1972.
22. Boen ST. Kinetics of peritoneal dialysis. Medicine 40:243–287, 1961.
23. Popovich RP, Moncrief JW, Decherd JB, et al. The definition of a novel portable/wearable equilibrium peritoneal dialysis technique (abstr). Trans Am Soc Artif Intern Organs 5:64, 1976.
24. Popovich RP, Moncrief JW, Nolph KD, et al. Continuous ambulatory peritoneal dialysis. Ann Intern Med 88:44–56, 1978.
25. Oreopoulos DG, Robson, M, Izatt S, et al. A simple and safe technique for CAPD. Trans Am Soc Artif Int Organs 24:484–489, 1978.
26. Oreopoulos DG, Khanna R, Williams P, et al. Efficacy of and clinical experience with CAPD in Canada. In Atkins R, Thomson N, Farrel PC, eds. Edinburgh: 1981: 114–125.
27. Diaz-Buxo JA, Walker PJ, Farmer CD, et al. Continuous cyclic peritoneal dialysis (CCPD). Trans Am Soc Artif Intern Organs 27:51–53, 1981.
28. Diaz-Buxo JA, Farmer CD, Walker PJ, et al. Continuous cyclic peritoneal dialysis—A preliminary report. Artif Organs 5:157–161, 1981.
29. Nakagawa D, Price C, Stinebaugh B, Suki W. Continuous cyclic peritoneal dialysis: A viable option in the treatment of chronic renal failure. Trans Am Soc Artif Intern Organs 27:55–57, 1981.
30. Price C, Suki W. New modifications of peritoneal dialysis: Options in the treatment of patients with renal failure. Am J Nephrol 1:97–104, 1981.
31. Putiloff PV. Materials for the study of the laws of growth of the human body in relation to the surface area: The trial on Russian subjects of planigraphic anatomy as a mean of exact anthropometry. Presented at the Siberian Branch of the Russian Geographic Society, Omsk, 1886.
32. Esperanca MJ, Collins DL. Peritoneal dialysis efficiency in relation to body weight. J Pediatr Surg 1:162–169, 1966.
33. Rubin JL, Cloauson M, Planch A, Jones Q. Measurements of peritoneal surface area in man and rat. Am J Med Sci 295:453–458, 1988.
34. Gosselin RE, Berndt WD. Diffusional transport of solutes through mesentery and peritoneum. J Theor Biol 3:487–495, 1962.
35. Gotloib L, Digenis GE, Rabinovich S, et al. Ultrastructure of normal rabbit mesentery. Nephron 34:248–255, 1983.
36. Odor L, Observations of the rat mesothilium with the electron and phase microscopes. Am J Anat 95:433–465, 1954.
37. Gotloib L, Shustack A. Ultrastructural morphology of the peritoneum: New findings and speculations on transfer of solutes and water during peritoneal dialysis. Perit Dial Bull 7:119–129, 1987.
38. Baradi AF, Hope J. Observations on ultrastructure of rabbit mesothelium. Exp Cell Res 34:33–44, 1964.
39. Fukata H. Electron microscopic study on normal rat peritoneal mesothelium and its changes in absorption of particulate iron dextran complex. Acta Pathol Jpn 13:309–325, 1963.
40. Whitaker D, Papadimirtriou JM, Walters MNI. The mesothelium and its reactions: A review. CRC Crit Rev Toxicol 10:81–144, 1982.

41. Dobbie JW. Morpho-functional correlations in human mesothelium. In La Greca G, Ronco C, Feriani M, et al., eds. Peritoneal Dialysis: Proceedings of Fourth International Course on Peritoneal Dialysis, Vicenza, Italy, 1991:33–39.

42. Dobbie JW. Ultrastructural similarities between mesothelial and type II pneumocytes and their relevance to phospholipid surfactant production by the peritoneum. In Dhanna R, Nolph KD, Prowant B, eds. Advances in Continuous Ambulatory Peritoneal Dialysis. Toronto: University of Toronto Press; 1988, pp 32–41.

43. Dobbie JW. Morphology of the peritoneum in CAPD. Blood Purif 7:74–85, 1989.

44. Laurent TC. The ultrastructure and physical-chemical properties of intersitial connective tissue. Pfluegers Arch (Suppl) 336:S21–S42, 1972.

45. Ausprunk DH, Boudreau CL, Nelson DA. Proteoglycans in the microvasculature. II. Histochemical localization in proliferating capillaries of the rabbit cornea. Am J Pathol 103:367–375, 1981.

46. Simionescu N, Simionescu M, Palade GE. Differentiated microdomians on the luminal surface of capillary endothelium. I. Preferential distribution of anionic sites. J Cell Biol 90:605–613, 1981.

47. Simionescu M, Simionescu N, Silbert J, Palade G. Differentiated microdomains on the luminal surface of the capillary endothelium. II. Partial characterization of their anionic sites. J Cell Biol 90:614–621, 1981.

48. Schneeberger EE, Hamelin M. Interactions of serum proteins with lung endothelial glycocalyx: Its effect on endothelial permeability. Am J Physiol 247:H206–H217, 1984.

49. Ryan US. The endothelial surface and responses to injury. Fed Proc 45:101–108, 1986.

50. Khanna R, Nolph KD. Peritoneal morphology and microcirculation. In Gokal R, ed. Continuous Peritoneal Ambulatory Peritoneal Dialysis. New York: Churchill Livingstone; 1986:23–26.

51. Von Recklinghausen: Das Lymph Gefassystem. In Stricker IM, ed. Handbuch der Lehre von den Geweben. Leipzig: Englemann; 1871.

52. Tsilibarry EC, Wissig SL. Absorption from the peritoneal cavity. SEM study of the mesothelium covering the peritoneal surface of the muscular portion of the diaphragm. Am J Anat 149:127–133, 1977.

53. Leak LV, Rahil K. Permeability of the diaphragmatic mesothelium: The structural basis for "stomata." Am J Anat 15:557–594, 1978.

54. Allen L. The peritoneal "stomata." Anat Rec 67:89–99, 1937.

55. French JE, Florey HW, Morris B. The absorption of particles by the lymphatics of the diaphragm. Q J Exper Physiol 45:88–103, 1960.

56. Allen L, Vogt E. A mechanism of lymphatic absorption from serous cavities. Am J Physiol 119:776–782, 1937.

57. Casley-Smith JR. Endothelial permeability—The passage of particles into and out of diaphragmatic lymphatics. Q J Exp Physiol 49:365–383, 1964.

58. (10)Brown KP. Peritoneal lymphatic absorption: An experimental investigation to determine the value of lymphaticostomy. Br J Surg 15:538–544, 1927–28.

59. Courtice FC, Steinbeck AW. Absorption of protein from the peritoneal cavity. J Physiol (London) 114:336–355, 1951.

60. Nylander G, Tjernberg B. The lymphatics of the greater omentum. An experimental study in the dog. Lymphology. 2:3–7, 1967.

61. DiPaolo N, Sacchi G, De Mia M, et al. Morphology of the peritoneal membrane during continuous ambulatory peritoneal dialysis. Nephron 44:204–211, 1986.

62. Gotliob L, Shostack A, Bar-Sella P, Cohen R. Continuous mesothelial injury and regeneration during long term peritoneal dialysis. Perit Dial Bull 7:148–155, 1987.

63. Dobbie JW, Zaki M, Wilson L. Ultrasturctural studies on the peritoneum with special reference to chronic ambulatory peritoneal dialysis. Scott Med J 26:213–223, 1981.

64. Dobbie JW, Lloyd JK, Gall CA. Categorization of ultrastructural changes in peritoneal mesothelium, stroma and blood vessels in uremia and CAPD patients. Adv Perit Dial 6:3–12, 1990.

65. Gotloib L, Bar-Sella P, Shostack A. Reduplicated basal lamina of small venules and mesothelium of human parietal peritoneum. Perit Dial Bull 5:212–215, 1985.

66. Di Paolo N, Sacchi G. Peritoneal vascular changes in continuous ambulatory peritoneal dialysis (CAPD): An in vivo model for the study of diabetic microangiophathy. Perit Dial Int 9:41–45, 1989.

67. Taylor AE, Granger DN. Exchange of macromolecules across the microcirculation. In Renkin EM, Michell CC, eds. Handbook of Physiology. Sec 2. The Cardiovascular System. American Physiological Society 1984:465.

68. Rippe B, Haraldsson B. Fluid and protein fluxes across small and large pores in the microvasculature. Applications of two-pore equations. Acta Physiol Scand 131:411–428, 1987.

69. Fox J, Galey F, Wayland H. Action of histamine on the mesenteric microvasculature. Microvasc Res 19:108–126, 1980.

70. Krediet RT, Koomen GCM, Koopman MG, et al. The peritoneal transport of serum proteins and neutral dextran in CAPD patients. Kidney Int 35:1064–1072, 1989.

71. Nolph KD, Miller FN, Pyle WK, et al. An hypothesis to explain the ultrafiltration characteristics of peritoneal dialysis. Kidney Int 20:543–548, 1981.

72. Leypoldt JK, Blindauer KM. Convection does not govern plasma to dialysate transport of protein. Kidney Int 42:1412–1418, 1992.

73. Schaeffer RC Jr, Bitrick MS, Holberg WC III, Katz MA. Macromolecular transport across endothelial monolayers. Int J Microcirc Clin Exp 11:181–201, 1992.

74. Popovich RP, Moncrief JW. Kinetic modeling of peritoneal transport. In Trevino-Bacerra A, Boen FST, eds. Today's art of peritoneal dialysis (Contributions to Nephrology, Vol. 17). Basel, Switzerland: Karger; 1979:59–72.

75. Lindholm B, Bergstrom J. Nutritional aspects on peritoneal dialysis. Kidney Int 42:165–171, 1993.

18

Patient Selection, Catheter Placement, and Dialysis Techniques

Dan Ihnat
The University of Arizona,
    Tucson, Arizona

W. Bradford Carter and Bruce E. Jarrell
The University of Maryland,
    Baltimore, Maryland

John Daller
University of Texas Medical Branch,
    Galveston, Texas

SELECTION OF PATIENTS FOR PERITONEAL DIALYSIS

In deciding whether to place a patient on peritoneal dialysis rather than hemodialysis, the long-term results of each treatment modality must be comparable. Although large multicenter randomized trials comparing peritoneal dialysis with hemodialysis have not been performed, nonrandomized comparisons of these two cohorts have found patient survival to be equivalent when adjusted for age, diabetes mellitus, and other comorbidities (1–5). Likewise, patients had similar hospitalization rates with peritoneal dialysis and hemodialysis (6).

As with hemodialysis, patients may be placed on peritoneal dialysis for either acute or chronic renal failure. Acutely, peritoneal dialysis is sometimes preferred to hemodialysis in patients with poor venous access, contraindications to heparinization, or marginal cardiovascular hemodynamics (7–12). Hypothermia is another indication for acute peritoneal dialysis (13–15). In patients with chronic renal failure, peritoneal dialysis is a suitable modality for renal replacement therapy if the patient or family members caring for them are willing to accept the added responsibility of performing dialysis and are able to maintain meticulous sterile technique in handling the catheter (16–21). Neonates and small children are especially suited for peritoneal dialysis (22). Although drug overdose was considered an acceptable indication for peritoneal dialysis in the past, hemodialysis is more effective in clearing drugs (23).

Contraindications

There are no absolute contraindications to peritoneal dialysis, but a number of relative contraindications exist:

1. Chronic obstructive pulmonary disease.
2. Gastroesophageal reflux disease.
3. Patients with inflammatory bowel disease or those taking steroids.
4. Patients with known abdominal adhesions or diffuse peritoneal malignancy.
5. Patients with acute surgical problems of the abdomen such as bowel obstruction, marked distention, or paralytic ileus.
6. Recent major abdominal surgery, especially in patients with abdominal drains.
7. Patients with enterostomies, ureterostomies, large abdominal wall hernias, or cellulitis of the abdominal wall that could result in peritonitis.
8. Marked obesity; these patients have an increased incidence of hernias, abdominal wall cellulitis and fungal infections.
9. Patients with hyperlipidemia, or protein malnutrition.
10. Patients with arthritis, blindness, or other neurological impairments that would preclude them from performing catheter exchanges.

CATHETER INSERTION TECHNIQUES

In general, catheters can be divided into two main groups, those designed for acute use (less than 3 days) or chronic use (greater than 3 days). Acute peritoneal dialysis catheters are straight, rigid and made of either nylon or polyethylene with numerous intraperitoneal side holes. They are inserted using the Seldinger technique and secured to the skin by suture. Because of the rigidity of the catheter and the lack of a barrier to bacterial invasion, a significant risk of peritonitis, peritoneal irritation, or bowel perforation exists if the catheter is used for more than 3 days.

Palmer designed the first permanent peritoneal dialysis catheter using a soft silicone rubber tube with a long subcutaneous portion (24). Tenchoff (25) subsequently added subcutaneous Dacron cuffs to the Palmer catheter, significantly decreasing the incidence of catheter-related infections and making long-term peritoneal access feasible. The majority of patients on peritoneal dialysis use the Tenckhoff catheter or one of its variations (26–28) (Figure 18.1).

Most peritoneal dialysis catheters have one or two Dacron cuffs. Although the incidence of leaks and exit site infections is similar (29), catheters with two cuffs have a longer survival (30) and are associated with a lower rate of peritonitis (26) than single-cuffed catheters. Single-cuffed catheters are preferred in neonates and infants to prevent cuff erosion through the skin. The intraabdominal portion of the catheter may be either straight or curled; a randomized trial demonstrated no difference in mechanical complications or infusion pain between straight and curled catheters (31).

Additional variations of the Tenckhoff catheter exist. The Toronto Western Hospital catheter has two additional flat silicon discs added to the intraabdominal portion of the catheter to prevent catheter migration and a disc at the base of the inner Dacron cuff to prevent leaks (32). A randomized prospective trial compared the Toronto Western catheter with both straight and coiled Tenckhoff catheters and found similar short-term outcomes in all three (33). The Swan-neck Missouri catheter has a 180-degree curve in the subcutaneous portion in order to direct both the internal and external exit sites downward and a flange at the inner cuff

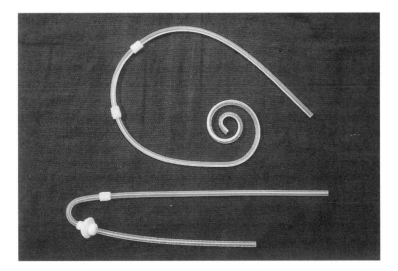

FIGURE 18.1   Examples of available peritoneal dialysis catheters.

to prevent leaks. A randomized trial comparing the Swan-neck catheter to the straight Tenckhoff catheter demonstrated no difference in 2-year catheter survival, peritonitis, or exit-site infection (34).

Other less commonly used catheters exist. The Lifecath catheter, which was designed to improve drainage, was found to have a higher incidence of drainage failure than the Tenckhoff catheter (35). Both the Cruz catheter, which has two 90-degree bends in the subcutaneous portion, and the Dermaport catheter are made of polyurethane. The Dermaport catheter was found to have a high incidence of catheter infection (36). Other catheters made of polyurethane have been reported to develop deformities with repeated exposure to alcohol or local antibiotics such as mupirocin (37,38). The Moncrief-Popovich catheter has its external segment left subcutaneously at the time of insertion (39). After 3 to 5 weeks of tissue ingrowth, it is exteriorized and attached to an adapter. Another modification of the Tenckhoff catheter is the Malpighi catheter, which has a 3.5-cm outer cuff positioned half extruded through the exit site (40). Theoretically, this retards bacterial ingrowth and decreases exit site infections.

Long-term peritoneal dialysis catheters may be placed either by open, Seldinger, or laproscopic techniques. All catheters are inserted in the operating room under sterile conditions, with either a local, regional, or general anesthetic. The catheter exit site is selected ahead of time in order to avoid placement in the belt line or skin folds and to choose a site that is easy for the patient to reach. Patients are given preoperative antibiotics to cover skin flora. If the catheter is placed by the open technique, a 2- to 3- in. transverse periumbilical incision is made over the rectus sheath and continued through to the peritoneum. A tunneler is used to bring the catheter out through a separate exit site, and the catheter tip is positioned in the pelvis. The inner Dacron cuff is sutured to the peritoneum using a nonabsorbable suture, the posterior and anterior rectus sheaths are closed around the catheter, the skin is closed, and the catheter is secured to the skin at the exit site. Finally, the catheter is irrigated with heparinized saline and drained by gravity to confirm proper function.

The peritoneal dialysis catheter can also be placed using either the Seldinger technique or laparoscopically. With the Seldinger technique, a trochar is inserted into the peritoneal cavity, a guidewire is inserted through the trochar, and the catheter is advanced over the wire. Certain catheters—including the Missouri, Toronto-Western and Lifecath—cannot be placed by the Seldinger technique owing to their configuration. In the laporoscopic technique, a trochar is placed into the peritoneal cavity and a pneumoperitoneum is created. A laparoscope is then used to place a guidewire into the pelvis under direct vision and the catheter is advanced into the pelvis over the guidewire.

Once the catheter has been inserted, it is helpful to test its function, particularly for chronic peritoneal dialysis catheters. A simple way to do this is to infuse 500 to 1000 mL of warm dialysate or Ringer's lactate into the peritoneal cavity at the time of insertion. One technique that we use is to start the infusion once the peritoneal cavity has been sealed around the catheter with a purse-string suture. By the time the wound is closed, the infusion will be complete. The infusate bag is then placed on the floor and passive drainage is tested. We like to see recovery of most of the 500- to 1000- mL infusion to know that the catheter is unobstructed. If the infusate is not recovered, the wound is reopened and the catheter repositioned and checked for obstruction again.

DIALYSIS TECHNIQUES

Peritoneal dialysis techniques vary with respect to volume, concentration, and timing of infusion of dialysate. Peritoneal dialysis is designed for use at home and can be performed in a variety of ways to meet individual social and physical needs. Two major modes of peritoneal dialysis exist: intermittent and continuous. Intermittent regimens are reserved primarily for patients who have high peritoneal transport rates or significant residual renal function. After early trials comparing hemodialysis with peritoneal dialysis demonstrated similar clinical and biochemical results, intermittent peritoneal dialysis gained broad support within the dialysis community (41). As experience grew, however, it became clear that dropouts, malnutrition, and poor control of hydration status occurred at a higher rate in patients receiving intermittent peritoneal dialysis compared to hemodialysis patients (42). Subsequently, either continuous peritoneal dialysis or hemodialysis have replaced intermittent peritoneal dialysis techniques. Clinical application of intermittent peritoneal dialysis techniques should generally be reserved for the following patients:

1. Patients awaiting renal transplant who have some clinically significant degree of residual renal function
2. Chronic and debilitated institutionalized patients requiring in-center peritoneal dialysis
3. Those in underdeveloped countries where the prevailing medical and economic factors rule out continuous peritoneal dialysis or hemodialysis

Continuous forms of peritoneal dialysis are based on the presence of dialysate within the peritoneal cavity around the clock except for instillation and drainage time. The advantage of continuous peritoneal dialysis is that both small and large molecules can be cleared efficiently and effectively over time while protein loss is similar to that in intermittent peritoneal dialysis. Furthermore, new developments in dialysate containers, tubing, and exchange equipment have made this technique of dialysis convenient, safe, and usable by a diversity of patients.

Two basic types of continuous peritoneal dialysis exist. Continuous ambulatory peritoneal dialysis is characterized by exchanging fluid within the peritoneal cavity four to five times per day and sleeping with dialysate dwelling in the peritoneal cavity. Alternatively, continuous cycler peritoneal dialysis is characterized by spending the waking hours with one unchanged volume of dialysate within the peritoneal cavity and having a machine (or cycler) fill and drain the peritoneal cavity on a regular basis several times throughout the night. Such machines have gone through tremendous improvements over the past decade, making for a user-friendly, independent technique of renal replacement therapy.

In determining the optimal dialysis solution for a patient, dextrose is the one solute that is provided in different concentrations to induce osmotic ultrafiltration from the blood. In the early days of dialysis, high sodium concentrations were used; current hemodialysate sodium concentrations are 132 meq/l. Higher sodium concentrations can induce severe thirst and result in excessive interdialytic fluid gains (43). The net transcapillary ultrafiltration rate is maximal at the beginning of an exchange and decreases exponentially as the glucose concentration is dissipated by absorption and dilution. The volume of ultrafiltrate produced peaks at about 2 to 3 h dwell time, when the forces of ultrafiltration and reabsorp-

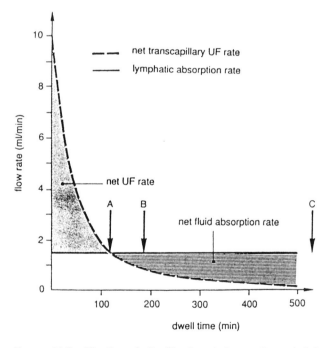

FIGURE 18.2 Kinetics of ultrafiltration during peritoneal dialysis. Arrow A: time at peak ultrafiltration; B: osmolar equilibrium; C: hypothetical glucose equilibrium. From Ref. 43a.

tion are equal (Figure 18.2) (43a). In order to replace the base requirement in the usually acidotic uremic patient, lactate must be used, since bicarbonate-containing solutes are hard to prepare and store (44). Other solutes such as magnesium, chloride and calcium are essentially in stable concentrations.

ADEQUACY OF PERITONEAL DIALYSIS

The use of peritoneal dialysis as a form of renal replacement therapy in end-stage renal disease continues to grow both in the United States and internationally. Assurance that these patients receive adequate dialysis remains a cardinal concern. Defining adequate dialysis in the setting of progressive loss of residual renal function and alterations in peritoneal membrane characteristics remains a controversial area. While a variety of clinical studies have tried to determine the best method of defining adequate dialysis, none of the published clinical studies have been performed as randomized clinical trials. Recently, the National Kidney Foundation published its Dialysis Outcomes Quality Initiative (DOQI) (45). As part of DOQI, 32 guidelines were published regarding the adequacy of peritoneal dialysis and appear in Table 18.1. A detailed discussion of these guidelines is beyond the scope of this text. Interested readers are referred to the DOQI publication for the details of the guidelines and an extensive reference list.

The use of urea kinetics to calculate the urea clearance per volume of urea distribution (Kt/V) has been applied in a variety of clinical dialysis studies to attempt to measure adequacy of dialysis. Early reports theorized that a Kt/V between 1.7 and 2.25 would be adequate weekly dialysis (46–49). Clinical experience demonstrated lower patient survival (44,50–54) and poorer clinical outcomes (55–57) with Kt/V < 1.5. A minimum Kt/V of 2.2/week is now widely accepted as a target goal for adequate dialysis. Furthermore, a total creatinine clearance of greater than 50 L/week/1.73 m^2 of body surface remains a second goal in developing a dialysis prescription (58,59). A multicenter study in Canada and the United States demonstrated that an increase of 0.1 Kt/V unit per week was associated with a 5% decrease in the relative risk of death, and an increase in creatinine clearance of 5 L/week/1.73 m^2 was associated with a 7% decrease in relative risk of death (60). No plateau was noted in this association up to a Kt/V of 2.3 or a creatinine clearance to 95 L/week/173 m^2.

In defining dialysis prescriptions, consideration of the patient's overall nutritional status is important. Adequate protein intake must be maintained, as clinical studies have shown that a protein catabolic rate below 0.8 g/kg normal body weight per day is associated with a high morbidity in the dialysis population. Patients who are well dialyzed have good appetites, eat well, and maintain normal serum albumin levels. Serum albumin remains a sensitive marker for morbidity and mortality in the dialysis population (44).

TABLE 18.1   Guidelines of the Dialysis Outcomes Quality Initiative

Guideline 1	When to initiate dialysis—Kt/V_{urea} criterion
Guideline 2	When to initiate dialysis—nPNA criterion
Guideline 3	Frequency of delivered PD dose and total solute clearance measurement within 6 months of initiation
Guideline 4	Measures of PD dose and total solute clearance
Guideline 5	Frequency of measurement of Kt/V_{urea}, Total C_{cr}, PNA, and total creatinine appearance
Guideline 6	Assessing residual renal function
Guideline 7	PD dose troubleshooting
Guideline 8	Reproducibility of measurement
Guideline 9	Estimating total body water and body surface area
Guideline 10	Timing of measurement
Guideline 11	Dialysate and urine collections
Guideline 12	Assessment of nutritional status
Guideline 13	Determining fat-free, edema-free body mass
Guideline 14	Use of modified Borah equation to assess nutritional status of pediatric PD patients
Guideline 15	Weekly dose of CAPD
Guideline 16	Weekly dose of NIPD and CCPD
Guideline 17	PD dose in subpopulations
Guideline 18	Use of empiric and computer modeling of PD dose
Guideline 19	Identify and correct patient-related failure to achieve prescribed PD dose
Guideline 20	Identify and correct staff-related failure to achieve prescribed PD dose
Guideline 21	Measurement of PD patient survival
Guideline 22	Measurement of PD technique survival
Guideline 23	Measurement of hospitalizations
Guideline 24	Measurement of patient-based assessment of quality of life
Guideline 25	Measurement of school attendance, growth, and developmental progress in pediatric PD patients
Guideline 26	Measurement of albumin concentration in PD patients
Guideline 27	Measurement of hemoglobin/hematocrit in PD patients
Guideline 28	Measurement of normalized PNA in PD patients
Guideline 29	Indications for PD
Guideline 30	Absolute containdications for PD
Guideline 31	Relative contraindications for PD
Guideline 32	Indications for switching from PD to HD

Source: From Ref. 45.

REFERENCES

1. Canadian Organ Replacement Registry: 1991 Annual Report, Hospital Medical Records Institute. Don Mills, Ontario, April 1993.
2. Maiorca R, Vonesh EF, Cavalli PL, et al. Continuous ambulatory peritoneal dialysis in the elderly. Perit Dial Int 11:118–127, 1991.
3. Gokal R, Jakubowski C, King J, et al. Outcome in patients on continuous ambulatory peritoneal dialysis and hemodialysis: 4-year analysis of a prospective multicenter study. Lancet 2:1105–1109, 1987.
4. Burton PR, Walls J. Selection-adjusted comparison of life expectancy of patients on continuous ambulatory peritoneal dialysis, hemodialysis and renal transplantation. Lancet 1:1115–1119, 1987.
5. Kurtz SB, Johnson WJ. A 4-year comparison of continuous ambulatory peritoneal dialysis and home hemodialysis: A preliminary report. Mayo Clin Proc 59:659–662, 1984.
6. Charytan C, Spinowitz BS, Galler M. A comparative study of continuous ambulatory peritoneal dialysis and center hemodialysis. Arch Intern Med 146:1138, 1986.
7. Posen GA, Luiscello J. Continuous equilibration peritoneal dialysis in the treatment of acute renal failure. Perit Dial Bull 1:6, 1980.
8. Firmat J, Zucchini A. Peritoneal dialysis in acute renal failure. Contrib Nephrol 17: 33–38, 1979.
9. Raja RM, Krasnoff SO, Moros JG, et al. Peritoneal dialysis in refractory congestive heart failure. Part I: Intermittent peritoneal dialysis. Perit Dial Bull 3:130–132, 1983.
10. Chopra MP, Gulati RB, Portal RW, et al. Peritoneal dialysis for pulmonary edema after acute myocardial infarction. Br Med J 3:77–80, 1970.
11. Maillox LU, Swartz CD, Onesti GO, et al. Peritoneal dialysis for refractory congestive heart failure. JAMA 199:873–878, 1967.
12. Rubin J, Bell R. Continuous ambulatory peritoneal dialysis as treatment of severe congestive heart failure in the face of chronic renal failure. Arch Intern Med 146: 1533–1538, 1986.
13. Reuler JB, Parker RA. Peritoneal dialysis in the management of hypothermia. JAMA 240:2289–2290, 1978.
14. Zawada ET Jr. Treatment of profound hypothermia with peritoneal dialysis. Dial Transplant 9:255–256, 1980.
15. O'Connor J. The treatment of profound hypothermia with peritoneal dialysis. Perit Dial Bull 2:171–173, 1982.
16. Ahmad S, Gallagher N, Shen F. Intermittent peritoneal dialysis: Status reassessed. Trans Am Soc Artif Intern Organs 25:86–88, 1979.
17. Diaz-Buxo JA, Walker PJ, Chandler JT, et al. Experience with intermittent peritoneal dialysis and continuous cyclic peritoneal dialysis. Am J Kidney Dis 4:242–248, 1984.
18. Popovich RP, Moncrief JW, Nolph KD, et al. Continuous ambulatory peritoneal dialysis. Ann Intern Med 88:449–456, 1978.
19. Oreopoulos DG, Robson M Izatt S, et al. A simple and safe technique for continuous ambulatory peritoneal dialysis. Trans Am Soc Artif Intern Organs 24:484–489, 1978.

20. Nolph KD, Sorkin M Rubin J, et al. Continuous ambulatory peritoneal dialysis: Three-year experience at one center. Ann Intern Med 92:609–613, 1982.
21. Diaz-Buxo JA, Walker PJ, Farmer CD, et al. Continuous cyclic peritoneal dialysis: A preliminary report. Artif Organs 5:157–161, 1981.
22. Fine RN. Choosing a dialysis therapy for children with end-stage renal disease. Am J Kidney Dis 4:249–252, 1984.
23. Wogan JM. Enhancement of elimination. In Noji EK, Kelen GD, eds. Manual of toxicologic Emergencies. Chicago, London, Boca Raton: Year Book; 1989.
24. Palmer RA, Newell JE, Gray EF, Quinton WE. Treatment of chronic renal failure by prolonged peritoneal dialysis. N Engl J Med 274:248–254, 1966.
25. Tenckhoff H, Schechter H. A bacteriologically safe peritoneal access device. Trans Am Soc Artif Intern Organs 14:181–186, 1973.
26. Lindblad AS, Hamilton RW, Nolph KD, Novak JW. A retrospective analysis of catheter configuration and cuff type: A national CAPD registry report. Perit Dial Int 8:129–133, 1988.
27. Port FK, Held PJ, Nolph KD, et al. Risk of peritonitis and technique failure by CAPD connection technique: A national study. Kidney Int 42:967–974, 1992.
28. Noph KD, Lindblad AS, Novak JW. Continuous ambulatory peritoneal dialysis. N Engl J Med 318:1595–1600, 1986.
29. Kim D, Burke D, Izatt S, et al. Single or double cuff peritoneal catheters? A prospective comparison. Trans Am Soc Artif Intern Organs 30:232–235, 1984.
30. Diaz-Buxo JA, Geissinger WT. Single cuff versus double cuff Tenckhoff catheter. Perit Dial Bull 4 (suppl):S100–S104, 1984.
31. Akyol AM, Porteous C, Brown MW. A comparison of two types of catheters for continuous ambulatory peritoneal dialysis (CAPD). Perit Dial Int 10:63–66, 1990.
32. Khanna R, Izatt S, Burke D, Mathews R, Vas S, Oreopoulos DG. Experience with the Toronto Western Hospital permanent peritoneal catheter. Perit Dial Bull 4:95–98, 1984.
33. Scott PD, Bakran A, Pearson R, et al. Peritoneal dialysis access. Prospective randomized trial of 3 different peritoneal catheters—Preliminary report. Perit Dial Int 14:289–290, 1994.
34. Eklund BH, Honkanen EO, Kala A-R, Kyllonen LE. Catheter configuration and outcome in patients on continuous ambulatory peritoneal dialysis: A prospective comparison of two catheters. Perit Dial Int 14:70–74, 1994.
35. Shah GM, Sabo A, Nguyen T, Juler GL. Peritoneal catheters: A comparative study of column disc and Tenckhoff catheters. Int J Artif Organs 13:267–272, 1990.
36. Hines WH, Smego DR, Longnecker RE. Failure of the Dermaport catheter as an access device in CAPD. (abstr). Am J Kidney Dis 15:A10, 1990.
37. Gokal R, Ash SR, Helfrich GB, et al. Peritoneal catheter and exit site practices: Toward optimum peritoneal access. Perit Dial Int 13:29–39, 1993.
38. Shyr YM. Complications of peritoneal catheters placed by a single surgeon. Perit Dial Int 14:401–403, 1994.
39. Moncrief JW, Popovich RP, Broadrick LJ, et al. The Moncrief-Popovich catheter. A new peritoneal access technique for patients on peritoneal dialysis. Am Soc Artif Intern Organs 39:62–65, 1993.
40. Han DC, Cha HK, So IN, et al. Subcutaneously implanted catheters reduce the inci-

dence of peritonitis during CAPD by eliminating infection by periluminal route. Adv Perit Dial 8:298–301, 1992.

41. Diaz-Buxo JA, Farmer CD, Chandler JT. Chronic peritoneal dialysis at home—An alternative for the patient with renal failure. Dial Transplant 6:64–70, 1977.

42. Ahmad S, Gallagher N, Shin F. Intermittent peritoneal dialysis: Status reassessed. ASAIO Trans 25:86–88, 1979.

43. Robson M, Oren H, Ravid M. Dialysate sodium concentration, hypertension and pulmonary edema in hemodialysis patients. Dial Transplant 7(7):678–679, 1978.

43a. Khanna R, Nolph KD, Oreopoulos DG. The Essentials of Peritoneal Dialysis. The Netherlands: Kluwer Academic Publishers, 1993, p 13.

44. Blake PG, Balaskas E, Blake R, Oreopoulos DG. Urea kinetics has limited relevance in assessing adequacy of dialysis in CAPD. Adv Perit Dial 8:65–70, 1992.

45. NKF-KDOQI. Clinical Practice Guidelines for Peritoneal Dialysis Adequacy. Am J Kidney Dis 37:S65–S136, 2001.

46. Popovich, RP, Moncrief, JW. Kinetic modeling of peritoneal transport. Contrib Nephrol 17:59–72, 1979.

47. Teehan BP, Schleifler CR, Sigler MH, Gilgore GS. A quantitative approach to the CAPD prescription. Perit Dial Bull 5:152–156, 1985.

48. Keshaviah PR, Nolph KD, Van Stone JC. The peak urea concentration hypothesis: A kinetic approach to comparing the adequacy of continuous ambulatory peritoneal dialysis and hemodialysis. Perit Dial Int 9:257–260, 1989.

49. Gotch FA. Application of urea kinetic modeling to adequacy of CAPD therapy. Adv Perit Dial 6:178–180, 1990.

50. Teehan BP, Schleifer CR, Brown JM, et al. Urea kinetic analysis and clinical outcome on CAPD. A five year longitudinal study. Adv Perit Dial 6:181–185, 1990.

51. Bland LA, Ridgeway MR, Aguero SM, et al. Potential bacteriologic and endotoxic hazards associated with liquid bicarbonate concentrate. ASAIO Trans 33:542–545, 1987.

52. Teehan BP, Scheleifer CR, Brown J. Urea kinetic modeling is an appropriate assessment of adequacy. Semin Dial 5:189, 1992.

53. DeAlvaro F, Bajo MA, Alvarez-Ude F, et al. Adequacy of peritoneal dialysis: Does Kt/V have the same predictive value as in HD? A multicenter study. Adv Perit Dial 8:93–97, 1992.

54. Lameire NH, Vanholder R, Veyt D, et al. A longitudinal five year survey of kinetic parameters in CAPD patients. Kidney Int 42:426–432, 1992.

55. Keshaviah PR, Nolph DK, Prowant B, et al. Defining adequacy of peritoneal dialysis with ureal kinetics. Adv Perit Dial 6:173–177, 1990.

56. Brandes JC, Piering WF, Beres JA, et al. Clinical outcome of continuous ambulatory peritoneal dialysis predicted by urea and creatinine kinetics. Am Soc Nephrol 2: 1430–1435, 1992.

57. Arkouche W, Delawwari E, My H, et al. Quantification of adequacy of peritoneal dialysis. Perit Dial Int (suppl 13): S215–S218, 1993.

58. Churchill DN. Adequacy of peritoneal dialysis: How much dialysis do we need? Kidney Int 46(suppl 28): S2–S6, 1994.

59. Twardowski ZJ, Nolph KD. Peritoneal dialysis: How much is enough? Semin Dial 1:75, 1988.

60. Churchill DN, Thorpe K, Taylor DW, Keshaviah P. For the CANUSA Study of Peritoneal Dialysis Adequacy: Adequacy of peritoneal dialysis. J Am Soc Nephrol 5:439, 1994.

19

Complications of Peritoneal Dialysis

Dan Ihnat
The University of Arizona,
  Tucson, Arizona

W. Bradford Carter
The University of Maryland, Baltimore, Maryland

Bruce E. Jarrell
The University of Maryland, Baltimore, Maryland

MECHANICAL COMPLICATIONS OF PERITONEAL DIALYSIS

In general, most patients tolerate dialysis without difficulty; however, some will develop complications related to peritoneal dialysis. These can be divided into mechanical and infectious complications. The performance of peritoneal dialysis changes the physiology of the peritoneal space by causing an increase in intraabdominal pressure. As expected, the intraabdominal pressure increases in proportion to the volume of dialysate instilled (1,2). The increased intraabdominal pressure predisposes the patient to hernias, rectoceles, cytoceles, gastroesophageal reflux, hiatal hernias, hemorrhoids, pleural effusions, and leakage of dialysate fluid.

Hernias are the most common complication, occurring in up to 11% of patients during a 5-year follow-up (3,4). The most common types of hernias are incisional, inguinal, and umbilical (3–8). The intraabdominal pressure measured in patients with hernias was found to be the same as that in patients without hernias (9), indicating that certain patients are predisposed to this complication.

Women have a higher incidence of recurrent hernias, especially multiparous women. There is some evidence that patients with polycystic kidney disease have a higher incidence of hernia formation (10). Finally, children, too, have been found to have a higher incidence of hernia formation (11,12). Hernias associated with peritoneal dialysis can become complicated with the same problems as in other individuals, including incarceration, strangulation, and obstruction.

Prevention of incisional hernias may be optimized by proper surgical technique during insertion. The use of a paramedian incision that traverses the rectus abdominis muscle may result in fewer hernias (13,14). In general, patients with preexisting hernias should undergo repair of the hernia prior to initiating peritoneal dialysis. After waiting several weeks for healing, peritoneal dialysis may be initiated with lower-volume dialysis for several more weeks to allow more complete wound healing.

Dialysate leaks most commonly occur at the peritoneal entrance of the catheter and can occur either internally or externally. While external leaks are easy to diagnose, internal leaks often present as genital or abdominal wall edema. This problem can be minimized if the use of new catheters can be delayed for approximately 2 weeks after insertion and low volumes are used initially. Leaks are treated conservatively and usually resolve with cessation of the peritoneal dialysis for 2 to 3 weeks. In general, it is preferable to switch the patient to hemodialysis until the leak seals, because approximately half of these patients will become infected if a persistent leak is present. Once the leak is sealed, low-volume dialysis is reinitiated prior to full-volume dialysis. Most of these leaks will resolve, although catheter removal is necessary on occasion (15,16).

Transdiaphragmatic leak resulting in hydrothorax is a serious complication that can occur at any time after starting peritoneal dialysis. The incidence is estimated to be less than 5% (17). Patients may be asymptomatic or may present with dyspnea, chest pain, hypotension, or atrial fibrillation. Acute effusions usually present within 48 h after the initiation of peritoneal dialysis and can be diagnosed by examining the thoracentesis fluid for a high glucose concentration. A pleuroperitoneal communication can be confirmed with isotope peritoneography (18). Methylene blue injection into the peritoneal cavity is not recommended, since it can lead to chemical peritonitis. Simply stopping peritoneal dialysis for a period of time often leads to spontaneous resolution (17,19,20). Obliteration of the pleural cavity with tetracycline or talc (17,20) and surgical repair of the diaphragmatic defect (21,22) have been reported to be successful; however, recurrent or refractory hydrothorax often leads to abandonment of peritoneal dialysis as a form of renal replacement therapy (20).

Peritoneal dialysis catheters are foreign bodies in the peritoneal cavity and can become obstructed, with a reported incidence of approximately 5 to 20% of all catheters placed (23). The frequency of immediate catheter failure is related to the experience of the physician inserting the catheter, and the amount of intraabdominal adhesions (24). Approximately 6 to 7% of catheters have inadequate flow rates immediately; 50% of these require replacement (25–26). If malfunction occurs, catheter position should be confirmed with plain film. In order to obtain optimal outflow of effluent, the tip of the catheter should lie in one of the pericolic gutters in the pelvis; location of the catheter tip in the upper abdomen is frequently associated with inadequate drainage (27,28).

Late catheter malfunction is associated with a number of factors. Catheter tip migration is associated with 5% of late drainage problems when straight catheters are used (25,26,29,30). Approximately 30 to 50% of these can be repositioned using either laparoscopic assistance or the a stiff guidewire and fluoroscopy (31–34). If the catheter repeatedly fails, however, it should be replaced. Other causes of late catheter failure include obstruction from clots, fibrin deposition, or omental adhesions (35,36). Flushing the catheter with fibrinolytic agents may achieve catheter salvage in these cases (37–41). Constipation is also associated with decreased rate of effluent flow and should be treated with laxatives.

Other less common complications of peritoneal dialysis can occur, including chronic low back pain due to increased lordotic curvature of the spine and a variety of GI disturbances such as gastroesophageal reflux, hemorrhoids, and early satiety. Vasovagal syncope remains a peritoneal complication of uncertain etiology but is probably related to increased intraabdominal pressure (42). Although pulmonary compromise due to increased abdominal pressure is a potential complication, patients with severe chronic obstructive pulmonary disease usually tolerate peritoneal dialysis fairly well (43). Finally, while sleep disturbance is common, particularly in patients using the cycler form of peritoneal dialysis, exacerbation of sleep apnea remains a potential complication (44).

INFECTIOUS COMPLICATIONS OF PERITONEAL DIALYSIS CATHETERS

Infection occurs in two specific locations, both intraperitoneally, with bacterial adherence to the intraperitoneal portion of the catheter, and at the exit site, with bacterial infection of the catheter and surrounding tissues. Peritonitis is the leading reason for patients to switch temporarily or permanently to hemodialysis (45) and is a major cause of their hospitalizations and death (46). Approximately 25 to 60% of patients ultimately discontinue peritoneal dialysis because of peritonitis and up to 15% of deaths occurring in patients on chronic ambulatory peritoneal dialysis (CAPD) are attributable to sepsis (47,48).

Peritonitis

Since its inception, peritonitis has plagued peritoneal dialysis as a frequent complication. The rate of peritonitis has fallen from 4 to 5 episodes per year in the late 1970s (49) to an episode every 24 to 36 months in the 1990s (50–53). The biggest contribution to this reduction has been the development of the Y-set system, which allows for infusion of new peritoneal dialysate fluid in the peritoneum after both draining the peritoneum and flushing the tubing with new, sterile dialysate with only one connection. The Y set has led to the delay of onset of the first attack of peritonitis after initiating peritoneal dialysis from an average of 11.4 months to 20.6 months (53). Despite these improvements, peritonitis occurs three to five times more frequently in patients on intermittent peritoneal dialysis than in patients on CAPD (54). This may be due to a decreased number of connections as well as improved host defense mechanisms during the periods when the peritoneal cavity is fluid-free.

The etiology of peritonitis has been extensively examined in the literature. Compromised host defenses have been implicated as a major factor in a patient's susceptibility to developing peritonitis. Dilution and acidification of opsonins and leukocytes by the dialysate as well as impaired lymphatic clearance have been reported (55–59). The piercing of the abdominal wall by the indwelling peritoneal catheter, of course, disrupts the integrity of the abdominal wall. Last, the uremic and malnourished metabolic milieu commonly found in end-stage renal disease patients leads to an impaired host immune response.

In addition to weakened host defense mechanisms, there are both exogenous and endogenous sources of bacterial contamination. Transluminal contamination through the peritoneal catheter by exogenous bacteria is the most common mechanism of peritoneal infection. Studies have shown patients to be at higher risk from their own skin and nasal flora than from bacterial flora from the environment or other people (60). Endogenous bacterial sources such as bowel, however, are the major cause of gram-negative peritoneal infections (61). Other endogenous sources of peritoneal infection such as bacteremia (49) or the female genital tract (62–65) are well-recognized but infrequent causes.

The diagnosis of peritonitis is made both on the basis of symptoms and on peritoneal dialysate findings. The most frequent symptom is a cloudy effluent (90% of patients), followed by abdominal pain (80 to 95% of patients). Approximately 60% of patients develop peritoneal signs, while fever is less common (approximately 30%) (54,66–68). Microscopic examination of the dialysate reveals greater than 100 leukocytes per deciliter with greater than 50% neutrophils (54). Normal dialysate has less than 50 leukocytes per deciliter. Gram's stain of the centrifuged sediment may reveal organisms in up to 20% of cases. A more useful method is culture of the sediment of a sample of 50 mL of the dialysate; this will be positive approximately 90% of the time (69–72). Culture of unconcentrated dialysate may frequently lead to false-negative results.

Approximately 70% culture-positive peritoneal infections are due to gram-positive organisms, with a predominance of coagulase-negative *Staphylococcus* followed by *Staphylococcus aureus* (60,73–78). Infection with *S. aureus* is more commonly associated with hypotension or septic shock and has a more virulent course than that due to coagulase-negative *Staphylococcus* (79,80). Another 20% of culture-positive peritoneal infections grow gram-negative organisms, with a predominance of *Pseudomonas* and Enterobacteriacae (60,73–78). *Pseudomonas* peritonitis is more difficult to eradicate and is associated with loss of the peritoneal cavity as well as ultrafiltration (81,82). Anaerobic peritonitis is frequently associated with bowel perforation and fecal leakage (54). Fungal peritonitis is more difficult to treat and requires early catheter removal (83).

Treatment of peritonitis should be initiated immediately when the signs and symptoms present. Gram's stain should guide antimicrobial treatment choice (Figure 19.1). If Gram's stain is negative, empiric therapy should cover gram-

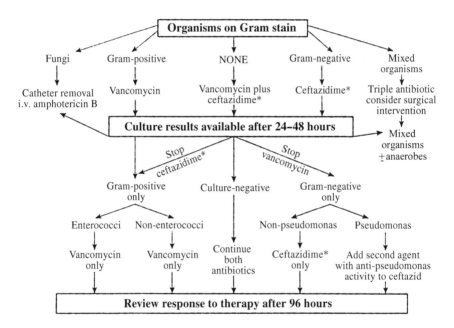

FIGURE 19.1 Decision analysis for initial antibiotic treatment of peritonitis. The recommended dose of antibiotics is intraperitoneal unless stated otherwise. LD, loading dose; MD, maintenance dose in each exchange; i.p., intraperitoneal; i.v., intravenous; p.o., orally. Vancomycin 30 mg/kg i.p. weekly or 1 g i.p. LD and 250 mg/L MD; ceftazidime 500 mg/L i.p. LD and 125 mg/L MD. *Tobramycin and gentamicin (1.5 to 2.0 mg/kg LD then 8 mg/L MD) is an alternative to ceftazidime. **Metronidazole 500 mg three times per day p.o. or i.v. in addition to vancomycin and ceftazidime or an aminogylycoside. ***Piperacillin 4 g i.v. twice daily and ciprofloxacin 750 mg p.o. twice daily; tobramycin or gentamycin 1.5–2.0 mg/kg LD then 8 mg/ kg MD.

positive and gram-negative organisms unless there is a previous history of infecting organisms. Antibiotics are typically administered intraperitoneally during dialysis (71,72). In general, both gram-negative and gram-positive infections are treated with a 2-week antibiotic course. *Pseudomonas* and *S. aureus* infections are perhaps the exception in that they typically require 3 to 4 weeks of treatment and probable catheter removal (71). Clinicians should be aware that the complications associated with antibiotics can still be seen with peritoneal administration. The ototoxicity notable with aminoglycoside administration can occur, particularly in the elderly.

Fungal infections are treated with amphotericin preferentially which can be given intraperitoneally or intravenously for 2 to 3 weeks for a total of 250 to 500 mg total dose. These patients should have a skin test prior to initiation and then be given the antibiotic daily. Unfortunately, amphotericin often fails to eradicate the infection, and catheter removal is necessary for complete eradication.

It is important to maintain the dialysis schedule in treating peritonitis. The large majority of patients can be treated as outpatients, but hospitalization may be necessary if multiple gram-negative organisms, *Pseudomonas*, or yeasts are present in the cultures. Patients need to keep a close eye on exchange volumes and weight, since peritoneal transport often increases with peritonitis, thus decreasing the dialysis drainage volume. The addition of heparin, 500 U/L, to the dialysate is indicated if there is evidence of fibrin deposition. Resistant peritonitis should alert the clinician to the possibility of fungal or resistant *Pseudomonas* infection. Although antibiotics can eradicate these organisms, persistent peritonitis requires catheter removal.

Exit-Site or Tunnel Infections

Infections can occur where the catheter exits the skin as well as along the tunnel in the subcutaneous route. This is usually recognized as erythema and induration of the skin overlying the catheter and purulent discharge at the exit site. The annual incidence of exit-site and tunnel infections is about 0.7 per patient per year (84). No clear relationship exists between the presence of exit-site infections and the type of catheter or the frequency of dialysis. It is probably best to prevent this complication with routine care of the exit site; local antibiotic ointments and povidone-iodine have been used successfully by many centers. Once a catheter becomes infected or a segment of exposed cuff is present, local procedures including cuff removal or exteriorization of the tunnel are generally unsuccessful (85–89). It is probably best to proceed with removal of the catheter. There have been some successful experiences with simultaneous removal of the infected catheter and insertion of a new catheter at a distant site.

Exit sites, tunnel, and catheter infections are usually associated with *Staphylococcus aureus* and *Pseudomonas aeruginosa* (90). *Staphylococcus epider-*

midis is commonly associated with exit-site infections but is a rare tunnel infection agent (48). Peritonitis in the absence of tunnel or catheter infection is highly responsive to antibiotic therapy; however, when peritonitis is associated with tunnel or catheter infections, removal of the catheter is invariably required.

SPECIAL PROBLEMS IN DIALYSIS

Peritoneal Dialysis in Children

Peritoneal dialysis can be done safely in children even under 1 year of age. Abdominal hernias appear to be more common, with up to 50% of children developing hernias (11,12) and a smaller number developing leaks. In one series, the majority of these were repaired surgically while the dialysis was continued. When inserting the catheter into a child, the surgeon should ascertain correct catheter position and ensure a watertight seal. Routine partial omentectomy has also been recommended in children and even bilateral groin exploration at the time of catheter insertion with ligation of a patent processus vaginalis has also been recommended.

Renal Transplant

Renal transplantation can be done safely with a peritoneal dialysis catheter in place. In planning a future transplant procedure, it is worthwhile to place the peritoneal dialysis catheter on the side opposite the planned transplant. For example, if most transplants are performed in the right iliac fossa, the dialysis catheter should be placed in the left side of the pelvis. Prior to proceeding with the transplant, one should document the absence of peritonitis by performing a white blood cell count of the peritoneal dialysate in addition to performing a history and physical examination. Posttransplantation, the dialysis catheter may be used for treatment of acute renal failure providing the peritoneum was not violated during the transplant procedure. If the peritoneum was entered during transplantation, hemodialysis is preferred. After stable renal function has been attained, the catheter may be removed. Most physicians recommend removal within 3 months following the transplant if adequate renal function is present. Patients should be instructed on catheter care with periodic flushes until the catheter is removed. In children, it may be prudent to remove the catheter at the time of discharge from the hospital.

Chronic Liver Failure

Peritoneal dialysis catheters can be used in patients with chronic liver failure. Catheter placement should be performed using the open technique to avoid injury to a patent umbilical vein. If unrecognized, this would be catastrophic in the presence of portal hypertension. Ascitic leaks are of concern, so particular attention should be paid to creating a watertight seal. Patients with ascites and liver failure are prone to significant protein loss in the dialysate; thus one should closely monitor the patient's nutritional status.

Abdominal Catastrophes

Abdominal catastrophes such as diverticulitis, perforated ulcers, acute cholecystitis, appendicitis and pancreatitis occur in peritoneal dialysis patients but fortunately are rare. The peritoneal dialysis fluid reflects abdominal events and can aid with diagnosis. Early catastrophes can occur at the time of catheter insertion due to perforation of the colon, bladder, or other viscus and should be recognized and treated promptly. Some diseases—such as cholecystitis, pancreatitis, uncomplicated incarcerated hernias, and early mesenteric ischemia—tend to produce a clear dialysate; large bowel inflammatory processes usually produce a cloudy dialysate due to a leukocytosis. Nonperforated diverticulitis usually responds to antibiotic treatment and discontinuance of the peritoneal dialysis, but complicated diverticulitis with perforation or abscess requires surgery.

Aside from the common abdominal problems, a number of more obscure problems may occur. Sclerosing peritonitis, which is a more chronic inflammatory process of the peritoneum, can cause intermittent crampy pain, adhesions, and fibrosis and may be demonstrable on computed tomography as a thickened peritoneum. These patients demonstrate loss of ultrafiltration capability. Hemoperitoneum is also seen and is usually a benign process. This commonly occurs initially after catheter insertion but can occur in chronic dialysis patients. One may also see blood in the dialysate with menstruation, ovulation, and even after colonoscopy. A third disorder, peritoneal dialysis eosinophilia, is noted by both peritoneal dialysate and peripheral blood eosinophilia and is associated with elevated levels of IgE. It usually occurs at the initiation of peritoneal dialysis, is poorly understood, and is usually asymptomatic and self-limited. If it persists, it may be treated with steroids, but catheter removal is not usually necessary.

REFERENCES

1. Gotloib L, Mines M, Garmizo L, Varka I. Hemodynamic effects of increasing intra-abdominal pressure in peritoneal dialysis. Perit Dial Bull 1:41, 1981.
2. Twardowski Z, Khanna R, Nolph KD, et al. Intra-abdominal pressures during natural activities in patients treated with CAPD. Nephron 44:129–135, 1986.
3. O'Connor J, Rigby R, Hardie I, et al. Abdominal hernias complicating CAPD. Am J Nephrology 6:271–274, 1986.
4. Digenis GE, Khanna R, Matthews R, et al. Abdominal, hernias in patients undergoing CAPD. Perit Dial Bull 2:115–118, 1982.
5. Rubin J, Raju S, Teal N, et al. Abdominal hernia in patients undergoing continuous ambulatory peritoneal dialysis. Arch Intern Med 142:1453–1455, 1982.

6. Rocco MV, Stone WJ. Abdominal hernias in chronic peritoneal dialysis patients: A review. Perit Dial Bull 5:171–174, 1985.

7. Wetherington G, Leapman S, Robinson R, Filo RS. Abdominal wall and inguinal hernias in CAPD. Am J Surg 150:357–360, 1985.

8. Wise M, Manos J, Gokal R. Small umbilical hernias in patients on CAPD. Perit Dial Bull 4:270–271, 1984.

9. Durand PY, Chanliau J, Gamberoni J, et al. Routine measurement of hydrostatic intraperitoneal pressure. Adv Perit Dial 8:108–112, 1992.

10. Modi KB, Grant AC, Garret A, Rodger RSC. Indirect inguinal hernia in CAPD patients with polycystic kidney disease. Adv Perit Dial 5:84–86, 1989.

11. Tank ES, Hatch DA. Hernias complicating CAPD in children. J Pediatr Surg 21: 41–42, 1986.

12. Von Lilien T, Salusky IB, Yap HK, et al. Hernias: A frequent complication in children treated with continuous peritoneal dialysis. Am J Kidney Dis 10:356–360, 1987.

13. Gokal R, Ash S, Helfrich GB, et al. Peritoneal catheters and exit site practices: Towards optimum peritoneal access. Perit Dial Int 13:29–39, 1993.

14. Spence P, Mathews R, Khanna R, Oreopoulos DG. Improved results with a paramedian technique for the insertion of peritoneal dialysis catheters. Surg Gynecol Obstet 161:585–587, 1985.

15. Nolph KD, Cutler SJ, Steinberg SM, et al. Factors associated with morbidity and mortality among patients on CAPD. ASAIO Trans 33:57–65, 1987.

16. Orfei R, Seybold K, Blumberg A. Genital edema in patients undergoing continuous ambulatory peritoneal dialysis. Perit Dial Bull 4:251–252, 1984.

17. Nomoto Y, Suga T, Nakajima K, et al. Acute hydrothorax in CAPD—A collaborative study of 161 centres. Am J Nephrol 9:363–367, 1989.

18. Spadero JJ, Thakur V, Nolph KD. Technetium-99m-labelled macroaggregated albumin in demonstration in transdiaphragmatic leakage of dialysate in peritoneal dialysis. Am J Nephrol 2:36–38, 1982.

19. Vezina D Winchester JF, Rakowski TA. Spontaneous resolution of a massive hydrothorax in a CAPD patient. Perit Dial Bull 7:212–213, 1987.

20. Green A, Logan M, Medawar W, et al. The management of hydrothorax in continuous ambulatory peritoneal dialysis. Perit Dial Int 10:271–274, 1990.

21. Pattison C, Rodger R, Adu J, et al. Surgical treatment of hydrothorax complicating CAPD. Clin Nephrol 21:191, 1984.

22. Allen S, Matthews HR. Surgical treatment of massive hydrothorax complicating CAPD. Clin Nephrol 36:299, 1991.

23. Khanna R, Wu G, Vas S, et al. Mortality and morbidity on continuous ambulatory peritoneal dialysis. ASAIO J 6:197–204, 1983.

24. Odor A, Alessio-Robles L, Luchter JL, et al. Experience with 150 consecutive permanent peritoneal catheters in patients on CAPD. Perit Dial Bull 5:226–229, 1985.

25. Schwartz R, Messana J, Rocher L, et al. The curled catheter: Dependable device for percutaneous peritoneal access. Perit Dial Int 10:231–235, 1990.

26. Robison RJ, Leapman SB, Wetherington GM, et al. Surgical considerations of continuous ambulatory peritoneal dialysis. Surgery 96:723–730, 1984.

27. Twardowski ZJ. Malposition and poor drainage of peritoneal catheters. Semin Dial 3:57, 1990.

28. Joffe P, Christensen AL, Jensen C. Peritoneal catheter tip location during non-complicated continuous ambulatory peritoneal dialysis. Perit Dial Int 11:261–264, 1991.
29. Yeh TJ, Wei CF, Chin TW. Catheter-related complications of continuous ambulatory peritoneal dialysis. Eur J Surg 158:277–279, 1992.
30. Schleifer CR, Ziemek H, Teehan BP, et al. Migration of peritoneal catheters: Personal experience and a survey of 72 other units. Perit Dial Bull 7:189–190, 1987.
31. Moss JS, Minda SA, Mewman GE, et al. Malpositioned peritoneal dialysis catheters: A critical reappraisal of correction by stiff-wire manipulation. Am J Kidney Dis 15: 305–308, 1990.
32. Wilson JAP, Swartz RD. Peritoneoscopy in the management of catheter malfunction during continuous ambulatory peritoneal dialysis. Dig Dis Sci 30:465–467, 1985.
33. Gibson DH, Heasley RN, Price JH, et al. Laparoscopic repositioning of blocked peritoneal dialysis catheters in patients on CAPD. Clin Nephrol 33:208, 1990.
34. Smith DW, Rankin RA. Value of peritoneoscopy for non-functioning continuous ambulatory peritoneal dialysis catheters. Gastrointest Endosc 35:90–92, 1989.
35. Lovinggood JP. Peritoneal catheter implantation for CAPD. Perit Dial Bull 4(suppl 3):S106, 1984.
36. Diaz-Buxo J. Mechanical complications of chronic peritoneal dialysis catheters. Semin Dial 4:106–109, 1991.
37. Benevent D, Peyronnet P, Brignon P, Leroux-Robert C. Urokinase infusion for obstructed catheters and peritonitis. Perit Dial Bull 5:77, 1985.
38. Wiegmann TB, Stuewe B, Duncan KA, et al. Effective use of streptokinase for peritoneal catheter failure. Am J Kidney Dis 6:119–123, 1985.
39. Palacios M, Schley W, Dougherty JC. Use of streptokinase to clear peritoneal catheters. Dial Transplant 11:172, 1982.
40. Bergstein JM, Andreoli SP, West KW, Grosfeld JL. Streptokinase therapy for occluded Tenckhoff catheters in children of CAPD. Perit Dial Int 8:137–139, 1988.
41. Scalamogna A, Castelnovo C, Cataluppi A. Intraperitoneal infusion of streptokinase in the treatment of a total (inflow-outflow) peritoneal catheter obstruction. Perit Dial Bull 6:41, 1986.
42. Diaz-Buxo JA. Clinical use of peritoneal dialysis. In Nissenson AR, Fine RN, Gentile DE, eds. Clinical Dialysis. Norwalk, CT: 1995:376–425.
43. O'Brien AAJ, Power J, O'Brien L, et al. The effect of 2 L dialysate on respiratory function. Perit Dial Bull 7:S57, 1987.
44. Wadhwa NK, Seliger M, Greenberg HE, et al. Sleep-related respiratory disorders in end-stage renal disease patients on peritoneal dialysis. Perit Dial Int 12:51–56, 1992.
45. Steinberg S, Cutler SJ, Nolph KD, Novak JW. A comprehensive report on the experience of patients on continuous ambulatory peritoneal dialysis for the treatment of end-stage renal disease. Am J Kidney Dis 4:233–241, 1984.
46. Tzamaloukas AH, Murata GH, Fox L. Peritoneal catheter loss and death in continuous ambulatory peritoneal dialysis peritonitis: Correlation with clinical and biochemical parameters. Pert Dial Int 13(suppl 2):S338–S340, 1993.
47. Wu G. A review of peritonitis episodes that caused interruption of continuous ambulatory peritoneal dialysis. Perit Dial Bull (suppl)3:S11–S13, 1983.
48. Piraino B. Bernardini J. Sorkin M. The influence of peritoneal catheter exit site

infections on peritonitis, tunnel infections, and catheter loss in patients on continuous ambulatory peritoneal dialysis. Am J Kidney Dis 8:436–440, 1986.

49. Popovich RP, Moncrief JW, Nolph KD, et al. Continuous ambulatory peritoneal dialysis. Ann Intern Med 88:449–456, 1978.

50. Buoncristiani C, Bianci P, Cozzani M, et al. A new safe simple connection system for CAPD. Int J Urol Nephrol 1:45, 1980.

51. Maiorca R, Cantaluppi A, Cancarini GC, et al. Prospective controlled trial of a Y connector and disinfectant to prevent peritonitis in CAPD. Lancet 2:642–644, 1983.

52. Canadian CAPD Clinical Trials Group/Peritonitis in CAPD: A multi-center randomized clinical trial comparing the Y connector disinfectant system to standard systems. Perit Dial Int 9:159, 1989.

53. VI Catheter related factors and peritonitis risk in CAPD patients. USRDS 1992 Annual Report. Am J Kidney Dis 20(suppl 2):48–54, 1992.

54. Mion C, Slingeneyer A, Canuad B. Peritonitis. In Gokal R, ed. Continuous Ambulatory Peritoneal Dialysis, Edinburgh: Churchill Livingstone; 1986:163.

55. Lamperi S, Carozzi S. Defective opsonic activity of peritoneal effluent during continuous ambulatory peritoneal dialysis (CAPD): Importance and prevention. Perit Dial Bull 6:87–92, 1986.

56. Lamperi S, Carozzi S. Immunological defenses in CAPD. Blood Purif 7:126–143, 1989.

57. Vas SI, Suwe A, Weatherhead J. Natural defense mechanisms of the peritoneum: The effect of peritoneal dialysis fluid on polymorphonuclear cell. In Atkins RC, Thomson NM, Farrell PC, eds. Peritoneal Dialysis. Edinburgh: Churchill Livingstone, 1981:41–51.

58. Verbrugh HA, Keane WF, Hoidal JR, et al. Peritoneal macrophage and opsonins: Antibacterialdefense in patients on chronic peritoneal dialysis. J Infect Dis 147:1018–1029, 1983.

59. Peresecenschi G, Blum M, Aviram A, et al. Impaired neutrophil response to acute bacterial infection in dialyzed patients. Arch Intern Med 141:1301–1302, 1982.

60. Eisenberg ES, Ambalu M, Szlagi G, et al. Colonization of skin and development of peritonitis due to coagulase-negative staphylococci in patients under-going peritoneal dialysis. J Infec Dis 156:478–482, 1987.

61. Keane WF, Peterson PK. Host defense mechanisms of the peritoneal cavity and continuous ambulatory peritoneal dialysis. Perit Dial Bull 4:122–127, 1984.

62. Oreopoulos DG, Robson M, Izatt S, et al. A simple and safe technique for continuous ambulatory peritoneal dialysis. ASAIO Trans 24:484–489, 1978.

63. Nolph KD, Sorkin M, Rubin J, et al. Continuous ambulatory peritoneal dialysis: Three-year experience at one center. Ann Intern Med 92:609–613, 1980.

64. Diaz-Buxo JA, Walker PJ, Farmer CD, et al. Continuous cyclic peritoneal dialysis: A preliminary report. Artif Organs 5:157–161, 1981.

65. Twardowski Z, Ksiazek A, Majdan M, et al. Kinetics of continuous ambulatory peritoneal dialysis (CAPD) with four exchanges per day. Clin Nephrol 15:119–130, 1981.

66. Males BM, Walshe JJ, Amsterdam D. Laboratory indices of clinical peritonitis, total leukocyte count, microscopy and microbiological culture of peritoneal dialysis effluent. J Clin Microbiol 25:2367–2371, 1987.

67. Fenton SS, Wu G, Cattran D, et al. Clinical aspects of peritonitis in patients on CAPD. Perit Dial Bull 1(suppl 1):S4, 1981.
68. Keane WF, Vas SI. Peritonitis. In Gokal R, Nolph KD, eds. The Textbook of Peritoneal Dialysis. Dordrecht: Kluwer, 1994:473.
69. Vas SI. Microbiological aspects of chronic ambulatory peritoneal dialysis. Kidney Int 23:83–92, 1983.
70. Fenton P. Laboratory diagnosis in patients undergoing CAPD. J Clin Pathol 35: 1181–1184, 1982.
71. Keane WF, Everett ED, Gloper TA, et al. Peritoneal dialysis related peritonitis— Treatment recommendations—1993 update. Perit Dial Int 13:14–28, 1993.
72. Report of a Working Party of the BSAC. Diagnosis and management of peritonitis in CAPD. Lancet 1:845–848, 1987.
73. Walshe JJ, West TE, West MR, et al. Carriage of staphylococci among CAPD patients and the significance of adherence and exopolysaccharide production. Tenth International Congress on Nephrology. London, 1987:203.
74. Rault R. Candida peritonitis complicating peritoneal dialysis. A report of five cases and review of the literature. Am J Kidney Dis 2:544–547, 1983.
75. Johnson RJ, Ramsey PJ, Gallagher N, et al. Fungal peritonitis in patients on peritoneal dialysis: Incidence, clinical features and prognosis. Am J Nephrol 5:169–175, 1985.
76. Rubin J. Management of fungal peritonitis. Perspect Perit Dial 4:10–11, 1986.
77. Khanna R, McNeeely DJ, Oreopoulos DG, et al. Treating fungal infections. Fungal peritonitis in CAPD. Br Med J 280:1147–1148, 1980.
78. Kerr CM, Perfect JR, Craven PC, et al. Fungal peritonitis in patients on continuous ambulatory peritoneal dialysis. Ann Intern Med 99:334–337, 1983.
79. Gregory MC, Duffy DP. Toxic shock following staphylococcal peritonitis. Clin Nephrol 20:101–104, 1983.
80. Kim D, Tapson J, Wu G, et al. Staphylococcus aureus peritonitis in patients on CAPD. ASAIO Trans 30:494–497, 1984.
81. Chan MK, Chan PC, Cheng IP, et al. Pseudomonas peritonitis in CAPD patients: Characteristics and outcome of treatment. Nephrol Dial Transplant 4:814–817, 1989.
82. Gokal R, Ramos JM, Francis DMA, et al. Peritonitis in continuous ambulatory peritoneal dialysis. Lancet 2:1388–1391, 1982.
83. Tapson JS, Mansy H, Freeman R, Wilkinson R. The high morbidity of CAPD fungal peritonitis—Description of 10 cases and review of treatment strategies. Q J Med 61:1047–1053, 1986.
84. Nolph KD, Cutler SJ, Steinberg SM, et al. CAPD in the US—A 3 year study. Kidney Int 28:198–205, 1985.
85. Twardowski ZJ, Khanna R. Peritoneal dialysis access and exit site care. In Gokal R, Nolph KD, eds. The Textbook of Peritoneal Dialysis. Dordrecht: Kluwer; 1994: 271.
86. Copley JB. Prevention of PD catheter related infections. Am J Kidney Dis 10:401–407, 1987.
87. Poirier VL, Daly BDT, Dasse KA, et al. Elimination of tunnel infection, in Maher JF, Winchester JF, eds. Frontiers in Peritoneal Dialysis. New York: Field, Rich and Associates; 1986:210–217.

88. Helfrich GB, Winchester JF. Shaving of external cuff of peritoneal catheter. Perit Dial Bull 2:183, 1982.
89. Piraino B, Bernardini J, Peitzman A, et al. Failure of peritoneal catheter. Perit Dial Bull 7:179–182, 1987.
90. Bernardini J, Holley JL, Johnston JR, et al. An analysis of 10-year trends in infections in adults on continuous ambulatory peritoneal dialysis (CAPD). Clin Nephrol 36:29–34, 1991.

Index

About the Editor

SCOTT S. BERMAN, M.D., F.A.C.S. is Chief of Vascular Surgery, Carondelet St. Mary's Hospital, Tucson, Arizona, and Research Professor of Biomedical Engineering at the University of Arizona, Tucson. He is a member of the vascular surgery teaching faculty at both the University of Arizona, Tucson, and the Arizona Heart Institute and Foundation, Phoenix. Dr. Berman is the author or coauthor of over 60 professional publications and a member of the Society for Vascular Surgery, the American Association of Vascular Surgery, the International Society of Endovascular Specialists, the Society of Cardiovascular and Interventional Radiology, the Society for Critical Care Medicine, and the American Medical Association. He received a B.Sc. degree (1983) in chemical engineering from the Pennsylvania State University, University Park, and the M.D. degree (1987) from Hahnemann University School of Medicine, Philadelphia, Pennsylvania. He completed a residency in general surgery at the Eastern Virginia Graduate School of Medicine, Norfolk, Virginia, and a fellowship in vascular surgery at the University of Arizona in Tucson.

ISBN 0-8247-0768-0